CONTENTS

Foundations of
Mental Health
Promotion

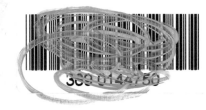

Manoj Sharma, MBBS, MCHES, PhD
Professor, Health Promotion and Education
Professor, Environmental Health
University of Cincinnati

Ashutosh Atri, MD, MS
Child and Adolescent Psychiatry Fellow
Department of Psychiatry and Behavioral Sciences
University of Texas Health Science Center

Paul Branscum, PhD, RD
Assistant Professor, Department of Health and Exercise Science
University of Oklahoma

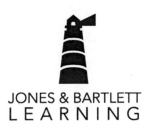

JONES & BARTLETT
LEARNING

World Headquarters
Jones & Bartlett Learning
5 Wall Street
Burlington, MA 01803
978-443-5000
info@jblearning.com
www.jblearning.com

Jones & Bartlett Learning books and products are available through most bookstores and online booksellers. To contact Jones & Bartlett Learning directly, call 800-832-0034, fax 978-443-8000, or visit our website, www.jblearning.com.

Production Credits

Publisher: Cathleen Sether
Senior Acquisitions Editor: Shoshanna Goldberg
Editorial Assistant: Sean Coombs
Production Manager: Julie Champagne Bolduc
Production Assistant: Emma Krosschell
Marketing Manager: Jody Yeskey
V.P., Manufacturing and Inventory Control: Therese Connell
Composition: Cenveo Publisher Services
Cover Design: Scott Moden

Photo Researcher: Sarah Cebulski
Permissions and Photo Research Assistant: Amy Rathburn
Cover Image: © Strakovskaya/ShutterStock, Inc.
Printing and Binding: Malloy, Inc.
Cover Printing: Malloy, Inc.

Some images in this book feature models. These models do not necessarily endorse, represent, or participate in the activities represented in the images.

Openers

Chapter 1 © Bassittart/ShutterStock, Inc.; **Chapter 2** © Jupiterimages/Comstock/Thinkstock; **Chapter 3** © Yuri Arcurs/ShutterStock, Inc.; **Chapter 4** © HannaMonika/ShutterStock, Inc.; **Chapter 5** © elwynn/ShutterStock, Inc.; **Chapter 6** © iStockphoto/Thinkstock; **Chapter 7** © Corbis; **Chapter 8** © forestpath/Fotolia.com; **Chapter 9** © mr.nico/Fotolia.com; **Chapter 10** © Monkey Business Images/Dreamstime.com; **Chapter 11** © iStockphoto/Thinkstock; **Chapter 12** © Hamera/Thinkstock

Library of Congress Cataloging-in-Publication Data
Sharma, Manoj.
    Foundations of mental health promotion / Manoj Sharma, Ashutosh Atri, Paul Branscum.
        p. ; cm.
    Includes bibliographical references and index.
    ISBN 978-0-7637-9341-8 (pbk.)
    I. Atri, Ashutosh. II. Branscum, Paul. III. Title.
    [DNLM: 1. Mental Health. 2. Health Promotion—methods. 3. Mental Disorders.
4. Mental Health Services. WM 101]
    362.2'2—dc23
                                                    2011035621
6048
Printed in the United States of America
15 14 13 12 11   10 9 8 7 6 5 4 3 2 1

PREFACE

We take great pleasure in presenting to our readers this textbook, *Foundations of Mental Health Promotion*. This book offers an introduction to the field of mental health promotion. It includes medical, epidemiological, behavioral, sociological, political, historical, developmental, and cultural perspectives on mental health. The goal of this book is to write an introductory text in the area of mental health for undergraduate students, introductory graduate classes, and practitioners interested in working in mental health. Currently such a text for health education and health promotion students does not exist.

In this book both individual-level and population-level approaches to dealing with mental health problems have been emphasized. Topics include mental health, mental illness, and historical perspectives; roles of health educators and health promoters in mental health promotion; determinants of mental health; stress and coping; understanding major psychotic disorders; understanding mood, anxiety, and personality disorders; alcohol dependence, tobacco use, and substance abuse; essentials of psychopharmacology and treatment of mental health disorders; mental health promotion for children and adolescents; mental health promotion for adults; mental health promotion for older adults; and mental health organizations.

Each chapter begins with key terms and a set of learning objectives. A thorough introduction and a concise summary have been included in each chapter. At least one boxed article called "Focus Feature" has been included in each chapter. These Focus Features deal with interesting discoveries, important aspects, anecdotes, or future directions being pursued on a particular topic that should help to consolidate interest on a topic and foster further reading. In addition to the Focus Features, important points and sometimes important quotations from each chapter have been pulled out into boxes to emphasize important topics. Each chapter includes a skill-building activity and review questions, as well as a detailed reference list and further readings. Each chapter also includes an annotated guide to reliable websites to explore. Each Web exercise provides interactive activities that directly relate to the chapter content and help students apply their new knowledge practically.

We hope you find this book useful. Please send us your comments and feedback so that it can be incorporated in subsequent editions of this work.

INSTRUCTOR RESOURCES

We have prepared a set of PowerPoint presentations and Test Bank questions for each chapter that instructors can use for classroom lectures. Please contact your sales representative for access.

ACKNOWLEDGMENTS

We would like to thank the following reviewers who read through this text and provided invaluable feedback and advice: Ari Fisher, MA, LSU; Dr. Amar Kanekar, East Stroudsburg University of Pennsylvania; Adam J. Mrdjenovich, PhD, The University of Toledo; and Jerry Thompson, RN, MSN, Samuel Merritt University.

We would also like to thank the Health team at Jones & Bartlett Learning: Shoshanna Goldberg, Senior Acquisitions Editor; Amy Bloom, Managing Editor; Julie Bolduc, Production Manager; and Jody Yeskey, Marketing Manager.

ABOUT THE AUTHORS

Manoj Sharma, MBBS, MCHES, PhD, is a professor in the Health Promotion and Education program and Department of Environmental Health at the University of Cincinnati. He is a physician by initial training and completed his doctorate in preventive medicine/public health from the Ohio State University. He has worked in community health for more than 25 years at all levels: local (Columbus Health Department, Omaha Healthy Start Program, Lead Safe Omaha Coalition); state (Nebraska Health and Human Services, Ohio Department of Health, Ohio Commission on Minority Health); national (American School Health Association, Centers for Disease Control and Prevention); and international (India, Italy, Mongolia, Nepal, United Arab Emirates, United Kingdom, Vietnam). His research interests are designing and evaluating theory-based health education and health promotion programs, alternative and complementary systems of health, and community-based participatory research.

Ashutosh Atri, MD, MS, is a fellow in the Department of Psychiatry and Behavioral Sciences at the University of Texas Health Sciences Center. He has completed postgraduate training in health education and health promotion from the University of Cincinnati. He has worked as a physician at SS Medical College, Rewa, India, and MGM Medical College, Indore, India. His research interests are in the field of international health, psychoeducation, mental health, and designing health education interventions for the mentally ill.

Paul Branscum, PhD, RD, is an assistant professor in the Department of Health and Exercise Science at the University of Oklahoma. He is a dietitian by initial training and has completed his doctorate in health promotion and education from the University of Cincinnati in 2011. His research interests include health promotion among children, survey design, mental health, and designing health promotion and education strategies to reduce childhood obesity.

CHAPTER 1

Mental Health, Mental Illness, and Historical Perspectives

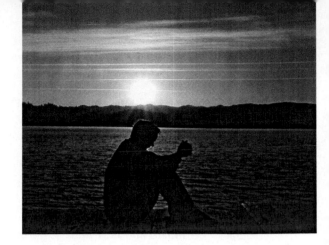

CHAPTER OBJECTIVES

After reading this chapter you should be able to
- Define health, mental health, and mental illness
- Describe common models of mental health
- Delineate the constituents of mental health education

- Discuss the concept of mental health promotion
- Trace the historical genesis of the field of mental health
- Explain some contemporary trends and standards in mental health

CONCEPT OF HEALTH

Before trying to understand the meaning of **mental health**, let us first begin by defining the meaning of **health**. Health is a very old term. In Old English it was used as *haelen* (to heal) and in Middle English as *helthe*, meaning to be sound in body, mind, or spirit. The word was related to the practice of medicine. In the ancient Greek civilization the definition of medicine was to "prolong life and prevent disease" or, in other words, to keep people healthy (Cook, 2004). Similarly, the term for medicine in ancient India was *Ayurveda*, or the science of life or health. By the 17th century in most medical textbooks the word *restoration* began to be used. By the end of the 19th century the word *health* was considered colloquial and was replaced with the word *hygiene*, which was considered more scientific (Cook, 2004).

After World War II interest in the word *health* again resurfaced with the formation of World Health Organization (WHO), a global entity. Around the same time the Hygienic Laboratory in the United States was renamed the National Institutes of Health. In 1948 the WHO defined health in its constitution as "a state of complete physical, mental, and social well-being and not merely the absence of disease or infirmity" (WHO, 1974, p. 1). However, this definition of health has received much criticism over the years.

First, the use of the word *state* in this definition is misleading. Health is dynamic and changes from time to time. For example, a person may be healthy in the morning, but in the afternoon he or she develops a headache and is thus not in the "state" of health. In the evening he or she may recover from the headache, thereby attaining the "state" of health again.

Second, the dimensions as mentioned in the definition are inadequate to capture variations in health. One such dimension is the political dimension. Do the rich get sick more often or the poor? Who controls greater resources for health? Which section of the population has a greater burden of mortality? All these and many more such questions pertain to the politics behind health. This dimension must be explicitly mentioned in the definition for it to be meaningfully complete. Another dimension not mentioned in the WHO's definition of health is the spiritual dimension (Perrin & McDermott, 1997). Bensley (1991) identified six different perspectives related to the spiritual dimension of health, namely, sense of fulfillment; values and beliefs of community and self; wholeness in life, well-being, God or a controlling power; and human–spiritual interaction. These perspectives are not mentioned in WHO's original definition.

Third, the word *well-being* is very subjective in its connotation. A definition must be objective, and subjectivity must be minimized. Fourth, the way health is defined makes it very difficult to measure. McDowell and Newell (1987) point out that "just as language molds the way we think, our health measurements influence (and are influenced by) the way we define and think about health" (p. 14); in other words, health and measurement are inextricably linked. Fifth, the way health is defined presents an idealistic or utopian view. It would be impossible to find someone who embodies all the attributes presented in the definition. Thus, the definition of health needs to be more realistic. Sixth, health is presented as an end product in the definition, whereas most people perceive health as a means for achieving something they value more. For example, a person may want to be healthy so he or she can raise a family. Finally, the WHO definition of health is written from an individualistic perspective in which health is defined for one person. It lacks the community orientation that is needed for something that is as complex as health.

Since the original WHO definition was published, it has been further modified in subsequent discussions at the world level. In November 1986 the first International Conference on Health Promotion was held in Ottawa, Canada (WHO, 1986). The conference culminated with the drafting of the Ottawa Charter for Health Promotion, wherein health was defined in a broader perspective:

> [H]ealth has been considered less as an abstract state and more as a means to an end which can be expressed in functional terms as a resource which permits people to lead an individually, socially, and economically productive life. Health is a resource for everyday life, not the object of living. It is a positive concept emphasizing social and personal resources as well as physical capabilities.

Keeping these aspects in mind, one can define health. We define health as a means to achieve desirable goals in life while maintaining multidimensional (physical, mental, social, political, economic, spiritual) equilibrium that is operationalized for individuals as well as for communities.

> *Health is defined as a means for achieving desirable goals in life while maintaining multidimensional (physical, mental, social, political, economic, spiritual) equilibrium that is operationalized for individuals as well as for communities.*

CONCEPTS OF MENTAL HEALTH AND MENTAL ILLNESS

We are beginning to understand that mental health is an integral part of the concept of health. A definition of health cannot be complete without the inclusion of mental health. Preston (1943) defines mental health as the ability to be happy and productive without being a nuisance to others. Guntrip (1961) defines mental health as the capacity to live life completely and realizing one's own natural potentials. The WHO defines mental health as "a state of well-being in which every individual realizes his or her own potential, can cope with the normal stresses of life, can work productively and fruitfully, and is able to make a contribution to her or his community" (WHO, 2009a, p. 1).

The Surgeon General's Report on mental health (U.S. Department of Health and Human Services [USDHHS], 1999) uses a "wide angle lens" to depict both mental health and mental illness. This report notes that in the past the mental health field primarily focused on people with mental illnesses, but more recently it is focusing on mental illness prevention and mental health promotion.

Is mental health an absence of mental illness? Some have suggested a **continuum model** with mental health on one end and mental illness on the other (Trent, 1993). Although there is some merit to this conceptualization, it looks at mental health as an absence of mental illness. This is not always true. For example, a person may suffer from depression. This person seeks treatment and is placed on antidepressant medication. This person may enjoy good mental health while still suffering from mental illness. Further, the continuum model represents a disease orientation to mental health. There are many myths and fears associated with mental illness and stigma attached to those who are mentally ill. The model also lends itself to victim blaming whereby it places responsibility of being mentally ill on the person. This may not always be the case as biological and genetic factors play an important role in causation of mental illness. All these reasons make this model less appealing to most people. Further, this model seeks to answer the question of what makes people sick, whereas the more important focus of a mental health model should be on what makes people healthy (Cattan, 2006).

Mental disorder or **mental illness** is defined in many ways. The *Diagnostic and Statistical Manual of Mental Disorders*, 4th edition, revised (DSM-IV-TR) is considered to be a well-known authority in this area. However, when it comes to defining mental illness the DSM-IV-TR states the following: "The concept of mental disorder, like many other concepts in medicine and science, lacks a consistent operational definition that covers all situations" (American Psychiatric Association, 2000, p. 13). The manual notes that it is very difficult to separate the physical aspects from mental aspects in causation of diseases and the body and mind are intricately linked to each other. However, it is difficult to define mental disorders in any other way but to focus on only mental aspects. The manual defines mental disorder as "clinically significant behavioral or psychological syndrome or pattern that occurs in an individual and that is associated with present distress (e.g., a painful symptom) or disability (i.e., impairment in one or more important areas of functioning) or with a significantly increased risk of suffering death, pain, disability, or an important loss of freedom" (American Psychiatric Association, 2000, p. 14). Therefore, mental disorder comprises behavioral or psychological signs and symptoms that cause misery to the patient; result in loss of physical, mental, social, or occupational functioning; and may lead to greater risk of morbidity, mortality, or loss of freedom.

Marie Jahoda developed a popular model for mental health using several criteria she considers essential for mental health (Jahoda, 1958). **Jahoda's model of mental health** comprises the following criteria (Seedhouse, 2002; Tengland, 2001):

- *Being realistic.* According to this criterion a mentally healthy person must be able to compare him- or herself with others in an objective fashion, and this assessment should lead to an image similar to that held by others.
- *Self-acceptance.* According to this criterion a mentally healthy person must accept himself or herself as he or she is without any complaints. To be mentally healthy one should not feel bad or inferior if one is not perfect.
- *Investment in living.* A mentally healthy person is positively concerned with other people and wants to be part of things around him or her. This also includes having long-term goals in life and having enough motivation to achieve those goals.
- *Independence.* A mentally healthy person is able to make independent decisions from a variety of environmental stimuli.
- *Environmental mastery.* In this criterion a mentally health person must be able to fulfill the following six factors: (1) demonstrate ability to love; (2) show adequacy in work, love, and play; (3) be adequate in interpersonal relationships; (4) be efficient in meeting situational necessities; (5) be able to adjust and adapt; and (6) be efficient in problem solving.

Per-Anders Tengland (2001) also discussed several criteria for mental health. **Tengland's model of mental health** defines 11 characteristics as essential for a mentally healthy person (pp. 137–138):

1. Ability to have high degree of correct memory
2. Ability to correctly perceive various stimuli
3. Exhibit high degree of rationality
4. Possess self-knowledge
5. Exhibit flexibility
6. Ability to experience emotions
7. Ability to feel empathy
8. Possess self-esteem and self-confidence
9. Demonstrate ability to communicate cognitive information
10. Identify what is appropriate in a communication
11. Ability to cooperate

MacDonald (2006) notes that Western authors have defined mental health and mental illness primarily from an individualistic perspective, which may not necessarily be accurate. This individualistic perspective is not depicted in other cultures. For example, Markus and Kitayama (1991) from Japan talk about "shared life space" instead of the "self." MacDonald (2006) advocates for a less individualistic and more social and ecological account of mental health. Social and cultural conditions and processes contribute to a large extent to the mental health of any person and must be included in defining and conceptualizing mental health. The structural inequalities contribute to mental health and mental illness and must be addressed. In this context we define mental health as the ability of an individual to fulfill his or her obligations to self and society while living in mutual harmony with the physical and social environment.

> *Mental health is defined as the ability of an individual to fulfill his or her obligations to self and society while living in mutual harmony with the physical and social environment.*

HEALTH EDUCATION AND HEALTH PROMOTION

Before we discuss mental health education and mental health promotion we need to understand health education and health promotion. **Health education** is the profession that deals with facilitation of modifying health behaviors. Health education has been defined in several ways. Downie, Fyfe, and Tannahill (1990) defined it as "[c]ommunication activity aimed at enhancing positive health and preventing or diminishing ill-health in individuals and groups through influencing the beliefs, attitudes and behavior of those with power and of the community at large" (p. 28). The 2000 Joint Committee on Health Education and Promotion Terminology (Gold & Miner, 2002) defined health education as "any combination of planned learning experiences based on sound theories that provide individuals, groups, and communities the opportunity to acquire information and the skills needed to make quality health decisions." The WHO (1998, p. 4) defined health education as "compris[ing] consciously constructed opportunities for learning involving some form of communication designed to improve health literacy, including improving knowledge, and developing life skills which are conducive to individual and community health." Green and Kreuter (2005, p. G-4) defined it as "any planned combination of learning experiences designed to predispose, enable, and reinforce voluntary behavior conducive to health in individuals, groups or communities."

From these definitions some things are clear. First, health education is a systematic, planned application, which would qualify it as a science. Second, the delivery of health education involves a set of techniques rather than just one, such as preparing health education informational brochures, pamphlets, and videos; delivering lectures; facilitating role plays or simulations; analyzing case studies; participating and reflecting in group discussions; self-reading; and interacting in computer-assisted training. In the past *health education* was used to encompass a wider range of functions, such as community mobilization, networking, advocacy, and so on. These methods are now embodied in the term *health promotion*; thus, health education is now perceived as more focused. Third, the primary purpose of health education is to influence antecedents of behavior so that healthy behaviors develop in a voluntary fashion (without any coercion). The common antecedents of behavior are awareness, information, knowledge, skills, beliefs, attitudes, and values. Finally, health education is performed at several levels. It can be done one-on-one, such as a counseling session; with a group of people, such as through a group discussion; at an organizational level, such as through an employee wellness fair; or at the community level, such as through a multiple-channel, multiple-approach campaign.

Since the publication of *Healthy People: The Surgeon General's Report on Health Promotion and Disease Prevention* (USDHHS, 1979), the term **health promotion** has gained popularity and continues to gain strength. This term has been used in the *Objectives for the Nation* (USDHHS, 1980), *Healthy People 2000* (USDHHS, 1990), *Healthy People 2010* (USDHHS, 2000), and *Healthy People 2020* (USDHHS, 2009) reports. Green and Kreuter (2005, p.G-4) defined health promotion as "any planned combination of educational, political, regulatory and organizational supports for actions and conditions of living conducive to the health of individuals, groups or communities." The 2000 Joint Committee on Health Education and Promotion Terminology (Gold & Miner, 2002, p. 4) defined health promotion as "any planned combination of educational, political, environmental, regulatory, or organizational mechanisms that support actions and conditions of living conducive to the health of individuals, groups, and communities." The *Ottawa Charter for Health Promotion* (WHO, 1986, p. 1) defined health promotion as "the process of enabling people to increase control over, and to improve their health." The Ottawa Charter identified five key action strategies for health promotion:

1. Building healthy public policy
2. Creating physical and social environments supportive of individual change
3. Strengthening community action
4. Developing personal skills such as increased self-efficacy and feelings of empowerment
5. Reorienting health services to the population and partnership with patients

These action areas were confirmed in the *Jakarta Declaration on Leading Health Promotion into the 21st Century* in 1997 (WHO, 1997). In addition, the Jakarta Declaration identified five priorities for health promotion:

1. Promote social responsibility for health
2. Increase investments for health development
3. Expand partnerships for health promotion
4. Increase community capacity and empower the individual
5. Secure an infrastructure for health promotion

Once again, all these depictions of health promotion have some things in common. First, just like health education, health promotion is also a systematic, planned application that would qualify as a science. Second, it entails methods beyond mere education. Such methods could consist of community mobilization, community organization, community participation, community development, community empowerment, networking, coalition building, advocacy, lobbying, policy development, formulating legislation, developing social norms, and so on. Third, unlike health education, it does not endorse voluntary change in behavior and uses measures that compel an individual's behavior change. These measures are uniform and mandatory. Often, the behavior change in health promotion comes from measures that an individual may not like, for example, an increase in insurance premium for a smoker. Finally, health promotion is done at the group or community level.

UNDERSTANDING MENTAL HEALTH EDUCATION AND MENTAL HEALTH PROMOTION

Mental health education deals with voluntarily modifying health behaviors to bring a person to be in harmony with his or her environment. Such behaviors include stress management behaviors, relaxation and adequate sleep behaviors, effective communication behaviors, anger management behaviors, anxiety reduction behaviors, healthy eating behaviors, healthy physical activity and exercise behaviors, time management behaviors, financial management behaviors, recreation and leisure management behaviors, and adequate work-performance behaviors (**Table 1.1**).

TABLE 1.1   Behaviors Addressed in Mental Health Education
Stress management behaviors
Relaxation and adequate sleep behaviors
Effective communication behaviors
Anger management behaviors
Anxiety reduction behaviors
Healthy eating behaviors
Healthy physical activity and exercise behaviors
Time management behaviors
Financial management behaviors
Recreation and leisure management behaviors
Adequate work-performance behaviors

Mental health education can be achieved one-on-one through a counseling session, with a group of people, at an organizational level, or at the community level, such as through a multiple-channel, multiple-approach campaign. Mental health behaviors are applicable at primary, secondary, and tertiary levels of prevention (Modeste & Tamayose, 2004; Pickett & Hanlon, 1998). **Primary prevention** refers to those preventive actions taken before the onset of a disease or injury with the intention of removing the possibility of its occurrence. All the behaviors mentioned above when done by healthy people can be considered primary prevention. **Secondary prevention** refers to actions that block the progression of an injury or disease at its incipient stage. When the abovementioned behaviors are practiced by people who are under stress, struggling with an anger problem, or experiencing anxiety, these can be considered as secondary prevention. **Tertiary prevention** refers to those actions taken after the onset of disease or injury with the intention of assisting diseased or disabled people. When the above behaviors are practiced by people who have been diagnosed with a mental illness to prevent relapses, these can be considered as tertiary prevention.

> *Mental health education deals with voluntarily modifying health behaviors to bring a person to be in harmony with his or her environment. It can be done one-on-one through a counseling session, with a group of people, at an organizational level, or at the community level.*

Mental health education can be practiced in schools with school children as primary target group, in worksites with employees as primary target group, in community settings with members of the community as primary target audience, in health care institutions with patients suffering from different ailments including mental illnesses as primary target audiences, and finally in colleges and universities with college students as primary audiences.

Mental health promotion entails developing policies, regulations, and environments that are conducive to making a person be in harmony with his or her environment. The scope of mental health promotion therefore is quite wide. It entails developing policies, regulations, and environments that reduce stress, ensure adequate work for all, foster relaxation opportunities for all, regulate anger and associated harms, reduce anxiety, provide adequate food for all, ensure adequate housing for all, provide sufficient supports for being physically active, and provide for enough recreation and leisure opportunities (**Table 1.2**).

Tilford (2006) notes that mental health promotion works in three ways: (1) by strengthening individuals by building healthy skills; (2) by strengthening communities by improving participation, environments, building mental health services, and so on; and (3) by reducing structural barriers to health by addressing discrimination, inequalities, and so on. Importantly, mental health promotion uses community-based approaches as opposed to individual-based approaches. In mental health promotion work is done at the community level using participatory approaches that in turn build the capacity of the community and empower the individuals that reside within those communities. Still,

> *Mental health promotion entails developing policies, regulations, and environments that are conducive to making a person be in harmony with his or her environment.*

much work in mental health promotion needs to be done. The WHO (2009b) notes that as many as 64% of countries around the world do not have any mental health legislation or have legislations that are more than 10 years old. Furthermore, most of the existing mental health legislation violates the rights of the mentally ill rather than protecting them.

TABLE 1.2   Focus of Mental Health Promotion

Developing policies, regulations, and environments that reduce stress

Developing policies, regulations, and environments that ensure adequate work for all

Developing policies, regulations, and environments that foster relaxation opportunities for all

Developing policies, regulations, and environments that regulate anger and associated harms

Developing policies, regulations, and environments that reduce anxiety

Developing policies, regulations, and environments that provide adequate food for all

Developing policies, regulations, and environments that ensure adequate housing for all

Developing policies, regulations, and environments that provide sufficient supports for being physically active

Developing policies, regulations, and environments that provide enough recreation and leisure opportunities

FOCUS FEATURE 1.1 MENTAL HEALTH PARITY AND ADDICTION EQUITY ACT OF 2008

Alternate name: Also known as Paul Wellstone and Pete Domenici Mental Health Parity and Addiction Equity Act of 2008.

Effective date: January 1, 2010

Purpose: The prime aim of the Act is to ensure mental illnesses are treated the same way as physical illnesses by insurance plans covering 50 or more employees (Luongo, 2008). Under this law it is estimated that 113 million people around the country will have access to nondiscriminatory mental health coverage (American Psychological Association Practice Organization, 2008).

Features:

- For health insurance the financial requirements applicable to mental health or substance use disorder benefits should be no more restrictive than the financial requirements applied to medical and surgical benefits covered by the insurance.
- The treatment limitations applicable to mental health or substance use disorder benefits should be no more restrictive than the treatment limitations applied to medical and surgical benefits covered by the insurance.
- The criteria for medical necessity determinations made under the plan with respect to mental health or substance use disorder benefits should be made available by the plan administrator (or the health insurance issuer offering such coverage) in accordance with regulations to any current or potential participant, beneficiary, or contracting provider upon request.

HISTORY OF MENTAL HEALTH

The history of mental health has predominantly focused on events related to mental illnesses. There are a few instances from history such as that from India in which yoga was used to improve and preserve mental health. The treatment of mental health disorders has undergone multiple changes over the years, including some major paradigm shifts. Over the course of history, mental illnesses and disorders have been approached essentially in three different ways: supernaturally, biologically, and psychologically. During most of early history the supernatural model was used to explain and attempt to remedy mental illnesses.

Primitive Times

There is evidence to indicate that mental illnesses existed during primitive times and that attempts were made to treat them. The supernatural concept of disease in general and mental illnesses in particular held that mental illness was created by divinities, demons, spirits, or magnetic fields emanating from the stars and moon (hence the term *lunatics*). It was widely believed that mental illnesses were created by evil spirits entering into and taking over the body. These evil spirits were forced out of the body by "medicine men" through magic and reincarnation. Records indicate that some primitive tribes even went so far as to drill holes in the skulls to let the evil spirits out, a technique called **trephining** (Horsley, 1888). Prayer and faith healing were also used, as was astrology. Exorcisms were widespread.

Ancient Civilization in India

In ancient India (2000–600 BCE) the period is characterized by the development of *Vedas* or the scriptures of teachings. Initially, the Vedas were transmitted orally from one generation to another. They were eventually written in Sanskrit and primarily consist of four collections called the *Rig-Veda*, the *Sama-Veda*, the *Yajur-Veda*, and the *Atharva-Veda* (Hines, 1999). Collectively, these are referred to as the *Samhitas*. It is believed that the system of *Ayurveda*, or the science of life or health, also originated during this time from *Atharva-Veda* (Park & Park, 1986; Subbarayappa, 2001). *Ayurveda* had eight branches: *Kayacikitsa* (internal medicine), *Salya tantra* (surgery), *Salakya tantra* (ophthalmology and ENT), *Kaumara brhtya* (pediatrics, obstetrics and gynecology), *Agada tantra* (toxicology), *Rasayana* (geriatrics and nutrition), *Vajikarana* (sexology), and *Bhuta Vidya* (psychiatry and demonology) (Subbarayappa, 2001). Two classical texts of *Ayurveda* are *Charaka* and *Susruta Samhita*. *Ayurveda* believes in *Pancha Bhutas*, or the five elements: space, air, fire, water, and earth.

The hallmark of *Ayurveda* is the **tridosha theory of disease**. The *doshas*, or humors, are *vata* (wind), *pitta* (gall), and *kapha* (mucus). Diseases were explained as disturbances in these three humors. In *Auyrveda* the mind is functionally divided into *ahankara* (ego), *ichha* (desire, will), and *buddhi* (intellect). *Ichha*, influenced by *ahankara*, dictates the mind and *buddhi* takes the decisions. Also linked to the *tridoshas* are the three *gunas*: *sattva* (truth, goodness), *rajas* (activity), and *tamas* (inertia). The ideal state of mind is in *sattvic guna*, whereas the agitated mind is in *rajas* and the lethargic or depressed mind is in *tamas*. *Bhuta Vidya* is the specialty within *Ayurveda* that deals with mental illnesses. Mental disorders are broadly classified into *doshonmada* (those disorders that have a physical basis) and *bhutonmada* (those disorders that have a purely mental basis).

The system of **yoga** also originated during this time. The word *yoga* is derived from the Sanskrit word meaning "union." It is an ancient system of physical and psychic practice to keep balance. In a more modern context yoga has been defined as "a systematic practice and implementation of mind and body in the living process of human beings to keep harmony within self, within society, and with nature" (Maharishi, 1992, p. 1). The first written records of this methodology appeared around 200 BCE in *Yogasutra* of Patanjali (Singh,

1983). The system consisted of the eightfold path, or *Asthangayoga*. The eight conventional steps of *Asthangayoga* consist of *Yama* (rules for living in society), *Niyama* (self-restraining rules), *Asaana* (low physical impact postures), *Pranayama* (breathing techniques), *Pratihara* (detachment of the mind from senses), *Dharana* (concentration), *Dhyana* (meditation), and *Samadhi* (complete union with super consciousness) (Romas & Sharma, 2010). The techniques of yoga are perhaps the most remarkable contributions of this era in the field of health. Yoga and meditation are now well-accepted forms of approaches for their beneficial role in preserving and improving mental health.

> *A*yurveda and yoga are perhaps the most remarkable contributions of Ancient India in the evolution of mental health.

Ancient Civilization in Egypt

In the Egyptian civilization (3000–300 BCE), which is known for its pyramids and sphinxes, issues of mental health can also be found. Because the Egyptians invented picture writing and recorded it on papyrus, much is known about this culture. The main sources for studying Egyptian civilization have been through surviving papyri, which have been translated into modern languages. Among papyri related to medicine, the most important to psychiatry are the Ebers and the Edwin Smith papyri (Nasser, 1987). In the Edwin Smith papyrus the brain is described as being enclosed in a membrane, with two hemispheres that are patterned with convolutions. There are descriptions of disorders such as hysteria, alcoholism, and sadness. There is no description of a physician who specialized in mental illnesses, but it seems the sorcerer was the psychiatrist (Nasser, 1987). It also seems that the sorcerer had some knowledge of hallucinogens such as mescaline.

Ancient Civilization in China

China is one of the world's oldest continuous civilizations, dating back more than 6,000 years. Around the 14th or 13th century BCE, during the Shang dynasty, it was believed that ailments were caused by the curses of dead ancestors, and methods of healing such as prayers, offerings, and incantations were performed (Subbarayappa, 2001).

An emperor physician, Huang Di, or the Yellow Emperor of China (2695–2589 BCE) is credited with initiating systematic Chinese medicine. Huang Di emphasized the importance of the principles of **yang** and **yin** everywhere in creation. *Yang* is the masculine principle and *yin* the feminine principle. Balance between these two signifies good health. *Yang* and *yin* generate five phases: water, fire, earth, wood, and metal. Chinese herbal therapy was based on these five phases. Huang Di also supported the use of acupuncture in Chinese medicine, which arose around 2600 BCE. This was the basis of treating mental illnesses. Huang Di emphasized prevention of diseases, quoting a Chinese proverb, "The superior doctor prevents diseases; the mediocre doctor attends to impending diseases; the inferior doctor treats full-blown diseases." Another concept of Chinese medicine is that of **qi**, which is the basis of activities of body and mind and is the primordial entity of both material (body) and nonmaterial (mind) things, gross and subtle (Subbarayappa, 2001).

Lao Tse, or Lao Tzu (which literally means Old Master), who lived around the 6th century BCE, developed the philosophy of **Taoism** (Khoo, 1998). His teachings disseminated the philosophy of the *Tao* (or the Way), which refers to a reality that naturally exists from primordial time and gives rise to all other things. *Tao* can be found by experiencing oneness in all things. Taoists introduced the idea of healing by drugs and used alchemy. Another well-known Chinese philosopher who influenced Chinese medicine and public health is Confucius (541–479 BCE). His philosophy emphasized correctness of social relationships along with personal and governmental morality. Regarding traditional and modern treatments, Confucius said, "Because the new methods of treatment are good, it does not follow that the old ones were bad; for if our honorable and worshipful ancestors had not recovered from their ailments, you and I would not be here today" (Huth & Murray, 2000, p. 359).

Ancient Civilization in Greece

It is believed that the roots of medicine, and the way it is practiced today, can be traced back to the Greek civilization in 5th century BCE, when Hippocrates (460–377 BCE) introduced a rational way of treating diseases (Cilliers & Retief, 2006). Hippocrates, often called the Father of Medicine, wrote a body of writings known as the **Corpus Hippocraticum**, a compilation of around 70 books. Classical Greek medicine involved four humors (blood, phlegm, black bile, and yellow bile), four elements (earth, air, fire, and water), and four qualities (hot, cold, moist, and dry). Any imbalance in these caused disease. Depression, for example, was caused by an excess of black bile. The system was rational because it was devoid of superstition and religion and was based on experimentation. Also, the training of a physician was done by apprenticeship under another physician. Another important feature of Greek civilization was the development of an ethical code of conduct for physicians. The Hippocratic Oath is still used today in many parts of the world by physicians. Most physicians in Greek civilization were men (*iatroi*), but there were also female doctors (*iatrinai*).

Hippocrates had concerns about how the mentally ill were treated. Hippocrates attempted to classify people by the way in which they behaved. The mentally ill were generally treated humanely by the ancient Greeks, and there was a movement away from belief in the supernatural origins of mental illnesses toward more rational explanations. Music, sedation with opium, activity, dietary measures, and hygiene were some means through which care was given (Alexander & Selesnick, 1966). A ritual of incubation in which a person was put to sleep in the temple and then his or her dreams were interpreted was a common practice (Evans, 2005).

Plato (427–327 BCE), a Greek philosopher, showed that medicine and philosophy were inextricably linked (Stempsey, 2001). He advocated holistic medicine, in which cure of the body alone without cure of the soul is not a whole cure. Holistic health involves uniting both body and soul; thus, along with medical technology, philosophy is needed for complete healing to take place. He also emphasized the role of personal responsibility in maintaining health and favored prevention rather than cure.

Ancient Roman Civilization

In earlier times medicine in Roman civilization was based on folk remedies, herbs, religious influences, and superstition. Around the 4th century BCE, Greek medicine started entering

Rome (Cilliers & Retief, 2006). To practice medicine in the Roman Empire, physicians only needed permission from a magistrate. Julius Caesar exempted physicians from paying tax and gave them citizenship. This practice was upheld by subsequent emperors such as Augustus, Vespasian, and Hadrian. The introduction of Greek practices also systematized medicine. The mentally ill were generally treated humanely by the Romans. **Aulus Cornelius Celsus** (25 BCE to 50 CE) was an important contributor to medicine in the Roman Empire. He differentiated between different types of the insane, such as those that are sad, those that are hilarious, and those that are violent and rebellious (Evans, 2005). He was humane in prescribing treatment for the insane and advocated for treatment with entertaining stories, persuasion, and diversion therapy.

> *Greeks and Romans were humane in prescribing treatment for those that were mentally ill.*

Middle Ages or Dark Ages (Between 500 CE and 1500 CE)

With the fall of the Roman Empire in 476 CE, the rational and humanitarian approaches to mental illnesses were forgotten and eventually replaced with witchcraft, shamanism, superstition, and mysticism. During this period the influence of the Church and associated dogma increased in the lives of common people. Great expenditures were made on Crusades, or Holy Wars. The average life expectancy was a mere 31 years (Glasscheib, 1964). Usually, the mentally ill were locked in asylums, where they were treated harshly— flogged, starved, and often tormented. Occasionally, however, families would hide the mentally ill, or they were left to roam the streets. During the later part of the Dark Ages (476–1000 CE), religious influences in Europe mainly dictated the treatment administered to the mentally ill. Burnings at the stake and the practice of witchcraft were fairly common during this period (Alexander & Selesnick, 1966).

While Europe was passing through the Dark Ages, the Arabs, borrowing from the Greeks and Romans, developed their own medical system, known as the **Unani system of medicine**. Unani medicine is still practiced widely in the south and southeast parts of Turkey to Saudi Arabia and in other parts of Asia, such as India and Pakistan (Yesilada, 2005). The Unani system uses herbs and folk remedies and is also influenced by Ayurveda (Subbarayappa, 2001). Abu Bakr Muhmad Ibn Zakariya al-Razi (also known as Rhazes) (865–925 CE) wrote the book *Kitab al-hawi fi al-tibb*, also known as *Liber continens*, which became a standard reference medical compendium (Browne, 1921). Rhazes did not believe in the dichotomy between the mind and body. He gave the concept of mental health and self-esteem as necessary to a patient's welfare (Stolyarov, n.d.). Another well-known physician of those times was Abu Ali al-Husayn ibn Abd Allah ibn Sina (980–1037 CE), who is also known as Avicenna in the West. He wrote the book *Kitab al-Qanun fi al-tibb*, or *Canon of Medicine* (Shah, 1966). In this book he described several mental illnesses. He believed in a close relationship between emotions and physical conditions and advocated the therapeutic role of music on physical and psychological well-being of patients. According to the Unani system, the human body and health were made up of seven components: elements (*Al-Arkan*), temperament (*Al-Mizaj*), four humors (*Al-Akhlat*), organs (*Al-A'da*), vital spirit (*Al-Arwah*), faculties (*Al-Quwa*), and functions (*Al-Afal*). The four elements were earth, fire, water, and air, and the four humors were blood, bile, phlegm, and black bile.

The Renaissance

The Renaissance (derived from French *renaissance*, meaning "rebirth") was a cultural movement spanning from 1420 to 1630 in which a revival of science, art, and culture occurred. It encompassed a revival of learning based on classical sources, the development of linear perspective in painting, and educational reform (Shorter, 1997). Unfortunately, in this period the approach to mental illnesses and the mentally ill changed little. The Middle Age belief that mental illnesses were caused by evil spirits carried on into this period. The mentally ill were frequently imprisoned or locked away in mental asylums and denied any professional care. Mental illnesses were mostly considered irreversible. The methods used to cure mental illnesses during this time were all rooted in ignorance and included purging, bleeding, and blistering. Viewed as demon-possessed or characterized as senseless animals, the mentally ill were subjected to appalling treatments. The widespread use of physical restraints—straitjackets and heavy arm and leg chains—often deprived patients of their self-respect and freedom (Shorter, 1997).

René Descartes (1596–1650), a French mathematician and philosopher, dichotomized mind and body. He looked upon the mind as being completely separate from the body. He advocated that the mind was under the purview of religion and the body was to be treated by physicians. This distinction shaped medicine for many years and was responsible for distinction between "physical health" and "mental health." However, in the 20th century this notion was challenged and the inseparable nature of the body and mind was established.

Paracelsus (1493–1541), a Swiss physician, did not believe evil spirits caused mental illness. This, however, did not change the general treatment of the mentally ill. Cotton Mather (1663–1728), a Puritan preacher in Boston, took a stance against the methods used in the Salem witchcraft trials (1692–1693) in which 19 women were tried and executed for witchcraft. He also advocated for physical examinations for mental illnesses (Lutz, 2000; Silverman, 1984). However, no real advancements in the care of the mentally ill were made before the 18th century (Alexander & Selesnick, 1966; Shorter, 1997; Trimble, 1996).

> *The thinking of Rene Descartes, which influenced Western medicine, dichotomized the body from the mind. He advocated that the mind was under the purview of religion and the body was to be treated by physicians.*

The 18th Century

Frank Mesmer (1733–1815), an Austrian physician, initiated a therapeutic approach to behavior. Mesmer believed that human body contained fluids similar to magnetic forces. He postulated that mental illnesses were due to misdistribution or deficiency of magnetism (Munson, 2001). Mesmer suggested that the mentally ill could be cured by holding rods filled with iron filings in water. He based his treatment on the idea that it would give people a balance in the universe. Even though Mesmer's technique proved to be wrong, it heralded a major paradigm shift in the perception and treatment of mental illnesses.

Benjamin Rush (1745–1813), an American physician, educator, writer, and humanitarian, wrote the book, *Medical Inquires and Observations upon the Diseases of the Mind* (Rush, 1812). The book advocated for humane treatment of mentally ill and is considered as the first textbook of psychiatry in America. The chapters of the book included topics such as intellectual derangement; remote, exciting, and predisposing causes of mental illness; hypochondriasis or tristimania; amenomania, mania, and remedies for mania; manalgia; means of improving the condition of mad people; dissociation; derangement in the will; derangement in the principle of faith; derangement of memory; fatuity; somnambulism; illusions; absence of mind; derangement of passions; morbid state of sexual appetite; and derangement in moral faculties. Many of the terms and topics used above are no longer used in modern terminology.

In 1793 **Philippe Pinel** (1745–1826), a French physician, challenged the traditional wisdom of keeping the mentally ill restrained when he removed the chains from patients at the Asylum de Bicetre in Paris (Shorter, 1997). He divided the patients and categorized them according to different disorders, replacing purging, bleeding, and blistering with simple and humane psychological treatments, along with observing and talking to the patients. Pinel's approach focused on close and friendly contact with the mentally ill, discussion about their personal difficulties, and a regimen of purposeful activities. He wrote a book, *Traité médico-philosophique sur l'aleniation mentale; ou la manie* (Medico-Philosophical Treatise on Mental Alienation or Mania), in 1801 in which he elaborates his psychologically oriented approach. His approach can be considered as the first psychotherapeutic approach to mentally ill patients. Pinel divided all mental illnesses into four categories—mania, melancholia, dementia, and idiocy—which was a revolutionary stride for those times. His theories on mental illness were the first to span both physiological and psychological explanations. He suggested that mental illnesses were either the result of having sustained excessive social or psychological stress or the consequence of hereditary causes or damage to the body. Pinel is credited as the first person to maintain written case studies on patients, which focused on their long-term treatment (Alexander & Selesnick, 1966; Shorter, 1997).

Pinel saw asylums as places for treatment and not places to hide the mentally ill. They were to be places where patients were seen as sick human beings deserving of dignity, compassion, and medical treatment. It was Pinel who first thought that those suffering from mental illness could be rehabilitated and returned to society. He oversaw the conversion of a residence for the mentally ill from a mad house into a hospital during his lifetime. Soon, Pinel's reforms were being imitated throughout the rest of Europe.

The 19th Century

Jean-Martin Charcot (1825–1893) was a French neurologist and professor of anatomical pathology, nicknamed "the Napoleon of the neuroses" (Jay, 2000). His work greatly influenced the mental health movement. Charcot's most impressive work was on hypnosis and hysteria. Charcot maintained that hysteria was a neurological disorder caused by hereditary problems in the nervous system. He used hypnosis to induce hysterical states in patients and scrutinized the results. Charcot was responsible for changing the French medical community's outlook regarding the validity of hypnosis (the practice had been previously rejected as Mesmerism).

Dorothea Lynde Dix (1802–1887) was an American activist on behalf of the indigent insane who is credited with the creation of the first generation of American mental asylums. During the Civil War she served as superintendent of army nurses. Dix traveled throughout the country and, through a vigorous program of lobbying state legislatures and the U.S. Congress, was able to effect legislation for better care of the mentally ill.

Reports from Australia mention that in the 19th century mentally ill people were treated like criminals and those found guilty of lunacy were imprisoned (Sands, 2009). Madness at that time was viewed to be a result of possession, "bad blood," or inherent character flaws rather an illness (Happell, 2007; Singh, Benson, Weir, Rosen, & Ash, 2001). The view at that time in Australia was that mental conditions were incurable. The first "lunatic asylum" (as was known in those days) was built in 1811 in Castle Hill (what is now known as New South Wales) (Happell, 2007). In 1848 the second asylum was built in Melbourne in Victoria (Sands, 2009).

Other important strides were made during his time. In the United States the first psychiatric training program was established at McLean Hospital in Waverly, Massachusetts. Research was conducted on the effects of the venereal disease (now called sexually transmitted illnesses) syphilis on the mind, and a generally humane approach was reinstituted toward the mentally ill.

The 20th Century

Clifford Beers (1876–1943), a Yale graduate and young businessman, was largely responsible for ushering in 20th century reforms in psychiatric care. After having suffered an acute breakdown brought on by the death of his brother, Beers was hospitalized in a private mental institution (Alexander & Selesnick, 1966; Shorter, 1997). He was subjected to the degrading treatment and mental and physical abuses typical of those times. The deplorable treatment he received over the next couple of years in multiple mental health institutions led Beers to publish his autobiography, *A Mind That Found Itself*. The need for better care of the mentally ill was thus made public. The book had an immediate impact, spreading his vision of a massive mental health reform movement around the world. The execution of the movement began soon thereafter when Beers founded the Connecticut Society for Mental Hygiene. The society expanded the following year, forming the National Committee for Mental Hygiene. The society, both in Connecticut and eventually nationally, set forth the following goals:

- To improve attitudes toward mental illness and the mentally ill
- To improve services for the mentally ill
- To work for the prevention of mental illness and promote mental health

The mental health movement was fairly well established by the time Beers died in 1943.

Sigmund Freud (1856–1939), an Austrian neurologist and psychiatrist, founded the psychoanalytic school of psychology (Shorter, 1997). Freud is best known for his theories of the unconscious mind, which probe deeply into the psychological side of the individual. He is also well known for his redefinition of sexual desire as the primary motivational energy of human life that is directed toward a wide variety of objects. Because of his seminal work on psychoanalysis, Freud is commonly referred to as the Father of Psychoanalysis. Freud's work has been highly influential, popularizing

Sigmund Freud was the originator of the psychoanalytic school of psychology.

such notions as the unconscious; the id, superego, and ego; the Oedipus complex; defense mechanisms; Freudian slips; and dream symbolism.

Another important person in the history of mental health movement is **Emil Kraepelin** (1856–1926), a German psychiatrist, who classified hundreds of mental disorders. He called the traditional view of looking at mental illnesses "symptomatic" and called his new approach "clinical." Kraepelin was among the first mental health workers who advocated that the origins of mental illness were rooted in biology and genetics. A contemporary of Kraepelin was Alois Alzheimer (1864–1915), a German neuropathologist and psychiatrist. He worked on histological features of a type of dementia known as Alzheimer's disease.

Australia during this time also saw improvements in the care of the mentally ill. In 1933 The Mental Hygiene Act of 1933 was passed that changed the title of "hospitals for the insane" to "mental hospitals" and "lunatics" to "mental patients" (Sands, 2009). But the mental hospitals suffered from the problem of overcrowding and were under-staffed (Reischel, 2003).

Among other pivotal incidents of the 20th century that helped shape the path of mental health care were three unrelated discoveries: use of **psychosurgery** as a treatment for certain mental health disorders, the introduction of **electroconvulsive therapy** (ECT) as a treatment for certain mental illnesses, and the introduction of **neuroleptic drugs**, which included antipsychotics and tranquilizers.

Psychosurgery was completely revolutionized in the 20th century by Antonio Egas Moniz (1874–1955), a Portuguese neurologist who introduced the psychosurgical technique of **lobotomy** (the removal or severing of certain connections in the brain) in 1936 (Micale & Porter, 1994; Shorter, 1997). He was awarded the Nobel Prize in 1949. In the United States a modified version of the procedure developed by Moniz was introduced by a neurologist named Walter Freeman and his associate, neurosurgeon James Watts, called a "prefrontal lobotomy" (Diefenbach, Diefenbach, Baumeister, & West, 1999). Lobotomies were used in the past to treat a wide range of severe mental illnesses, including schizophrenia, clinical depression, and various anxiety disorders. It is estimated that between 1936 and the mid-1950s some 20,000 frontal lobotomies were performed on mental patients in United States (Janssen, 2007). The procedure had many side effects and made the patient listless and dull, without drive or initiative. This procedure was banned by several countries in the 1950s and ultimately fell out of use after neuroleptics were introduced.

Another important discovery of the 20th century was ECT. In 1938 Ugo Cerletti, an Italian psychiatrist, first tested ECT on human patients (Alexander & Selesnick, 1966; Shorter, 1997). In the years after Cerletti and others experimented with ECT on a much broader scale and were able to establish its utility and safety in clinical practice. Today, even though arguments persist regarding whether ECT is therapy or cruelty, it is established as a therapeutic option for mental conditions such as acute schizophrenia, manic-depressive illness, and episodes of major depression.

The introduction of neuroleptic drugs, including antipsychotics and major tranquilizers, starting in the 1950s marked the beginning of a new chapter in the annals of mental health. The use of these drugs led to a markedly reduced need for physical restraints. The first traditional antipsychotic drug, chlorpromazine, was introduced to treat patients with schizophrenia and other major mental disorders in 1952 (Janssen, 2007). In the 1960s haloperidol and lithium were discovered. Haloperidol provided calmness to agitated patients, and lithium revolutionized the treatment of mania. Over the past decades substantial interest in the research and development of novel neuroleptic drugs has led to the introduction of newer, relatively safer alternatives to the original medications.

In the United States in the 1960s hospitalization was quite common for mentally ill patients. It is estimated that 422,000 patients were hospitalized for mental illness in 1962 in the United States (Janssen, 2007). In the 1970s the trend for deinstitutionalization became the norm. In 1970 the term "health maintenance organization" (HMO) was introduced by Paul Ellwood who was a health policy advisor in the Nixon Administration (Druss, 2002; Luft, 1981). Health maintenance organizations were a response toward curtailing rising costs of health care by reducing hospitalizations. In the 1980s health plans began developing "managed care" mechanisms. **Managed care** refers to a system of financing and providing health care that seeks to cut costs and to improve quality of care. With the introduction of managed care since the 1980s short-duration hospital stay with early reentry into the community has become the standard care for mentally ill (Janssen, 2007). In 1990s use of brain imaging and atypical antipsychotic drugs have further improved understanding and treatment of mental illnesses. **Table 1.3** summarizes the key events in the timeline of the history of mental health.

TABLE 1.3	History of Mental Health: A Timeline
Time Period	**Event**
Primitive	Some primitive tribes were drilling holes in the skulls to let the evil spirits out, called trephining.
2000–600 BCE	*Bhuta vidya* as part of *Ayurveda* used for prevention and treatment of mental illnesses in India.
200 BCE	Origin of yoga in India to help in mental health.
3000–300 BCE	Ebers and Edwin Smith papyri had records of mental illnesses.
2695–2589 BCE	Huang Di in China talked about balance between *yang* (masculine principle) and *yin* (feminine principle) for mental health. Acupuncture was used to treat mental illnesses.
460–377 BCE	Hippocrates practiced Greek medicine that involved four humors (blood, phlegm, black bile, and yellow bile), four elements (earth, air, fire, and water), and four qualities (hot, cold, moist, and dry).
25 BCE to 50 CE	Aulus Cornelius Celsus, a physician in the Roman Empire, was humane in prescribing treatment for the insane and advocated for treatment with entertaining stories, persuasion, and diversion therapy.
476–1000 CE	During the Dark Ages in Europe religious influences dictated the treatment administered to the mentally ill.
865–925 CE	During the Middle Ages the Unani system was developed in the Arab world. Rhazes, a Unani physician, introduced the concept of mental health and self-esteem as necessary to a patient's welfare.

(continued)

TABLE 1.3	History of Mental Health: A Timeline *(Continued)*
Time Period	**Event**
1420–1630	During this period of Renaissance the treatments of mentally ill were rooted in ignorance and included purging, bleeding, and blistering.
1733–1815	Frank Mesmer suggested the mentally ill could be cured by holding rods filled with iron filings in water.
1745–1813	Benjamin Rush advocated for humane treatment of the mentally ill and wrote the book, *Medical Inquires and Observations upon the Diseases of the Mind*, the first textbook on psychiatry in America.
1745–1826	Philippe Pinel advocated simple and humane psychological treatments for the mentally ill. He wrote a book, *Traité médico-philosophique sur l'aleniation mentale; ou la manie* (Medico-Philosophical Treatise on Mental Alienation or Mania). His approach can be considered as the first psychotherapeutic approach to mentally ill patients.
1825–1893	Jean-Martin Charcot, a French neurologist, applied hypnosis for treatment of mentally ill.
1802–1887	Dorothea Lynde Dix, through a vigorous program of lobbying state legislatures and the U.S. Congress, was able to effect legislation for better care of the mentally ill.
1876–1943	Clifford Beers, who suffered from mental disease, wrote the book, *A Mind That Found Itself*, that underscored the need for better care of the mentally ill. He founded the Connecticut Society for Mental Hygiene that later expanded to the National Committee for Mental Hygiene.
1856–1939	Sigmund Freud, an Austrian neurologist and psychiatrist, described psychoanalysis.
1856–1926	Emil Kraepelin, a German psychiatrist, classified hundreds of mental disorders. He advocated that the origins of mental illness were rooted in biology and genetics.
1874–1955	Antonio Egas Moniz, a Portuguese neurologist, introduced the psychosurgical technique of lobotomy.
1938	Ugo Cerletti, an Italian psychiatrist, first tested ECT on human patients.
1950s	Introduction of neuroleptic drugs, including antipsychotics and major tranquilizers
1960s	Haloperidol, which calmed agitated patients, and lithium, which treated mania, were discovered. Hospitalization was quite common for mentally ill.
1970s	Health maintenance organizations were introduced. The trend for deinstitutionalization of mentally ill became the norm in the United States.
1980s	Managed care became the norm. Short-duration hospital stays with early reentry into the community became the standard care for the mentally ill.
1990s	Brain imaging and atypical antipsychotic drugs further improved the understanding and treatment of mental illnesses.

CONTEMPORARY TRENDS AND STANDARDS IN MENTAL HEALTH

Multiple trends over the course of the past several decades have shaped the evolution of mental health as a field. Some of these trends have been molded by social influences, whereas others have been ushered in due to the economic forces at play. The field has also diversified with the arrival of a range of disciplines that address different aspects of an individual's mental health in a variety of settings. Perhaps the most important trends have been the move toward deinstitutionalization, legislation to support mental health, the rapid development of managed care, and a general movement toward biological underpinnings of mental health disorders.

Deinstitutionalization

Deinstitutionalization, the process of replacing long-stay psychiatric hospitals with less isolated community mental health service for those diagnosed with mental disorder or developmental disability, first began in the 1960s. The major factors that propelled the trend of deinstitutionalization in United States were a community mental health philosophy that it is better to treat the mentally ill nearer to their families, jobs, and communities; the effectiveness of newer psychopharmacological agents; the increasing importance of legal, judicial, and legislative actions in defining where and under what circumstances mental patients could be treated; and funding opportunities under Medicaid, Medicare, and Supplemental Security Income that allowed states to shift the fiscal burden of the mentally ill to federal care if they moved patients out of state facilities (Talbott, 2004). Even though the trend of deinstitutionalization was based on compassionate mental health care, it resulted in multiple problems for the chronically mentally ill patient. Two new syndromes were described as an aftermath of deinstitutionalization: "falling between the cracks," indicating a total lack of follow-up and aftercare for patients discharged into the community, and the "revolving door phenomenon," referring to the continued readmissions of discharged patients (Talbott, 2004).

Legislation

The **Americans with Disabilities Act** was signed into effect on July 26, 1990 by then President George Bush (Information and Technical Assistance on the Americans with Disabilities Act, 2009). This first of a kind comprehensive law prohibited private employers, state and local governments, employment agencies, and labor unions from discriminating against qualified individuals with disabilities in job application procedures, hiring, firing, advancement, compensation, job training, and other terms, conditions, and privileges of employment. The Act also included employment agencies and labor organizations.

The **mental health parity law (The Wellstone-Domenici Parity Act)** was enacted into law on October 3, 2008 and became effective on January 1, 2010 (American Psychological Association Practice Organization, 2008). This law purported to end health insurance benefit inequities between mental health/substance use disorders and medical-surgical benefits for group health plans with more than 50 employees. Equity in coverage applies to all financial requirements, including lifetime and annual dollar limits, deductibles, copayments, coinsurance and out-of-pocket expenses, and to all treatment limitations, including frequency of treatment, number of visits, days of coverage, and other similar limits. Please refer to Focus Feature 1.1 for further details.

Growth of Managed Care

Managed care, which emerged in 1980s, refers to a system of financing and providing health care that seeks to cut costs and improves quality of care. Due to major cuts in health programs, managed care systems currently provide most of the mental health care. Because of the inherent focus on cost containment, managed care attempts to set strict limits for mental health care both for inpatient and outpatient treatment settings. **Capping,** the practice of limiting the dollar amount for an individuals' lifetime psychiatric care, has been criticized by practitioners and patients. The managed care approach has also drastically reduced the number and kind of psychotherapy sessions for which an individual can be reimbursed. As mentioned above, some recent legislative enactments have addressed the bias managed care creates in the field of mental health.

Biological Approach Toward Mental Health

Technological advances have helped unravel new information about the physiology and chemistry of the brain. Studies have focused extensively on the connection between the anatomy and physiology of the human brain with mental health and behavior. So profound were some of these developments that then president George Bush designated the 1990s as the Decade of the Brain: "to enhance public awareness of the benefits to be derived from brain research" (Library of Congress, 2000). **Biological psychiatry**, an approach to understand mental disorders in terms of the biological functions of the nervous system, has gained favor in current times, and there is an increasing pressure on mental health providers to focus on psychopharmacology or drugs that can produce rapid resolution of some symptoms of mental disorders. Regrettably, this has also resulted in neglect and, occasionally, discouragement of other forms of treatment approaches such as psychotherapy (Barry, 2002).

FOCUS FEATURE 1.2 WHO'S FRAMEWORK ON MENTAL HEALTH, HUMAN RIGHTS, AND LEGISLATION

WHO (2009b) identifies common human rights violations of mental ill people as

- Insufficient access to essential mental health care
- Unsuitable forced admission in mental health facilities
- Violations within mental institutions such as use of shackles, filthy living conditions, and so on
- Discrimination and violations of basic rights outside of mental institutions
- Inappropriate detentions in prisons

Therefore, WHO (2009b) recommends the following:

- Mental health care must be available at the community level for anyone who may need it.
- Countries must set up monitoring bodies to make certain human rights are being respected in all mental health institutions.
- People with mental illnesses have the same human rights as others. Countries must protect them from discrimination.
- People with mental illnesses must be steered away from the criminal justice system and toward mental health services.

SKILL-BUILDING ACTIVITY

Several functionaries work in the area of mental health. A mental health functionary or mental health professional is a person who provides services for either improving an individual's mental health or for treating mental illness in a person. Some of the mental health

			Tasks	Approximate
TABLE 1.4 Professional Distinctions Between Mental Health Providers				
Professional	**Degree(s)**	**License**	**Performed**	**Annual Income**
Psychiatrist				
Clinical psychologist				
Internist				
Family physician				
Physician assistant				
Psychiatric (clinical) social worker				
Psychiatric nurse				
Psychiatric aide				
Mental health counselor or psychotherapist				
Art therapist				
Mental health educator				
Mental health advocate				

professionals are psychiatrists, clinical psychologists, internists, family physicians, physician assistants, psychiatric (clinical) social workers, psychiatric nurses, psychiatric aides, mental health counselors/psychotherapists, art therapists, mental health educators, mental health advocates, and others. Use the Internet and other sources to complete **Table 1.4**.

SUMMARY

Health is defined as a means to achieve desirable goals in life while maintaining multidimensional (physical, mental, social, political, economic, spiritual) equilibrium that is operationalized for individuals as well as for communities. *Mental health* is defined as the ability of an individual to fulfill his or her obligations to self and society while living in mutual harmony with the physical and social environment. *Mental health education* deals with voluntarily modifying health behaviors that are conducive to making a person be in harmony with his or her environment. Such behaviors include stress management behaviors, relaxation and adequate sleep behaviors, effective communication behaviors, anger management behaviors, anxiety reduction behaviors, healthy eating behaviors, healthy physical activity and exercise behaviors, time management behaviors, financial management behaviors, recreation and leisure management behaviors, and adequate work-performance behaviors. *Mental health promotion* entails developing policies, regulations, and environments that are conducive to making a person be in harmony with his or her environment. It entails developing policies, regulations, and environments that reduce stress, ensure adequate work for all, foster relaxation opportunities for all, regulate anger and associated harms, reduce anxiety, provide adequate food for all, ensure adequate housing for all, provide sufficient supports for being physically active, and provide for enough recreation and leisure opportunities.

Ancient civilization in India (2000–600 BCE) introduced the practices of *Ayurveda* and yoga, which have provided important contributions to mental health. In the Egyptian civilization (3000–300 BCE) the Ebers and the Edwin Smith papyri are most important to mental illness and mental health. Ancient civilization in China is credited with developing the Chinese system of medicine based on *qi, yang,* and *yin.* The mentally ill were generally treated humanely by the ancient Greeks and Romans. During the Middle ages (500–1500 CE) the Arabs originated a system of medicine called the Unani system. During the Renaissance Rene Descartes (1596–1650), a French philosopher, dichotomized mind and the body. In the 18th century Frank Mesmer (1733–1815) suggested that the mentally ill could be cured by holding rods filled with iron filings in water, which was later found to be erroneous. Benjamin Rush (1745–1813) wrote the book, *Medical Inquires and Observations upon the Diseases of the Mind,* which advocated for humane treatment of mentally ill; it is considered as the first textbook on psychiatry in America. In 1793 Philippe Pinel (1745–1826), a French physician, challenged the traditional wisdom of keeping the mentally ill restrained when he removed the chains from patients at the Asylum de Bicetre in Paris. He wrote a book, *Traité médico-philosophique sur l'aleniation mentale; ou la manie* (Medico-Philosophical Treatise on Mental Alienation or Mania) in 1801 in which he elaborates his psychologically oriented approach. His approach can be considered as the first psychotherapeutic approach to mentally ill patients. In 19th century Jean-Martin Charcot (1825–1893) worked on hypnosis and hysteria, and Dorothea Lynde Dix (1802–1887), an American activist on behalf of the indigent insane, is credited with the creation of the first generation of American mental asylums.

Clifford Beers (1876–1943), after being confined to multiple mental health institutions, wrote his autobiography, *A Mind That Found Itself,* thereby making the need for better care of the mentally ill a public issue. Sigmund Freud (1856–1939) founded the psychoanalytic school of psychology. Emil Kraepelin (1856–1926) classified mental disorders and advocated that the origins of mental illness were rooted in biology and genetics. Psychosurgery (lobotomy) was initiated by Antonio Egas Moniz (1874–1955) and was popular between 1936 and mid-1950s, after which it was discontinued. In 1938 Ugo Cerletti, an Italian psychiatrist, first tested ECT on human patients. The introduction of neuroleptic drugs starting in the 1950s marked the beginning of a new chapter in the annals of mental health. In the 1970s the trend for deinstitutionalization became the norm. In the 1980s health plans began developing "managed care" mechanisms. In 1990s use of brain imaging and atypical antipsychotic drugs further improved the understanding and treatment of mental illnesses. Contemporary trends are the move toward deinstitutionalization, legislation to support mental health, the rapid development of managed care, and a general movement towards biological underpinnings of mental health disorders.

REVIEW QUESTIONS

1. Define health, mental health, and mental illness.
2. Describe Jahoda's model of mental health.
3. Identify the key aspects of Tengland's model of mental health.
4. What are the constituents of mental health education?
5. Differentiate between mental health education and mental health promotion.

6. Discuss the contributions of the ancient civilization of India to mental health.
7. Explain the contributions of Greco-Roman civilization to mental health.
8. Identify the salient contributions of the 18th century physicians Frank Mesmer, Benjamin Rush, and Philippe Pinel in the care of mentally ill.
9. Describe the contributions of Emil Kraepelin and Sigmund Freud to mental health.
10. Differentiate between psychosurgery and electroconvulsive therapy.
11. Discuss some contemporary trends in the field of mental health.

WEBSITES TO EXPLORE

Electroconvulsive Therapy

http://www.mayoclinic.com/health/electroconvulsive-therapy/MY00129

This website from Mayo Clinic defines electroconvulsive therapy (ECT), why it is done, the risks associated with it, how to prepare, what to expect, and results. *The website also has links to a video about a woman's experience with ECT. Watch the video. Would you recommend ECT for a loved one who has been prescribed it? Why or why not?*

History of Mental Illness

http://www.mentalwellness.com/mentalwellness/sch_history.html#top

This website provides a timeline of key events in the history of mental health and mental illnesses. The timeline contains significant events from the 1600s to 1997. *Review this timeline. Find out more about an event mentioned in the timeline by doing a Google search on that topic.*

History of Mental Illness

http://www.bipolarworld.net/Bipolar%20Disorder/History/mental_illness.htm

This website has some interesting links to persons and events related to history of mental illness, particularly bipolar disorder. Some of these links are pictorial histories, Pharaoh to Freud, history of DSM, Emil Kraepelin, history of self-help movement, Dorothea Dix, and so on. *Visit one of the links and make a fact sheet on a topic of your interest.*

Internet Mental Health

http://www.mentalhealth.com/

This website, developed by a Canadian psychiatrist, Dr. Phillip Long, has useful information about mental health and mental illnesses. The website is intended for mental health professionals, patients with mental illness, families of patients, mental health support groups, students, and members from the general public. *The website toolbar has search, index, and glossary features. Using the search feature, find out more about a mental illness.*

Psychosurgery

http://www.psychosurgery.org/about-lobotomy/

This website is about psychosurgery, commonly referred to as lobotomy, that was practiced between 1936 and the mid-1950s to treat mentally ill patients. The website has information on three common forms of psychosurgery: prefrontal leucotomy, prefrontal lobotomy, and transorbital lobotomy. *The website has oral histories from relatives of people who were lobotomized. Read an oral history. What is your opinion of psychosurgery?*

REFERENCES AND FURTHER READINGS

Alexander, F., & Selesnick, S. T. (1966). *The history of psychiatry: An evaluation of psychiatric thought and practice from prehistoric times*. New York: Harper & Row.

American Psychiatric Association. (2000). *Diagnostic and statistical manual of mental disorders* (4th ed., text revision). Arlington, VA: Author.

American Psychological Association Practice Organization. (2008). *Summary of the Wellstone-Domenici Mental Health Parity and Addiction Equity Act of 2008*. Retrieved from http://www.apapractice.org/apo/in_the_news/parity_summary.GenericArticle.Single.articleLink.GenericArticle.Single.file.tmp/SummaryOfTheNewParityLaw.pdf.

Barry, P. B. (2002). *Mental health and mental illness*. New York: Lippincott.

Bensley, R. J. (1991). Defining spiritual health: A review of the literature. *Journal of Health Education, 22*(5), 287–290.

Browne, E. G. (1921). *Arabian medicine*. London: Cambridge University Press.

Cattan, M. (2006). Introduction. In M. Cattan & S. Tilford (Eds.), *Mental health promotion. A lifespan approach* (pp. 1–8). Berkshire, UK: Open University Press.

Cilliers, L., & Retief, F. P. (2006). Medical practice in Graeco-roman antiquity. *Curationis, 29*(2), 34–40.

Cook, H. (2004). Historical keywords: Health. *Lancet, 364*, 1481.

Diefenbach, G. J., Diefenbach, D., Baumeister, A., & West, M. (1999). Portrayal of lobotomy in the popular press: 1935–1960. *Journal of the History of Neurosciences*, 8(1), 60–69.

Downie, R., Fyfe, C., & Tannahill, A. (1990). *Health promotion: Models and values*. Oxford, UK: Oxford University Press.

Druss, B. G. (2002). The mental health/primary care interface in the United States: History, structure, and context. *General Hospital Psychiatry, 24*, 197–202.

Evans, K. (2005). Historical foundations. In R. Elder, K. Evans, & D. Nizette (Eds.), *Psychiatric and mental health nursing* (pp. 28–44). Marrickville, NSW, Australia: Elsevier.

Glascheib, H. S. (1964). *The march of medicine: The emergence and triumph of modern medicine*. New York: G. P. Putnam's Sons.

Gold, R. S., & Miner, K. R., for the 2000 Joint Committee on Health Education and Promotion Terminology. (2002). Report of the 2000 Joint Committee on Health Education and Promotion Terminology. *Journal of School Health, 72*, 3–7.

Green, L. W., & Kreuter, M. W. (2005). *Health program planning: An educational and ecological approach* (4th ed.). Boston: McGraw-Hill.

Guntrip, H. (1961). *Personality structure and human interaction the developing synthesis of psychodynamic theory*. London: Hogarth.

Happell, B. (2007). Appreciating the importance of history: A brief historical overview of mental health, mental health nursing and education in Australia. *The International Journal of Psychiatric Nursing Research, 12*(2), 1439–1445.

Hines, R. (1999). *Ancient Indian religion. The Vedas*. Retrieved from http://www.wsu.edu/~dee/ANCINDIA/VEDAS.htm.

Horsley, V. (1888). Trephining in the Neolithic period. *Journal of the Anthropological Institute of Great Britain and Ireland, 17*(1888), 100–106.

Huth, E. J., & Murray, T. J. (2000). *Medicine in quotations: Views of health and diseases through the ages* (p. 359). Philadelphia: American College of Physicians.

Information and Technical Assistance on the Americans with Disabilities Act. (2009). *Americans with Disabilities Act*. Retrieved from http://www.ada.gov/.

Jahoda, M. (1958). *Current concepts of positive mental health*. New York: Basic Books.

Janssen (2007). *History of mental illness*. Retrieved from http://www.mentalwellness.com/mental wellness/sch_history.html#top.

Jay, V. (2000). The legacy of Jean-Martin Charcot. *Archives of Pathology and Laboratory Medicine, 124*(1), 10–11.

Khoo, K. K. (1998). The Tao and the Logos: Lao Tzu and the Gospel of John. *International Review of Mission, 87*(344), 77–84.

Library of Congress. (2000). *Project on the decade of the brain*. Retrieved from http://www.loc.gov /loc/brain/.

Luft, H. S. (1981). *Health maintenance organizations, dimensions of performance*. New York: Wiley.

Luongo, T. (2008). *The Mental Health Parity and Addiction Equity Act of 2008: Equal footing for those suffering from mental health and addiction disorders*. Retrieved from http://www.hrtutor.com/en /news_rss/articles/2008/12-02-Mental-Health-Parity-and-Addiction-Equity-Act-of–2008.aspx.

Lutz, N. J. (2000). *Cotton Mather*. Philadelphia: Chelsea House Publishers.

MacDonald, G. (2006). What is mental health? In M. Cattan & S. Tilford (Eds.), *Mental health promotion. A lifespan approach* (pp. 8–32). Berkshire, UK: Open University Press.

Maharishi, Y. V. (1992). *Journey of consciousness*. New Delhi: Macmillan India Limited.

Markus, H. R., & Kitayama, S. (1991). Culture and the self: Implications for cognition, emotion, and motivation. *Psychological Review, 98*, 224–253.

McDowell, I., & Newell, C. (1987). The theoretical and technical foundations of health measurement. In I. McDowell & C. Newell (Eds.), *Measuring health: A guide to rating scales and questionnaires* (pp. 10–42). New York: Oxford University Press.

Micale, M. S., & Porter, R. (1994). *Discovering the history of psychiatry*. New York: Oxford University Press.

Modeste, N. M., & Tamayose, T. (Eds.). (2004). *Dictionary of public health promotion and education. Terms and concepts* (2nd ed.). San Francisco: Jossey Bass.

Munson, C. E. (2001). *The mental health diagnostic desk reference: Visual guides and more for learning to use the Diagnostic and Statistical Manual (DSM-IV TR)*. Binghamton, NY: Haworth Press.

Nasser, M. (1987). Psychiatry in ancient Egypt. *Bulletin of the Royal College of Psychiatrists, 11*, 420–422.

Park, J. E., & Park, K. (1986). *Textbook of preventive and social medicine* (11th ed.). Jabalpur, India: Banarasidas Bhanot Publishers.

Perrin, K. M., & McDermott, R. J. (1997). The spiritual dimension of health: A review. *American Journal of Health Studies, 13*(2), 90–99.

Pickett, G., & Hanlon, J. J. (1998). *Public health: Administration and practice* (10th ed.). St. Louis, MO: Mosby.

Preston, G. H. (1943). *The substance of mental health*. New York: Farrar & Rinehart.

Reischel, H. J. (2003). *The care that was* (2nd ed.). Burleigh, Australia: Poseidon Books.

Romas, J. A., & Sharma, M. (2010). *Practical stress management. A comprehensive workbook for promoting health and managing change through stress reduction* (5th ed.). San Francisco: Benjamin Cummings.

Rush, B. (1812). *Medical inquires and observations upon the diseases of the mind.* Philadelphia: John Grigg.

Sands, N. M. (2009). Round the bend: A brief history of mental health nursing in Victoria, Australia 1848 to 1950's. *Issues in Mental Health Nursing, 30,* 364–371.

Seedhouse, D. (2002). *Total health promotion. Mental health, rational fields and the quest for autonomy.* West Sussex, UK: John Wiley and Sons.

Shah, M. H. (1966). *The general principles of Avicenna's canon of medicine.* Karachi, Pakistan: Naveed Clinic.

Shorter, E. (1997) *A history of psychiatry: From the era of the asylum to the age of Prozac.* New York: John Wiley & Sons.

Silverman, K. (1984). *The life and times of Cotton Mather.* New York: Harper & Row.

Singh, B., Benson, A., Weir, W., Rosen, A., & Ash, D. (2001). The history of mental health services in Australia. In G. Meadows & B. Singh (Eds.), *Mental health in Australia: Collaborative community practice.* South Melbourne, Australia: Oxford University Press.

Singh, K. (1983). *Religions of India.* New Delhi: Clarion Books.

Stempsey, W. E. (2001). Plato and holistic medicine. *Medicine, Health Care, and Philosophy, 4*(2), 201–209.

Stolyarov G. II, (n.d.). *Rhazes: The thinking Western physician.* Retrieved from http://www.liberal institute.com/IslamicPhysicianRhazes.html.

Subbarayappa, B. V. (2001). The roots of ancient medicine: An historical outline. *Journal of Biosciences, 26*(2), 135–143.

Talbott, J. A. (2004). Deinstitutionalization: Avoiding the disasters of the past. *Psychiatric Services, 55,* 1112–1115.

Tengland, P. (2001). *Mental health. A philosophical analysis.* Dordrecht, The Netherlands: Kluwer Academic.

Tilford, S. (2006). Mental health promotion. In M. Cattan & S. Tilford (Eds.), *Mental health promotion. A lifespan approach* (pp. 33–63). Berkshire, UK: Open University Press.

Trent, D. (1993). *Promoting mental health: Everyone's business.* Surrey, United Kingdom: NW Surrey Health Authority.

Trimble, M. R. (1996). *Biological psychiatry.* New York: Wiley.

U.S. Department of Health and Human Services (USDHHS). (1979). *Healthy People: The Surgeon General's report on health promotion and disease prevention.* Washington, DC: Author.

U.S. Department of Health and Human Services (USDHHS). (1980). *Promoting health—preventing disease. Objectives for the nation.* Washington, DC: Author.

U.S. Department of Health and Human Services (USDHHS). (1990). *Healthy People 2000. National health promotion and disease prevention objectives.* Washington, DC: Author.

U.S. Department of Health and Human Services (USDHHS). (1999). *Mental health: A report of the Surgeon General—Executive summary.* Rockville, MD: Author.

U.S. Department of Health and Human Services (USDHHS). (2000). *Healthy People 2010* (Vols. 1–2). Washington, DC: Author.

U.S. Department of Health and Human Services (USDHHS). (2009). *Healthy People 2020: The road ahead.* Retrieved from http://www.healthypeople.gov/HP2020/

World Health Organization (WHO). (1974). Constitution of the World Health Organization. *Chronicle of the World Health Organization, 1,* 29–43.

World Health Organization (WHO). (1986). *Ottawa Charter for Health Promotion, 1986.* Geneva: Author.

World Health Organization (WHO). (1997). *The Jakarta Declaration on leading health promotion into the 21st century.* Geneva: Author.

World Health Organization (WHO). (1998). *Health promotion glossary.* Available from http://www.who.int/hpr/NPH/docs/hp_glossary_en.pdf.

World Health Organization (WHO). (2001). *The World Health Report 2001. Mental health: New understanding, new hope.* Retrieved from http://www.who.int/whr2001/.

World Health Organization (WHO). (2009a). *Mental health.* Retrieved from http://www.who.int/mental_health/en/.

World Health Organization (WHO). (2009b). *WHO's framework on mental health, human rights and legislation.* Retrieved from http://www.who.int/mental_health/policy/fact_sheet_mnh_hr_leg_2105.pdf.

Yesilada, E. (2005). Past and future contributions to traditional medicine in the health care system of the Middle-East. *Journal of Ethnopharmacology, 100*(1–2), 135–137.

CHAPTER 2

Roles of Health Educators and Health Promoters in Mental Health Promotion

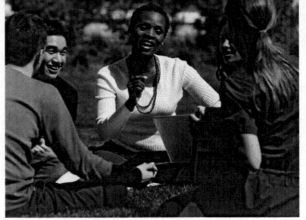

KEY CONCEPTS

- acculturation
- Certified Health Education Specialist (CHES)
- code of ethics for health educators
- cultural competence
- cultural sensitivity

- McCollum's model of mental health education
- mental health educator
- mental health promoter
- National Commission for Health Education Credentialing (NCHEC)

CHAPTER OBJECTIVES

After reading this chapter you should be able to
- List the responsibilities of certified health education specialists
- Identify the settings for mental health promotion
- Apply McCollum's model of mental health education
- Describe the role of health educators and health promoters in mental health promotion
- Discuss the role of cultural competency in mental health promotion
- Describe the attributes of a culturally competent mental health educator and mental health promoter
- Define national standards on culturally and linguistically appropriate services

RESPONSIBILITIES AND COMPETENCIES OF HEALTH EDUCATORS

The history of health education dates to the late 19th century, when the first academic programs emerged for developing school health educators (Allegrante et al., 2004). Since that time the field has expanded and grown substantially. The 2003 "Directory of Institutions Offering Undergraduate and Graduate Degree Programs in Health Education" listed 258 institutions offering baccalaureate, master's, and doctoral degrees in health education (American Association for Health Education [AAHE], 2003).

As the profession of health education has grown, greater interest has arisen in establishing standards and holding professionals accountable to those standards. In February 1978 a conference for health educators was convened in Bethesda, Maryland to analyze the similarities and differences in preparation of health educators from different practice settings and discuss possibilities for developing uniform guidelines (National Commission for Health Education Credentialing [NCHEC], Society for Public Health Education [SOPHE], & AAIIE, 2006; U.S. Department of Health, Education and Welfare, 1978). Soon after, the Role Delineation Project was implemented, which looked at the role of the entry-level health education specialist and identified the desirable responsibilities, functions, skills, and knowledge for that level. These were verified by a survey of practicing health educators. The process led to the formation of a document entitled *A Framework for the Development of Competency-Based Curricula for Entry-Level Health Educators* (NCHEC, 1985).

In 1986 the second Bethesda Conference was held, which provided consensus for the certification process; in 1988 the **National Commission for Health Education Credentialing (NCHEC)** was established. In 1989 a charter certification phase was introduced, during which health educators could become certified by submission of letters of support and academic records. From 1990 onward the NCHEC has conducted competency-based national certification examinations. An individual who meets the required health education training qualifications, successfully passes the certification exam, and meets continuing education requirements is known as a **Certified Health Education Specialist (CHES)**. In 2006 there were 12,000 such certified individuals (NCHEC, SOPHE, & AAHE, 2006).

National Commission for Health Education Credentialing is the official organization that attests Certified Health Education Specialists.

In 1992 efforts were undertaken to determine graduate-level competencies by the AAHE and SOPHE. A Joint Committee for the Development of Graduate-Level Preparation standards was formed. *A Competency-Based Framework for Graduate Level Health Educators* was published in 1999 (AAHE, NCHEC, & SOPHE, 1999).

In 1998 the profession launched the National Health Educator Competencies Update Project (CUP), a 6-year project to reverify the entry-level health education responsibilities, competencies, and subcompetencies and to verify the advanced-level competencies and subcompetencies (Airhihenbuwa et al., 2005; Gilmore, Olsen, Taub, & Connell, 2005). The CUP model identifies three levels of practice: (1) entry (competencies and subcompetencies performed by health educators with a baccalaureate or master's degree and less than 5 years of experience), (2) advanced 1 (competencies and subcompetencies performed by health educators with a baccalaureate or master's degree and more than 5 years of experience), and (3) advanced 2 (competencies and subcompetencies performed by health educators with a doctoral degree and 5 years or more of experience). The CUP model contains seven areas of responsibility, 35 competencies, and 163 subcompetencies, many of which are similar to previous models. Research and advocacy have been combined to form area IV and communication and advocacy have been combined in area VII.

Health education is an important and integral function of public health. The Institute of Medicine (1988) defined three core functions of public health in its *Future of Public Health* report:

1. *Assessment*: Every public health agency should regularly and systematically collect, assemble, analyze, and make available information on the health of the community.
2. *Policy development*: Every public health agency should assist in the development of comprehensive public health policies.
3. *Assurance*: Every public health agency should ensure that services necessary to achieve agreed-upon goals in communities are provided either directly or by regulations or by other agencies.

Building on these identified functions, the Public Health Functions Steering Committee (1994) identified six public health goals and 10 essential public health services. The six goals are to (1) prevent epidemics and the spread of disease, (2) protect against environmental hazards, (3) prevent injuries, (4) promote and encourage healthy behaviors, (5) respond to disasters and assist communities in recovery, and (6) ensure the quality and accessibility of health services. The 10 essential public health services are to (1) monitor health status to identify community health problems; (2) diagnose and investigate health problems and health hazards in the community; (3) inform, educate, and empower people about health issues; (4) mobilize community partnerships to identify and solve health problems; (5) develop policies and plans that support individual and community health efforts; (6) enforce laws and regulations that protect health and ensure safety; (7) link people to needed personal health services and ensure the provision of health care when it is otherwise unavailable; (8) ensure the availability of a competent public health and personal health care workforce; (9) evaluate the effectiveness, accessibility, and quality of personal and population-based health services; and (10) research new insights and innovative solutions to health problems. It can be seen from both these lists that health education is a core and integral function of public health and that health educators are key public health functionaries.

> *The three core functions of public health functionaries are assessment, policy development, and assurance.*

The Institute of Medicine (2002) published another report, *The Future of the Public's Health in the 21st Century*, which echoed the vision expressed in *Healthy People 2020* (U.S. Department of Health and Human Services, 2009). It emphasized the following key areas of actions:

- Adopting a focus on population health that includes multiple determinants of health
- Strengthening the public health infrastructure
- Building partnerships
- Developing systems of accountability
- Emphasizing evidence
- Improving communication

Once again, all these functions underscore the inextricable linkage between public health and health education. Health education is an important subset of public health.

CODE OF ETHICS FOR THE HEALTH EDUCATION PROFESSION

In recent years there has been an increasing interest regarding ethics in all walks of life. Ethics is a major area of philosophy that deals with the study of morality. Practicing ethical behavior provides a standard for performance in any profession. In health education the earliest effort to develop a code of ethics appears to be the 1976 code of ethics developed by the Society for Public Health Education (Taub, Kreuter, Parcel, & Vitello, 1987). A coalition of national health education organizations, composed of the American Academy of Health Behavior, the AAHE, the American College Health Association, the American Public Health Association's Public Health Education and Health Promotion Section and School Health Education and Services Section, the American School Health Association, the Directors of Health Promotion and Education, Eta Sigma Gamma, the SOPHE, and the Society of State Directors of Health, Physical Education and Recreation, has developed a unified **code of ethics for health educators** (Coalition of National Health Education Organizations, 2004).

SETTINGS FOR MENTAL HEALTH PROMOTION

It is in this backdrop of health education and public health we recognize that health educators are an important public health functionary that are also responsible for mental health education and promotion. A **mental health educator** works in the area of mental health education by teaching health behavior modification so a person can be in harmony with his or her environment. Such behaviors include stress management behaviors, relaxation and adequate sleep behaviors, effective communication behaviors, anger management behaviors, anxiety reduction behaviors, healthy eating behaviors, healthy physical activity and exercise behaviors, time management behaviors, financial management behaviors, recreation and leisure management behaviors, and adequate work-performance behaviors. A **mental health promoter** develops policies, regulations, and environments that are conducive to making an individual be in harmony with his or her environment. Such policies, regulations, and environments include procedures that reduce stress, ensure adequate work for all, foster relaxation opportunities for all, regulate anger and associated harms, reduce anxiety, provide adequate food for all, ensure adequate housing for all, provide sufficient supports for being physically active, and provide for enough recreation and leisure opportunities.

A mental health educator works in the area of mental health education by teaching health behavior modification so a person can be in harmony with his or her environment.

Mental health educators work in a variety of settings: *community settings*, such as a public health department, a not-for-profit organization, a faith-based organization, or another community-based organization; *schools*, as school health educators where they could be looking at all aspects of health education along with mental health; *health care settings*, such as hospitals or mental health facilities; and *worksites*, such as businesses or industrial organizations where they could be looking at all aspects of health education along with mental health.

A mental health promoter develops policies, regulations, and environments that are conducive to making an individual be in harmony with his or her environment.

Mental health promoters could work with *government* where they develop policies, regulations, and environments that are conducive to mental health. They could also work in *community settings* where they help in promoting policies, regulations, and environments that are conducive to mental health. They could also work in *international settings* with international organizations promoting mental health.

At present there are rather limited opportunities for exclusive mental health education or promotion work. Most mental health work is done by general health educators who also have responsibilities in other areas. There are three reasons for this. First, a lot of stigma is associated with mental illnesses, and communities do not want to directly address mental health issues. It rarely makes it to a community-identified priority list despite being a very important epidemiologically identified priority. It is encouraging to note, however, that in recent years this stigma has reduced a little. Second, there is a lack of funding. The funding for public health is as such rather limited as compared with medical expenditures. In this context money is not readily available for prevention activities. Finally, health education has limited course work and training in the area of mental health, which limits health educators from solely doing mental health work.

MCCOLLUM'S MODEL OF MENTAL HEALTH EDUCATION

The field of mental health is dominated by functionaries who work with mentally ill patients. McCollum (1981) envisioned mental health educators who would work with "normal" people to teach principles and skills of positive mental health. She mentioned that such mental health educators would serve as teachers of cognitive, emotional, and behavioral approaches for healthy people in order for them to cope with stresses of daily living. Such mental health educators would be conversant in one or more areas such as stress, child management, drugs and alcohol, or communication and would use established educational methods. She proposed a six-step model for mental health educators based on the adult education model of Bergevin, Morris, and Smith (1963). However, we call it **McCollum's model of mental health education** because she applied it to mental health education:

1. *Population selection*: In this step the mental health educator selects the target population with whom he or she will work. Ideally, such groups should be small and homogenous, and members from the target population must be actively involved in addressing the issue.
2. *Need identification*: This step entails identifying the interests and needs of the target population. A mental health educator must explore with the group how they developed interest in their chosen topic and then identify ways of serving that interest in the best possible way.
3. *Goal setting*: The next step for the mental health educator is to set short-term and long-term goals for changes in knowledge, beliefs, attitudes, and behaviors.
4. *Selection of resources*: Next, the mental health educator selects resources that are needed to address the chosen issue(s). A number of educational tools, such as videos, DVDs, films, case studies, books, and pamphlets, are available on different topics from which the mental health educator can select the resources.
5. *Selection of instructional techniques*: There are several educational techniques such as lecture, group discussion, demonstration redemonstration, case study, role playing, psychodrama, simulation, panel discussion, open forum, colloquium, and symposium from which the mental health educator can select his or her approach.

6. *Evaluation*: This process of knowing whether the intervention achieved what it intended to achieve is done at three levels. The first level is to evaluate the planning and implementation of each step. The second level is to ascertain consumer satisfaction and immediate effects of education. The third level is application of learned skills in future situations. Some informal methods for evaluation are participant reaction sheet, participant interviews, use of an observer, and group discussion. More formal methods include evaluations of behavior change using quasi-experimental and experimental designs.

ROLES OF MENTAL HEALTH EDUCATORS AND MENTAL HEALTH PROMOTERS IN MENTAL HEALTH PROMOTION

The following discussion is based on areas of responsibility for health educators based on the CUP model applied to mental health educators and mental health promoters. The first area for mental health education and mental health promotion pertains to assessing individual and community needs related to mental health. One of the roles in this category is to retrieve mental health–related literature using databases such as Medline (PubMed), ERIC, CINAHL, Google Scholar, and PsycINFO. Mental health educators develop mental health education surveys to conduct needs assessment in the area of mental health, identify behaviors and their antecedents that either promote or hinder mental health, assess learning styles and environments for their target audiences in imparting mental health education, ascertain factors that augment or retard mental health education in the setting in which they are working, and, finally, analyze the mental health needs assessment data.

The second area for mental health education and mental health promotion pertains to planning mental health education strategies, interventions, and programs. The first role in this category is to involve people and organizations in planning mental health education programs. There is a lot of stigma associated with mental illnesses, and this needs to be removed by the mental health educator to generate support. Involvement of organizations for a common purpose is called a coalition. Formation of coalitions around mental health issues is an important task for the mental health promoter. In planning mental health education programs the mental health educator must incorporate research results, results of needs assessment, and principles of community organization. The mental health educator must develop measurable and appropriate program objectives. An easy way to remember how to make effective objectives is through the acronym SMART (Specific, Measurable, Action verb, Realistic, and Time frame). Wherever possible the mental health educator must make efforts that the mental health education programs are based on behavioral theories and have a logical scope and sequence plan. The mental health programs must be an integral part of all other health education efforts. A mental health educator must design mental health strategies, programs, and approaches that are consistent with the objectives. Mental health educators must use a variety of educational methods such as lecture, case study, small group discussion, role play, psychodrama, and simulation. Mental health educators must use appropriate technology, methods, and media for different groups and aim for culturally competent programs. Finally, a mental health educator must ascertain the resources and plan strategies to overcome barriers in implementation of the mental health education program.

The third area for mental health education and mental health promotion pertains to implementing mental health education strategies, interventions, and programs. Mental health educators must be able to apply community organization principles, collect baseline data pertaining to mental health objectives, deliver mental health programs, and conduct group facilitation. Mental health educators must be well versed with technology, capable of using a variety of educational methods, and be able to decide which method to use when. Mental health educators must use the code of ethics as described earlier in this chapter. Mental health educators must be well versed with theory-based methods, be culturally sensitive, and be able to deal with controversial mental health topics. Finally, a mental health educator must be able to conduct training programs using instructional resources for a variety of mental health topics such as stress management, relaxation and adequate sleep, effective communication, anger management, anxiety reduction, healthy eating, healthy physical activity and exercise, time management, financial management, recreation and leisure management, and adequate work-performance.

The fourth area for mental health education and mental health promotion pertains to conducting evaluation and research of mental health education programs. The mental health educator develops plans for evaluation and research that entails synthesizing information from the literature, choosing research designs and qualitative or quantitative paradigms, and locating existing valid and reliable instruments. If instruments are not available, then the mental health educator develops valid and reliable instruments. Mental health educators implement evaluation plans, analyze evaluation data, and apply appropriate evaluation technology. Mental health educators interpret results from evaluation and research by data analysis, comparison of evaluation findings to other projects, developing recommendations based on evaluation results, and writing reports. Finally, the mental health educator develops plans for implementing suggestions resulting from evaluation, sustains and improves mental health programs, and comes up with explanations for the findings from evaluation.

The fifth area for mental health education and mental health promotion pertains to administering mental health education strategies, interventions, and programs. Mental health educators must be able to demonstrate leadership in their organizations. Some characteristics of this attribute entail ability to conduct strategic planning, develop synchrony between organizational culture and programmatic goals, develop collegiality among program personnel, and ensure compliance of programs with laws and regulations. Mental health educators or promoters must be able to obtain and manage monetary resources by grant writing or other efforts. Mental health educators or promoters must be able to manage human resources by involving volunteers, demonstrating leadership, applying human resource policies, delineating qualifications for personnel on projects, fostering staff development, and implementing appropriate conflict resolution. Finally, the mental health educator or promoter must obtain support and acceptance for the mental health program by applying public relation concepts, developing cooperation among personnel, and providing support for individuals who deliver professional development courses.

The sixth area for mental health education and mental health promotion pertains to serving as a health education resource person in mental health. This category requires use of mental health–related information resources, including computerized ones. The other attribute in this category requires the mental health educator to be able to respond to requests for mental health information by either providing the information or referring to an appropriate source. A mental health educator must also be able to select resource materials for dissemination. Finally, a mental health educator or promoter must be able to establish consultative relationships by acting as a liaison between the mental health program and other organizations and clients, applying networking skills, and facilitating collaborative training efforts.

The seventh area for mental health education and mental health promotion pertains to communicating and advocating for mental health and mental health education. Mental health educators or promoters must be able to analyze and respond to current and future needs in mental health. He or she must be cognizant of factors that influence decision makers and challenges facing mental health programs. He or she must be able to implement advocacy initiatives. He or she must be able to implement a variety of communication methods by assessing appropriate language and use of culturally relevant materials. A mental health educator must promote the field of mental health education by having a personal plan as well as a collective plan. He or she must be familiar with mental health organizations. Finally, the mental health educator or promoter must be able to influence policies related to mental health.

CULTURAL COMPETENCY IN MENTAL HEALTH PROMOTION

The United States is a land of immigrants. We have a lot of diversity in our country, and this diversity is valued in our culture. However, diversity presents unique challenges when it comes to designing mental health education programs. Over the years this diversity has increased. Today, a number of people in the United States do not speak English at home; a substantial proportion of the U.S. population was not born here; minority groups have grown in numbers; the population of disabled people who are living is quite high; and there is a growing segment of gay, lesbian, bisexual, and transgender individuals (Perez & Luquis, 2008). All these diverse segments of the population have mental health needs. If we consider the entire population to be homogenous, we will not be able to reach out to the diverse needs of these segments.

Acculturation is the psychosocial adjustment and adaptation to a new culture of a person from another culture. Traditionally, acculturation has been defined as the behavioral and psychological changes in an individual that occur as a result of contact between people belonging to different cultural groups (Berry, 1997). Other researchers have approached acculturation in a slightly broader manner, calling it the social and psychological exchanges that take place when there is continuous contact and interaction between individuals from different cultures (Berry, 1997; Redfield, Linton, & Herskovits, 1936; Ryder, Alden, & Paulhus, 2000). Irrespective of how we define it, acculturation is often visualized as the individual's psychosocial adjustment and adaptation to a new culture. The specific set of difficulties an individual immigrant faces could be physical (new climatic conditions and a search for an abode), biological (changes in diet and diseases), social (dislocation of friends and formation of new relationships), cultural (sudden changes in political, economic, and religious contexts), and psychological (a need to change attitudes, values, and mental health connotations).

Berry's (1997) four classifications of acculturation has gained widespread acceptance despite limited research-based evidence. The four modes of acculturation he proposed are integration, assimilation, separation, and marginalization. *Integration* is the identification and involvement of an immigrant with both cultures, the mode that is linked with the most optimal mental health outcome. *Assimilation* is the state in which the immigrant identifies solely with the new culture. *Separation* is the situation in which the individual is involved only in his or her native culture, and *marginalization* is lack of involvement in either cultures and rejection of both.

The phenomenon of acculturation has assumed immense importance in contemporary times because more and more people are migrating from their native countries to others. A simple way of defining migration is to picture it as a phenomenon of individuals moving from one country, place, or locality to another. It can include the entire gamut of situations, from individuals who move to study, to seek better employment, to better their future, to avoid political and religious harassment, and to marry as well as family units that move to better their lives or join their established family members elsewhere. Avoidance of persecution is a relatively uncommon but nonetheless important reason for migration. Needless to say, once having been through the process of migration, the individuals who migrated undergo the closely related process of acculturation.

Programs are often developed to facilitate the process of acculturation. This is especially important when dealing with mental health programs. In this context two terms need to be understood: cultural sensitivity and cultural competence. Resnicow, Soler, Braithwaite, Ahluwalia, and Butler (2000, p. 271) defined **cultural sensitivity** as "the extent to which ethnic/cultural characteristics, experiences, norms, values, behavioral patterns, and beliefs of a target population as well as relevant historical, environmental, and social forces are incorporated in the design, delivery, and evaluation of targeted health promotion materials and programs." In the planning, implementation, and evaluation of mental health programs the characteristics of different ethnic compositions of target populations are very important.

There are two structures of cultural sensitivity, which can be thought of in terms of two primary dimensions (Resnicow, Baranowski, Ahluwalia, & Braithwaite, 1999): surface structure and deep structure. The former involves matching intervention materials and messages to the visible social and behavioral characteristics of a target population. It also includes an identification of the channels of communication and settings that would work best for a target group. For audiovisual materials, surface structure may involve using brand names and languages familiar to, and chosen by, the target audience. For example, a mental health program attempting to reach out to inner-city African American women might best be executed in a church setting.

> *Cultural sensitivity entails paying attention to and incorporating the cultural beliefs, attitudes, behaviors, values, historical aspects, social dimensions, and ecological characteristics of different ethnic compositions of target population in planning, implementation, and evaluation of mental health programs.*

Deep structure is the second dimension of cultural sensitivity and takes into account the manner in which cultural, social, environmental, psychological, and historical factors influence health behaviors across different racial/ethnic populations. Comprehension of how the target population perceives the cause and effect of an intervention is included in the deep structure. For example, some ethnic groups ascribe certain diseases to paranormal phenomena, and a health intervention targeting one of those conditions is bound to fail if it does not consider how that ethnic group will perceive the individual elements of the program. To sum up, the surface structure of an intervention can increase the receptivity, understanding, or acceptance of messages, whereas deep structure conveys salience and consequently determines the program's impact (Simons-Morton, Donohew, & Crump, 1997).

Regarding **cultural competence**, the health care industry has to be flexible enough to be able to meet the needs of an increasingly diverse population and discard the idea of one-size-fits-all health care. Cultural competence goes beyond either cultural awareness or cultural sensitivity. A more generic approach is to define it as the possession of cultural knowledge and respect for different cultural perspectives and possessing and using skills effectively in cross-cultural situations (Cross, Bazron, Dennis, & Isaacs 1989; Orlandi, 1995). Andrulis, Delbanco, and Shaw-Taylor (1999) presented the concept as a continuum, recognizing the fact that individuals and institutions can differ in the effectiveness of their responses to cultural diversity.

> *Cultural competence is possession of cultural knowledge and respect for different cultural perspectives and possessing and using skills effectively in cross-cultural situations.*

A mental health educator or mental health promoter must possess several qualities to be culturally competent. First, he or she must have basic cultural knowledge of all the major diverse groups represented in his or her target population. He or she must know their language; customs; common beliefs, attitudes, and practices regarding mental health and mental health issues; and important historical, social, and ecological dimensions about their culture. Second, he or she must genuinely respect the diversity in the target population. The more diverse the population, the greater its strength because it can look at any problem from multifarious perspectives and then choose the best solution. A mental health educator must be aware of his or her own biases in dealing with people from other cultures and must be able to remain respectful of the differences. Third, the mental health educator must have skills to linguistically understand and communicate with different members of the target population. If the educator does not possess these skills, then he or she must be able to hire the services of a translator/interpreter. Finally, the mental health educator or mental health promoter must be in possession of cross-cultural skills for communication and must be able to use them in cross-cultural situations.

NATIONAL STANDARDS ON CULTURALLY AND LINGUISTICALLY APPROPRIATE SERVICES

The Office of Minority Health (2007) developed 14 national standards on culturally and linguistically appropriate services (CLAS) directed toward health care organizations. They are arranged by three themes (culturally competent care, language access services, and organizational supports for cultural competence) and three types (mandates, guidelines, and recommendations).

A. Culturally competent care

1. It is a guideline that proposes health care organizations should ensure their patients receive effective, comprehensible, and respectful care that is provided in a way that is well matched with their language and culture.
2. It is a guideline that proposes health care organizations should hire and maintain staff and leadership that is representative of the demographics of that area.

3. It is a guideline that proposes health care organizations should ensure that all staff must receive ongoing education and training in CLAS delivery.

B. Language access services

4. It is a mandate that requires health care organizations to give language assistance services that include free bilingual staff and interpreter services at all times to patients with limited proficiency in English.
5. It is a mandate that requires health care organizations to provide patients both verbally and through written means about their right to receive language assistance services.
6. It is a mandate that requires health care organizations to ensure the competence of language assistance provided to patients with limited English proficiency patients/consumers by interpreters and bilingual staff.
7. It is a mandate that requires health care organizations to make available signage and easy to understand patient-related materials in the languages of the demographic groups.

C. Organizational supports for cultural competence

8. It is a guideline that proposes health care organizations must have a written strategic plan to provide CLAS.
9. It is a guideline that proposes health care organizations must conduct baseline and ongoing organizational self-assessments of CLAS-related activities and must integrate cultural and linguistic competence–related measures into their audits, quality improvement programs, patient satisfaction instruments, and evaluations.
10. It is a guideline that proposes health care organizations should ensure patient data related to race, ethnicity, and spoken and written languages be collected and updated on health records and linked with management information systems.
11. It is a guideline that proposes health care organizations should retain a current demographic, cultural, and epidemiological profile of the community along with a needs assessment to correctly plan and implement services that meet the cultural and linguistic characteristics of the region.
12. It is a guideline that proposes health care organizations should develop mutual partnerships with communities and involve patients and communities in planning and implementing CLAS.
13. It is a guideline that proposes health care organizations ensure culturally and linguistically sensitive conflict and grievance resolution processes for patients/consumers.
14. It is a recommendation that health care organizations must regularly make available to the public their efforts toward providing CLAS.

FOCUS FEATURE 2.1 HYPOTHETICAL JOB DESCRIPTION OF A MENTAL HEALTH EDUCATOR

John Doe graduated with a bachelor's degree in Health Promotion and Education from the University of Cincinnati. He has also passed the CHES exam. For his internship he worked as an intern in the

(continued)

Behavioral and Mental Health Unit at a local hospital because he was interested in pursuing a career in mental health education and mental health promotion. Upon completion of his internship he has been offered a position to work as mental health educator with the unit at the hospital. His job responsibilities are as follows:

- To design and conduct stress management and relaxation workshops for patients suffering from mental illnesses, chronic diseases, and terminal illnesses
- To assist in facilitating support groups for patients suffering from schizophrenia, bipolar disorder, anxiety and depression-related disorders, and other mental illnesses
- To assist in facilitating support groups for family members of patients suffering from mental illnesses
- To assist in supervision of volunteers and psychiatric aides who want to work in the Behavioral and Mental Health Unit at the hospital
- To organize monthly educational forums in the city of Cincinnati and Hamilton County with community partners that reduce stigma associated with mental illness and promote understanding toward people suffering from mental illnesses
- To collaborate with psychiatrists, psychologists, mental health counselors, and social workers in effective functioning of the Behavioral and Mental Health Unit
- To participate in writing grants for conducting mental health education

He reports to the Director of the Behavioral and Mental Health Unit at the hospital. Let us see what kind of course work and skills helped him get this job. He completed several courses related to health education:

- Introduction to Health Promotion
- Health Promotion Planning and Development
- Health and Human Behavior
- Evaluation of Health and Fitness Programs
- Implementing and Promoting Health Programs
- Chronic and Communicable Diseases

He also completed several courses related to mental health:

- Drugs and Society
- Stress Reduction
- Mental health

In addition, he completed a job-specific internship that helped him learn the skills needed for the job.

FOCUS FEATURE 2.2 CASE STUDY EXEMPLIFYING THE IMPORTANCE OF CULTURALLY COMPETENT INTERVENTIONS FOR MENTAL HEALTH CARE

Victor Garcia is a first-generation Cuban immigrant who migrated to New York City at the age of 25. Presently, he goes to college for an undergraduate degree and also works part time at a restaurant. He is single and lives with his mother. The rest of his family is in Cuba, and he has limited contact with them. He has a limited social support, confined to few school friends and some "acquaintances" from work.

(continued)

He has a very limited English proficiency and has consequently had difficulties at school and at social situations. For the past year and a half he has struggled with multiple physical symptoms. He has seen numerous internists, has had a thorough cardiologic and endocrinology workup, and has ended up in the emergency room on more than one occasion. He was referred for a psychiatric workup. He describes his symptoms as "random pains all over the body, constipation, tightness in chest, poor sleep, tingling sensation down the spine, sensation of choking and nausea accompanied by crying and a general feeling of hopelessness." The treating physician does not speak any Spanish and proceeds to conduct the entire clinical interview and examination in English. He diagnoses the patient with mood disorder unspecified and recommends psychotherapy. Simultaneously, he prescribes an antidepressant and asks the patient to follow up in 3 to 4 weeks. The treating physician believes he has followed the "standard of care." The patient, however, believes he has not been properly understood and that his doctor is trying to "throw medicines at him."

Because of his strong cultural bias against psychotropic medications the patient does not comply with the treatment. He misses several of his consecutive appointments, deteriorates clinically, and is eventually admitted to an inpatient psychiatric hospital where he is diagnosed with "severe major depression."

The following are important points:

- Utilizing the services of a translator/interpreter might have helped avert a wrong diagnosis in the above vignette.
- Addressing the patient's strongly rooted cultural bias against psychiatric medications may have helped ensure compliance and follow-up.
- Psychiatric illnesses may manifest with somatic or physical rather than psychological symptoms in certain cultures. For instance, patients with depression may present with pain in almost any part of the body. It may have helped if the treating clinician had focused on this aspect of culturally competent care.
- The affiliation for the family unit varies across different cultures. This should have been addressed or at least explored more in the example above. With this individual's consent his mother could also be involved in the treatment plan, to gather collateral information and to possibly help improve the treatment compliance.
- Finally, the social support of certain populations (migrants etc.) may be suboptimal and may need to be addressed.

SKILL-BUILDING ACTIVITY

In this chapter you were introduced to McCollum's model of mental health education. The first step in this model is population selection. Imagine you work with African American women who are pregnant in the inner city of a large city in the United States. A recent survey shows that perinatal depression is on the rise in this community. Perinatal depression includes a suppression of the mood that can affect a woman during pregnancy and after the birth of her newborn. It includes conditions such as prenatal depression, the "baby blues," postpartum depression, and postpartum psychosis. Your task is to apply McCollum's model of mental health education and to develop a culturally competent program to prevent the occurrence of this condition. You can also plan for early diagnosis and treatment in your application.

SUMMARY

The NCHEC certifies health educators who are then known as CHES. The National Health Educator CUP model identified seven areas of responsibility for health educators: (1) assess individual and community needs for health education; (2) plan health education strategies, interventions, and programs; (3) implement health education strategies, interventions, and programs; (4) conduct evaluation and research related to health education; (5) administer health education strategies, interventions, and programs; (6) serve as a health education resource person; and (7) communicate and advocate for health and health education. The Coalition of National Health Education Organizations developed a "code of ethics for health educators" that has six areas: (1) responsibility to the public, (2) responsibility to the profession, (3) responsibility to the employers, (4) responsibility in the delivery of health education, (5) responsibility in research and evaluation, and (6) responsibility in professional preparation. A mental health educator works in the area of mental health education by teaching health behavior modification so a person can be in harmony with his or her environment. A mental health promoter is a person who develops policies, regulations, and environments that are conducive to making an individual be in harmony with his or her environment. Mental health educators and promoters work in community settings, school settings, worksite settings, health care settings, and international settings.

McCollum's model of mental health education is a six-step model developed in 1981 for mental health education: (1) population selection, (2) need identification, (3) goal setting, (4) selection of resources, (5) selection of instructional techniques, and (6) evaluation. Mental health programs and educators must be culturally sensitive and culturally competent. Cultural sensitivity refers to paying attention to and incorporating the cultural beliefs, attitudes, behaviors, values, historical aspects, social dimensions, and ecological characteristics of different ethnic compositions of target population in planning, implementation, and evaluation of mental health programs. Cultural competence is the possession of cultural knowledge and respect for different cultural perspectives and having skills and being able to use those skills effectively in cross-cultural situations.

REVIEW QUESTIONS

1. Discuss the role of the National Commission for Health Education Credentialing.
2. What seven areas of responsibilities for health educators are identified in the CUP model?
3. What are the six responsibilities in the code of ethics for health educators?
4. What do mental health educators and mental health promoters do? What are some settings in which they can work?
5. Describe McCollum's model of mental health education. Can you apply this model to stress reduction in college students?
6. Describe the role of health educators and health promoters in mental health promotion.
7. Differentiate between cultural sensitivity and cultural competence.

8. List any five national standards on culturally and linguistically appropriate services (CLAS).
9. Discuss the attributes of a culturally competent mental health educator.

WEBSITES TO EXPLORE

Cultural Competence

http://cecp.air.org/cultural/default.htm

This website raises some questions on cultural competence and answers them. Some of the questions are: What is cultural competence? Why is cultural competence important? What does research say? What are others doing? How is cultural competence integrated into education? How does cultural competence differ from cultural sensitivity? How does cultural competence benefit children? Where can I find more information? Who should be involved? *Read the answers to these questions and prepare a table that differentiates cultural sensitivity and cultural competence.*

Mental Health Continuing Education

http://www.athealthce.com/

Most mental health professionals are required to have some sort of certification, licensure, or registration. To maintain these credentials they have to undertake continuing education courses. This website lists some of the continuing education credits available for mental health professionals. *Click on the catalog. Read about some courses that interest you. Which courses would you like to take if you had to take continuing education credits?*

Mental Health Education Consortium Project

http://www.lahc.edu/MentalHealth/

This website describes a collaborative project between Los Angeles County Department of Mental Health and Los Angeles Community College District. Its aim is to propagate mental health information to colleges all over the state of California. The links are home, project overview, mission, booklets, and training tips. *Click on booklets and download the two booklets. Read and review any one of these booklets summarizing the strengths and weaknesses.*

National Commission for Health Education Credentialing, Inc.

http://www.nchec.org/

This website credentials Certified Health Education Specialists (CHES). If you are not a CHES then you cannot see all the links but you can see the links (1) about NCHEC that describes mission and purpose, leadership, history, strategic plan, staff links, and frequently asked questions about it; (2) NCHEC news that has the CHES bulletin, latest news from NCHEC, and why health education has been in the news; (3) details about health education credentialing; (4) details about the CHES exam; (5) details about renewal and recertification; and (6) designated continuing education providers. *Browse this website and find out about the CHES exam. Do you believe you would be eligible for this exam? If so, do you have any plans to take it?*

Office of Minority Health: Cultural Competency Section

http://minorityhealth.hhs.gov/templates/browse.aspx?lvl=1&lvlID=3

This is a website of the Office of Minority Health that deals with cultural competency. Links on this website consist of (1) a guide to assist health care organizations use effective language access services geared toward limited-English-proficient patients with limited English proficiency; (2) a curriculum on cultural competency for emergency responders; (3) an online educational program for nurses on cultural competency; (4) National Standards on Culturally and Linguistically Appropriate Services; (5) a guide for physicians on cultural competency; and (6) a patient-centered guide for implementing language access services in healthcare organizations. *Choose any one of these sections and prepare a summary and critique.*

REFERENCES AND FURTHER READINGS

Airhihenbuwa, C. O., Cottrell, R. R., Adeyanju, M., Auld, M. E., Lysoby, L., & Smith, B. J. (2005). The National Health Educator Competencies Update Project: Celebrating a milestone and recommending next steps to the profession. *American Journal of Health Education, 36,* 361–370.

Allegrante, J. P., Airhihenbuwa, C. O., Auld, M. E., Birch, D. A., Roe, K. M., & Smith, B. J. (2004). Toward a unified system of accreditation for professional preparation in health education: Final report of the National Task Force on Accreditation in Health Education. *Health Education and Behavior, 31,* 668–683.

American Association for Health Education (AAHE). (2003). Directory of institutions offering undergraduate and graduate degree programs in health education. 2003 edition. *American Journal of Health Education, 34*(4), 219–235.

American Association for Health Education (AAHE), National Commission for Health Education Credentialing (NCHED), & Society for Public Health Education (SOPHE). (1999). *A competency-based framework for graduate-level health educators.* Allentown, PA: National Commission for Health Education Credentialing.

Andrulis, D. P., Delbanco, T. L, & Shaw-Taylor, Y. (1999). *Cross cultural competence in health care survey.* Washington, DC: National Public Health and Hospital Institute.

Bergevin, P., Morris, D., & Smith, R. M. (1963). *Adult education procedures: A handbook of tested patterns for effective participation.* New York: Seabury.

Berry, J. W. (1997). Immigration, acculturation, and adaptation. *Applied Psychology: An International Review, 46*(1), 5–33.

Coalition of National Health Education Organizations. (2004). *Code of ethics.* Retrieved from http://www.hsc.usf.edu/CFH/cnheo/ethics.htm.

Cross, T. L., Bazron, B. J., Dennis, K. W, & Isaacs, M. R. (1989). *Towards a culturally competent system of care: A monograph on effective services for minority children who are severely emotionally disturbed.* Washington, DC: CASSP Technical Assistance Center, Georgetown University Child Development Center.

Gilmore, G. D., Olsen, L. K., Taub, A., & Connell, D. (2005). Overview of the National Health Educator Competencies Update Project, 1998–2004. *Health Education and Behavior, 32,* 725–737.

Institute of Medicine. (1988). *Future of public health.* Washington, DC: National Academy Press.

Institute of Medicine. (2002). *The future of the public's health in the 21st century.* Washington, DC: National Academy Press.

McCollum, M. G. (1981). Recasting a role for mental health educators. *American Mental Health Counselors Association Journal, 3*(1), 37-47.

National Commission for Health Education Credentialing (NCHEC). (1985). *A framework for the development of competency based curricula for entry-level health educators.* New York: Author.

National Commission for Health Education Credentialing (NCHEC), Society for Public Health Education (SOPHE), & American Association for Health Education (AAHE). (2006). *Competency-based framework for health educators—2006.* Whitehall, PA: Author.

Office of Minority Health. (2007). National standards on culturally and linguistically appropriate services (CLAS). Retrieved from http://minorityhealth.hhs.gov/templates/browse.aspx?lvl=2&lvlID=15.

Orlandi, M. A. (Ed.). (1995). *Cultural competence for evaluators: A guide for alcohol and other drug abuse prevention practitioners working with ethnic/racial communities* (Vol. 1, 2nd ed.). OSAP Cultural Competence Series. Rockville, MD: U.S. Department of Health and Human Services.

Perez, M.A., & Luquis, R. R. (2008). *Cultural competence in health education and health promotion.* San Francisco: Jossey Bass.

Public Health Functions Steering Committee. (1994). Public health in America. Retrieved from http://www.health.gov/phfunctions/public.htm.

Redfield, R., Linton, R., & Herskovits, M. J. (1936). Memorandum for the study of acculturation. *American Anthropologist, 38,* 149–152.

Resnicow, K., Baranowski, T., Ahluwalia, J. S., & Braithwaite, R. L. (1999). Cultural sensitivity in public health: Defined and demystified. *Ethnicity and Disease, 9*(1), 10–21.

Resnicow, K., Soler, R., Braithwaite, R. L., Ahluwalia, J. S., & Butler, J. (2000). Cultural sensitivity in substance use prevention. *Journal of Community Psychology, 28,* 271–292.

Ryder, A. G., Alden, L. E., & Paulhus, D. L. (2000). Is acculturation unidimensional or bidimensional? A head to head comparison in the prediction of personality, self-identity, and adjustment. *Journal of Personality and Social Psychology, 79*(1), 77–88.

Simons-Morton, B. G., Donohew, L., & Crump, A. D. (1997). Health communication in the prevention of alcohol, tobacco, and drug use. *Health Education & Behavior, 24*(5), 544–554.

Taub, A., Kreuter, M., Parcel, G., & Vitello, E. (1987). Report from the AAHE/SOPHE Joint Committee on Ethics. *Health Education Quarterly, 14*(1), 79–90.

U.S. Department of Health, Education and Welfare. (1978). *Preparation and practice of community, patient, and school health educators: Proceedings of the workshop on commonalities and differences.* Washington, DC: Division of Allied Health Professions.

U.S. Department of Health and Human Services. (2009). Healthy People 2020: The road ahead. Retrieved from http://www.healthypeople.gov/HP2020/default.asp.

References and Further Readings

CHAPTER 3

Determinants of Mental Health

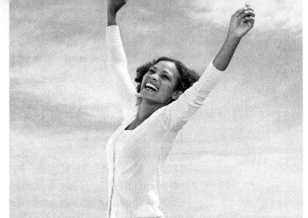

CHAPTER OBJECTIVES

After reading this chapter you should be able to
- Describe how mental health is measured
- Discuss the positive factors affecting mental health that include hardiness, sense of coherence, acculturation, social support, optimism, and self-esteem
- Define the components of hardiness and how it affects mental health
- Elaborate the components of sense of coherence and how it affects mental health
- Identify the negative factors affecting mental health such as socioeconomic factors, loneliness, negative familial factors, sleep problems, distress, and migration

MEASURING MENTAL HEALTH

Mental health has been measured in the literature in several ways, although most instruments rely on self-report. Kessler and colleagues (2002, 2003) developed the Kessler Psychological Distress Scales K-10 and K-6. There are two versions of these scales: self-administered and interviewer administered. These scales have been translated into Arabic, Chinese, Dutch, German, Hebrew, Italian, Japanese, Portuguese, and Spanish. The K-10 scale has been used by the World Health Organization in its World Mental Health surveys that include approximately 250,000 people in 30 countries. The K-6 scale is presented in Focus Feature 3.1.

Another instrument, SF-36 (Ware, Gandek, & the IQOLA Project Group, 1994; Ware, Kosinski, & Keller, 1994), is a short form with 36 questions that also measures physical health. This instrument provides an eight-scale profile of functional health and well-being scores and physical and mental health summary measures along with a preference-based health utility index (Ware, n.d.). It has been used in over 4,000 publications in 50 countries. The eight scales in this instrument are physical functioning, role-physical, bodily pain, general health, vitality, social functioning, role-emotional, and mental health. The first four scales comprise the summary measure of physical health, whereas the remaining four constitute the summary measure of mental health.

A shorter version of SF-36 has been developed, the SF-12, with just 12 items (Ware, Kosinski, & Keller, 1995), which can be self-administered and interview administered. This widely used instrument is especially suitable for large samples when the purpose is to monitor overall physical and mental health.

Berkman (1971) developed an eight-item Index of Psychological Well-Being used to measure mental health in a general population through a mail-questionnaire survey. Berkman (1971) also found this index was positively associated with physical health.

Mental health is mostly measured by self-reports.

FOCUS FEATURE 3.1 K6+ SELF–REPORT MEASURE

The following questions ask about how you have been feeling during the **past 30 days**. For each question please circle the number that best describes how often you had this feeling.

Q1. During the past 30 days, about how often did you feel...	**All of the time**	**Most of the time**	**Some of the time**	**A little of the time**	**None of the time**
a. nervous?	1	2	3	4	5
b. hopeless?	1	2	3	4	5
c. restless or fidgety?	1	2	3	4	5
d. so depressed that nothing could cheer you up?	1	2	3	4	5
e. that everything was an effort?	1	2	3	4	5
f. worthless?	1	2	3	4	5

Q2. The last questions asked about feelings that might have occurred during the past 30 days. Taking them altogether, did these feelings occur <u>more often</u> in the past 30 days than is usual for you, <u>about the same</u> as usual, or <u>less often</u> than usual? (If you <u>never</u> have any of these feelings circle response option 4.

More often than usual			**About the same as usual**	**Less often than usual**		
A lot	**Some**	**A little**		**A little**	**Some**	**A lot**
1	2	3	4	5	6	7

The next few questions are about how these feelings may have affected you in the past 30 days. You need not answer these questions if you answered "None of the time" to **all** of the six questions about your feelings.

Q3. During the past 30 days, how many days out of 30 were you <u>totally unable</u> to work or carry out your normal activities because of these feelings?

_____ **(Number of days)**

Q4. Not counting the days you reported in response to Q3, how many days in the past 30 were you able to do only <u>half or less</u> of what you would normally have been able to do because of these feelings?

_____ **(Number of days)**

Q5. During the past 30 days, how many times did you see a doctor or other health professional about these feelings?

_____ **(Number of times)**

	All of the time	Most of the time	Some of the time	A little of the time	None of the time
Q6. During the past 30 days, how often have physical health problems been the main cause of these feelings?	1	2	3	4	5

Source: Kessler, R. C., Barker, P. R., Colpe, L. J., Epstein, J. F., Gfroerer, J. C., Hiripi, E., Howes, M. J., Normand, S-L. T., Manderscheid, R. W., Walters, E. E., Zaslavsky, A. M. (2003). Screening for serious mental illness in the general population *Archives of General Psychiatry. 60*(2), 184–189. Used with permission.

POSITIVE FACTORS AFFECTING MENTAL HEALTH

Several factors foster mental health, such as hardiness, sense of coherence, acculturation, social support, optimism, and self-esteem. Each of these factors is discussed below.

Hardiness

The theory of hardiness originated in the 1970s. Suzanne Kobasa (1979a, 1979b) conducted an 8-year study of executives undergoing the major stress of losing their jobs or being reassigned and found that individuals who displayed a certain set of personality characteristics remained healthier and happier during the crisis. She labeled such personality traits **hardiness**. Hardiness has three constructs (Taylor & Aspinwall, 1996): control, commitment, and challenge (**Table 3.1**). **Control** refers to a person's belief that he or she causes the events of his or her life and can influence the environment. The greater a person's belief in his or her control, the better that person is able to endure the adverse effects of stress and has better mental health. **Commitment** refers to a person's tendency to become involved in whatever he or she encounters or to a feeling of deep involvement in the activities of life. The higher a person's commitment, the higher that person's ability to cope with stress and achieve better mental health. **Challenge** refers to a person's willingness to undertake change, confront new activities, and obtain opportunities for growth.

TABLE 3.1	Key Constructs of the Theory of Hardiness
Construct	**Definition**
Control	Belief that one causes the events of one's life and can influence the environment
Commitment	Tendency to involve oneself in whatever one encounters or a feeling of deep involvement in activities of life
Challenge	Willingness to undertake change and confront new activities and obtain opportunities for growth

The greater a sense of challenge a person has, the easier he or she is able to cope with stress and demonstrate better mental health.

People who exhibit hardiness traits are likely to have better mental health than those who are deficient in control, commitment, or challenge dimensions (Atri, Sharma, & Cottrell, 2006–2007; Ben-Zur, Duvdevany, & Lury, 2005; Lambert, Lambert, Petrini, Li, & Zhang, 2007; Maddi & Khoshaba, 1994; Ramanaiah, Sharpe, & Byravan, 1999). Higher hardiness scores are also linked to better sport performance (Sheard, 2009). Webster and Austin (1999) modified hardiness in a clinical nursing intervention and found it reduced distress, symptoms related to obsessive-compulsive behavior, hostility, and psychotic symptoms. In addition, it increased positive thoughts, feelings, and behaviors. Neria and colleagues (2001) found that the hardiness general score and commitment and control variables had significant association with the mental health scores, distress, and general psychiatric symptomatology. In this study the challenge component of hardiness was not found to be significantly associated with mental health scores.

Several mechanisms have been suggested by which hardiness could be contributing to mental health. According to Kobasa (1979b), appraisal and coping mediate the effects of hardiness on mental health. Florian, Mikulincer, and Taubman (1995) also support this idea. It appears from the available literature that hardiness alters appraisal in two ways.

The mechanism whereby stressful life events produce illness is presumably physiological. Whatever this physiological response is, the personality characteristics of hardiness may cut into it, decreasing the likelihood of breakdown into illness.

—Kobasa (1985, p. 187)

First, it reduces the appraisal of threat caused by potentially stressful events, and, second, it increases the expectations of successful coping. Further, it is argued that hardy persons prefer to adopt problem-focused strategies when faced with a potential stressor. Persons lacking in the hardiness personality trait adopt regressive techniques like denial, which can further compound stress and lead to more emotional maladjustment in the long run. Focus Feature 3.2 presents one scale that measures hardiness among college students.

FOCUS FEATURE 3.2 COLLEGE STUDENT HARDINESS MEASURE (CSHM)

Instructions:

For each statement below please circle the number which best represents your situation, choice or standpoint. The scale is divided into 4 choices from 1–4.

1 = Never true or not applicable to you

2 = Occasionally true/Sometimes applicable to you

3 = Oftentimes true/Frequently applicable to you

4 = Always true or applicable to you

Generally speaking,

1. I prefer not to make changes in my daily schedule.

    1   2   3   4

2. I really like and appreciate my work.

    1   2   3   4

3. A lot of events in life happen because they have to.

    1   2   3   4

4. No matter how hard I try, my efforts usually do not accomplish much.

    1   2   3   4

5. I like a lot of variety in my work.

    1   2   3   4

6. I often wake up eager to take up life wherever it left off.

    1   2   3   4

7. Lots of times, I am unsure of my own intentions and motives.

    1   2   3   4

8. I find life really exciting on most days.

    1   2   3   4

9. I am in a good mood most of the time.

    1   2   3   4

Scoring:

For questions 2, 3, 5, 6, 8, and 9 take the numbers you circled as your scores.

For questions 1, 7, and 4 change your score as per the following legend:

If you circled a 1 give yourself a 4

If you circled a 2 give yourself a 3

If you circled a 3 give yourself a 2

If you circled a 4 give yourself a 1

Summate all scores. Your score should range from 9 to 36. If you have scored less than 18 then your hardiness score is less and you must try to increase it.

Source: Atri, A. (2007). Role of social support, hardiness and acculturation as predictors of mental health among the international students of Asian Indian origin in Ohio. Master's thesis. Available from Ohio Link.

Sense of Coherence

Also in the 1970s, **a sense of coherence** originated as a theory (Antonovsky, 1979, 1987). This is a way of seeing the world that enhances mental health. The three constructs of the sense of coherence are comprehensibility, manageability, and meaningfulness (**Table 3.2**). **Comprehensibility** refers to the extent to which one perceives the stressors that confront him or her make cognitive sense, implying there is some set structure, consistency, order, clarity, and predictability. **Manageability** refers to the extent to which one believes the resources under one's control are adequate to meet the demands posed by the stressors. **Meaningfulness** refers to the extent to which one believes life makes sense emotionally and that at least some of the stressors in life are worth investing energy in and are worthy of commitment and engagement. It entails looking at challenges in life as welcome rather than burdensome.

A sense of coherence is measured in several ways. Erikson and Lindstrom (2005) conducted a systematic review of validity and reliability of Antonovsky's (1987) sense of coherence (SOC) scale and found the SOC scale has been used in about 33 languages in 32 countries with approximately 15 different versions. There are three main versions, one with 29 items, one with 13 items, and a recent one with just 3 items. SOC-29 and SOC-13 have acceptable reliability and validity and are cross-culturally applicable (Erikson & Lindstrom, 2005). Focus Feature 3.3 presents SOC-29 and SOC-13.

According to Antonovsky, sense of coherence is a "global orientation that expresses the extent to which one has a pervasive, enduring though dynamic feeling of confidence that (1) the stimuli deriving from one's internal and external environments in the course of living are structured, predictable and explicable; (2) the resources are available to one to meet the demands posed by these stimuli; and (3) these demands are challenges, worthy of investment and engagement."

—Antonovsky (1987)

A study on survivors of myocardial infarction was found that sense of coherence was an important predictor for quality of life after infarction (Norekvål et al., 2009). Quality of life was measured in physical domain, psychological domain, and environmental domain, and sense of coherence contributed in all three domains. In a study of nurses high sense of coherence was found to serve as a buffer in preventing mental distress (Malinauskiene, Leisyte, & Malinauskas, 2009). Another study of Hungarian medical students found that psychological distress was inversely related to sense of coherence (Bíró, Balajti, Adány, & Kósa, 2009). A study from Japan found that high sense of coherence helped workers to cope with their job demand and improved mental health (Urakawa & Yokoyama, 2009). Strengthening sense of coherence has also been suggested as an important strategy in mental health rehabilitation (Griffiths, 2009).

TABLE 3.2 Constructs of Sense of Coherence	
Construct	**Definition**
Comprehensibility	The extent to which one perceives the stressors that confront one make cognitive sense, implying some set structure, consistency, order, clarity, and predictability
Manageability	The extent to which one believes the resources under one's control are adequate to meet the demands posed by the stressors
Meaningfulness	The extent to which one believes life makes sense emotionally and that at least some of the stressors in life are worth investing energy in and are worthy of commitment and engagement

FOCUS FEATURE 3.3 SENSE OF COHERENCE QUESTIONNAIRE

Sense of coherence has three components: comprehensibility (C), manageability (MA), and meaning-fulness (ME). In the questionnaire the items that tap into each of these components is marked by the initials on the left side of each item. The questionnaire also has four facets: A. Modality (with three elements: 1. instrumental; 2. cognitive; 3. affective); B. Source (with three elements: 1. internal; 2. external; 3. both); C. Demand (with three elements: 1. concrete; 2. diffuse; 3. abstract); and D. Time (with three elements: 1. past; 2. present; 3. future). These elements are also indicated by four numbers on the left side of each item. An "R" marked on the 13 items signifies that before calculating the score these items should be reversed. Furthermore, 13 items have been marked with an asterisk (*). These asterisk-marked items constitute the short version SOC-13.

1.   C R 1312   When you talk to people, do you have the feeling that they don't understand you?
         1   2   3   4   5   6   7
never have this feeling   always have this feeling

2.   MA 1111   In the past, when you had to do something which depended upon cooperation with others, did you have the feeling that it:
         1   2   3   4   5   6   7
surely wouldn't get done   surely would get done

3.   C 1322   Think of the people with whom you come into contact daily, aside from the ones to whom you feel closest. How well do you know most of them?
         1   2   3   4   5   6   7
you feel that they're strangers   you know them very well

*4.   ME R 1222   Do you have the feeling that you don't really care about what goes on around you?
         1   2   3   4   5   6   7
very seldom or never   very often

*5.   C R 1221   Has it happened in the past that you were surprised by the behavior of people whom you thought you knew well?
         1   2   3   4   5   6   7
never happened   always happened

*6.   MA R 1221   Has it happened that people whom you counted on disappointed you?
         1   2   3   4   5   6   7
never happened   always happened

7.   ME R 2332   Life is:
         1   2   3   4   5   6   7
full of interest   completely routine

*8.   ME 2331   Until now your life has had:
         1   2   3   4   5   6   7
no clear goals or purpose at all   very clear goals and purpose

*9.   MA 1221   Do you have the feeling that you're being treated unfairly?
         1   2   3   4   5   6   7
very often   very seldom or never

10.   C 2331   In the past ten years your life has been:
         1   2   3   4   5   6   7
full of changes without your   completely consistent and clear
knowing what will happen next

(continued)

11.   ME R 1313   Most of the things you do in the future will probably be:
      1   2   3   4   5   6   7
completely fascinating   deadly boring

*12. C 2232   Do you have the feeling that you are in an unfamiliar situation and don't know
what to do?
      1   2   3   4   5   6   7
very often   very seldom or never

13.   MA R 2332   What best describes how you see life?
      1   2   3   4   5   6   7
one can always find a solution   there is no solution to painful things
to painful things in life   in life

14.   ME R 2132   When you think about your life, you very often:
      1   2   3   4   5   6   7
feel how good it is to be alive   ask yourself why you exist at all

15.   C 1112   When you face a difficult problem, the choice of a solution is:
      1   2   3   4   5   6   7
always confusing and hard to find   always completely clear

*16. ME R 1312   Doing the things you do every day is:
      1   2   3   4   5   6   7
a source of deep pleasure   a source of pain and boredom
and satisfaction

17.   C   2333   Your life in the future will probably be:
      1   2   3   4   5   6   7
full of changes without your knowing   completely consistent and clear
what will happen next

18.   MA 3211   When something unpleasant happened in the past your tendency was:
      1   2   3   4   5   6   7
"to beat yourself up" about it   to say "ok , that's that, I have to live
                                                         with it and go on"

*19. C   2122   Do you have very mixed-up feelings and ideas?
      1   2   3   4   5   6   7
very often   very seldom or never

20.   MA R 1113   When you do something that gives you a good feeling:
      1   2   3   4   5   6   7
It's certain that you'll go on   it's certain that something will
feeling good   happen to spoil the feeling

*21. C   3122   Does it happen that you have feelings inside you would rather not feel?
      1   2   3   4   5   6   7
very often   very seldom or never

22.   ME 2333   You anticipate that your personal life in the future will be:
      1   2   3   4   5   6   7
totally without meaning or purpose   full of meaning and purpose

23. MA R 1223   Do you think that there will *always* be people whom you'll be able to count on in the future?

    1   2   3   4   5   6   7
you're certain there will be   you doubt there will be

24. C   2233   Does it happen that you have the feeling that you don't know exactly what's about to happen?

    1   2   3   4   5   6   7
very often   very seldom or never

*25. MA R 3131   Many people—even those of strong character—sometimes feel like sad sacks (losers) in certain situations. How often have you felt this way in the past?

    1   2   3   4   5   6   7
never   very often

*26. C 1211   When something happened, have you generally found that:

    1   2   3   4   5   6   7
you overestimated or underestimated   you saw things in the right
importance   proportion

27. MA R 1313   When you think of difficulties you are likely to face in important aspects of your life, do you have the feeling that:

    1   2   3   4   5   6   7
you will always succeed in overcoming   you won't succeed in overcoming
the difficulties   the difficulties

*28. ME 1212   How often do you have the feeling that there is little meaning in the things you do in your daily life?

    1   2   3   4   5   6   7
very often   very seldom or never

*29. MA 3122   How often do you have feelings that you're not sure you can keep under control?

    1   2   3   4   5   6   7
very often   very seldom or never

Scoring

After reversing the 13 items total all the points. The higher the score, the stronger the sense of coherence is.

Source: Antonovsky, A. (1987). *Unraveling the mystery of health. How people manage stress and stay well* (pp. 189–194). San Francisco: Jossey-Bass Publishers.

Acculturation

Acculturation as a concept was introduced in Chapter 2. In this chapter its relationship to mental health is discussed. Acculturation entails the social and psychological exchanges that take place when there is continuous contact and interaction between individuals from different cultures (Berry, 1997; Redfield, Linton, & Herskovits, 1936; Ryder, Alden, & Paulhus, 2000). Acculturation has been seen as the psychosocial adjustment and adaptation to a new culture for people from another culture. Two distinct theoretical frameworks have dominated the study of this complex cultural phenomenon. One school of researchers believes that acculturation is a one-dimensional construct that can be conceptualized along a single continuum, ranging from the immersion in the person's culture of origin to immersion in the dominant or host culture (Gordon, 1995). A competing school of thought argues that acculturation consists of two distinct and independent dimensions, adherence to the dominant culture and maintenance of the culture of origin (Berry, 1997; Mann & Gamba, 1996; Rogler, Cortes, & Malgady, 1991; Ryder, Alden, & Paulhus, 2000). The use of these two models has produced a copious amount of literature that has explored the multiple changes that occur when individuals adapt to different cultural environments.

The specific set of difficulties that an individual immigrant has to face can be physical (new climatic conditions and search for abode), biological (changes in diet and diseases), social (dislocation of friends and formation of new relationships), cultural (sudden changes in political, economic, and religious contexts), and psychological (need to change attitudes, values, and mental health connotations). Acculturation is usually seen as the behavioral and psychological changes in an individual that occur as a result of contact between people belonging to different culture groups (Berry, 1997).

Berry (1997) provided four classifications of acculturation that has gained widespread acceptance despite limited research based evidence: (1) integration, (2) assimilation, (3) separation, and (4) marginalization. Integration is the identification and involvement of an immigrant with both native and new cultures. This mode is linked to the most optimal mental health outcomes. Assimilation is the condition where the immigrant identifies solely with the new culture. Separation is the situation where the individual is involved only in the native culture, and marginalization is the lack of involvement in either culture and rejection of both. Assimilation, separation, and marginalization have been associated with increasingly poorer mental health outcomes. Integration, as mentioned earlier, has been linked to the best mental health outcome.

Some literature supports the linkage between acculturation and mental health for some minority groups like Hispanic Americans and Chinese Americans. Rogler and colleagues (1991) in their literature analysis of research-based publications relevant to acculturation and mental health status in Hispanics found that although the amount of research done on the topic had magnified over the years, there was a paucity of integration of findings and a tendency not to "think outside the box." Berdahl and Torres Stone (2009) also found that acculturation was an important determinant among Latinos in their use of mental health care services. González and González (2008) in a study with Mexican Americans and Mexican immigrants found that respondents with low scores on acculturation reported significantly higher depressive symptoms. Shen and Takeuchi (2001) in their work on a structural model of acculturation and mental health status among Chinese Americans found that even though there was a significant relationship between acculturation and mental health status, the link was indirect and mediated through another variable such as socioeconomic status.

Acculturation has been proposed as a dynamic process of adaptation, and three types of direct relationships between acculturation and mental health have been speculated (Rogler et al., 1991). The first view embraces the idea that because acculturation was the adaptation of an individual to a new culture; a positive relationship must exist between acculturation and mental health. This view asserts that well-"acculturated" individuals maintain optimal mental health because they have successfully adjusted to their new environment and are optimally functioning in social and occupational arenas. The second view hypothesizes an inverse relationship between acculturation and mental health and bases it on the assumption that high levels of acculturation require significant attempts to strive for a bicultural balance that leads to heightened levels of psychological distress, which in turn adversely affect mental health. The third and final perspective proposes a curvilinear relationship between the two variables and implies that people halfway through the acculturation process are most susceptible to psychological disorders. The rationale offered for this line of reasoning is that people who are either fully integrated into an alien culture or those who remain entrenched in their parent culture would feel more content than those who were midway in the process and were still actively struggling to strike a balance between their two cultures.

Shen and Takeuchi (2001) in their review of empirical research exploring acculturation and mental health found conflicting results. They found six studies that demonstrated an inverse relationship between the two variables, three that yielded a positive relationship between mental health and acculturation, and four that failed to yield any relationship whatsoever. None of the existing studies supported the curvilinear relationship as tenable. These researchers found that studies yielding a positive correlation had smaller sample sizes and had not taken confounding variables into consideration, whereas the works that demonstrated no relationship had controlled for confounding factors and were on larger scales. It was believed that because a direct and predictable relationship between acculturation and mental health had not been demonstrated, an inclusion of other potentially relevant variables including but not limited to the demographic characteristics would better help the research. It was hoped that the direct and secondarily mediated effects of acculturation on mental health could be better predicted by the use of variables such as language proficiency.

Social Support

Another construct found to positively influence mental health is **social support**, which is the help obtained through social relationships and interpersonal exchanges (Heaney & Israel, 2008). House (1981) classified social support into four types: (1) emotional support, which entails providing understanding, love, caring, and reliance; (2) informational support, which entails providing information, guidance, and counsel; (3) instrumental support, which entails providing concrete assistance and support; and (4) appraisal support, which entails providing evaluative assistance. Social support can be naturally occurring, in the form of parents, spouse, other family members, and friends, or it can be created artificially by the health educator. Social support buffers the effect of stressors and shields a person from negative consequences. The process of demonstrating a causal linkage between social support and mental health is quite challenging for several reasons (Atri, 2007). First, there is a potential bias in retrospective recall of social support among currently symptomatic individuals. Second, even with prospective studies it would be difficult to distinguish between whether the lack of social support served as an antecedent to distress or as an attendant of distress. Finally, in longitudinal studies it is a potential difficulty in locating genuinely premorbid individuals because conditions such as subclinical depression in itself could lead to decreased social support.

Irrespective of how one differentiates social support and how a researcher goes about measuring and quantifying it, typically research has maintained that a positive correlation exists between social support and mental health (Barnett & Gotlib, 1988). Adding weight to these findings, Kawachi and Berkman (2001) found that smaller social networks, fewer relationships, and lower perceived adequacy of social support had all been linked to depressive symptomatology.

Two generic mechanisms have been proposed regarding how social support could have a bearing on health: main effects and stress buffering (Cohen & Wills, 1985; LaRocco, House, & French, 1980). Arguments have also been made that the models are possibly not exclusive and could be operating together under certain conditions of duress.

Main Effect Model

The main effect model maintains that social support and connectedness are advantageous irrespective of whether one is currently facing a life stressor or not. It describes direct routes through which social support has a bearing on the psychological well-being of an individual. Cohen (2004) explores the main effect and asserts that individuals who participate in a social network are subject to social controls and peer pressures that influence normative health behaviors and also that integration could engender feelings of responsibility for others, resulting in increased motivation to take care of oneself so that responsibility could be fulfilled. He further adds that social integration helps in the realization of one's sense of self and emotional tone because role concepts shared among different people provide guidance on how people should act in different roles.

Stress Buffering Model

The stress buffering model often used by psychologists asserts that social networks and connections benefit health by providing material resources and psychological supports needed to tide over a stressful situation and hence are of benefit only for people actually facing such a situation but not for other people without such stressful demands. Stress influences health both by promoting coping responses detrimental to health (such as use of smoking, alcohol, etc.) and by activation of physiological systems such as the sympathetic axis (Johnson, Kamilaris, Chrousos, & Gold, 1992). Continued activation of these systems could precipitate a range of physical and psychiatric disorders. The perceived ability of support from those comprising the social networks is thought to enhance a person's perceived coping abilities and help better deal with a stressful situation. The emotional and physiological responses to the stressors can also be diluted by the realization that help is close at hand. Further downhill, the support helps when that "close at hand help" is actually exploited to one's advantage. It has also been proposed that not all four subtypes of social support are equally potent in the wake of all possible stressors. Cohen (2004) argued that on analyzing the different subtypes of social support, only emotional support works in the face of a whole range of stressful events, whereas the other three subtypes are limited to responding to specific needs elicited by a stressor. For example, if a person became bankrupt both instrumental support (monetary gifts, loans, etc.) and emotional support (empathy, company of friends) could act as antistressors, but for a stressor like death instrumental supports hold little if any significance and it is the emotional component that provides all the relief. A study done in Spain on migrants from Ecuador and Romania found that social support provided by those living in one's home culture was an effective buffer against mental distress (González-Castro & Ubillos, 2009).

Kawachi and Berkman (2001) suggest that both models are not mutually exclusive but are complementary. Both models can actually explain the influences that specific facets of social relationships have on psychological well-being. These researchers suggest that the structural aspects of social relationships like social integration probably operate through the main effect, whereas the emotional component like perceived support operates through the stress buffering mechanism.

> *Social support buffers the effect of stressors and shields a person from negative consequences.*

Optimism

Another positive construct linked to good mental health is **optimism** (Scheier & Carver, 1985), which is the tendency to expect the best possible outcome or to think about the most hopeful aspects of any situation. It was originally measured by a scale called the Life Orientation Test (Scheier & Carver, 1985), which was later revised (Scheier, Carver, & Bridges, 1994). Several studies have linked optimism to better coping and mental health (Burris, Brechting, Salsman, & Carlson, 2009; Gruber-Baldini, Ye, Anderson, & Shulman, 2009; Segerstrom, 2007). Optimism acts by several pathways to ensure better health. First, optimism affects a person's efforts to avoid illness by increasing attention to information about potential health threats. Second, optimism directly improves coping. Optimism is linked to engagement coping (Carver & Connor-Smith, 2010). Third, optimism acts through its influence on the maintenance of positive mood. Martin Seligman spoke about the modifiability of this construct in his books, *Learned Optimism* (1990) and *What You Can Change and What You Can't* (1994). An Australian study with twins found that genes predispose one to high optimism, which in turn predisposes one to good mental health (Mosing, Zietsch, Shekar, Wright, & Martin, 2009).

Self-Esteem

Self-esteem is a popular concept both in mental health and common parlance. Classically, Rosenberg (1965) defined **self-esteem** as a favorable or unfavorable attitude toward oneself. Blascovich and Tomaka (1991) defined it as an individual's sense of one's own worth or the extent of an individual's approval, value, appreciation, or liking of oneself. Self-esteem is related to self-worth or self-concept and is somewhat similar to these terms. However, it is different from self-efficacy. Self-efficacy is the behavior-specific confidence that a person has in his or her ability to perform any given behavior (Bandura, 1986, 2004).

Self-esteem is an important component of mental health (Mann, Hosman, Schaalma, & de Vries, 2004; Veselska et al., 2009). In children it is also associated with academic success. It has been found that low self-esteem is associated with depression and academic failure. A cross-cultural study done with South East Asian refugees in the United States found that self-esteem is a predictor of depression and scholastic achievement (Fox, Burns, Popovich, Belknap, & Frank-Stromborg, 2004). In a study of nursing students self-esteem was found to be a predictor of mental health, particularly lower self-esteem being associated with depression (Furegato, Santos, & Silva, 2008). In a study of Korean adolescents low self-esteem was associated with mental health problems such as depression and anxiety (Kim, 2003). A study from Egypt found protective effects of self-esteem on suicide risk behaviors among at-risk adolescents (Sharaf, Thompson, & Walsh, 2009). Bovier, Chamot, and Perneger (2004) found that self-esteem is an important protective factor for mental health among young adults. In a study with homeless youth in Canada, self-esteem was found to be the most important protective factor that predicted levels of loneliness, feelings of being trapped, and suicidal ideation (Kidd & Shahar, 2008).

> *S*elf-esteem is defined as an individual's sense of one's own worth or the extent of an individual's approval, value, appreciation, or liking of oneself.
>
> —Blascovich and Tomaka (1991)

A popular way of measuring self-esteem is the Rosenberg self-esteem scale (Rosenberg, 1989). Originally, the scale used Guttman scaling but now uses Likert scaling. The scale is presented in Focus Feature 3.4.

FOCUS FEATURE 3.4 ROSENBERG SELF-ESTEEM SCALE

Instructions: Below is a list of statements dealing with your general feelings about yourself. If you strongly agree, circle **SA**. If you agree with the statement, circle **A**. If you disagree, circle **D**. If you strongly disagree, circle **SD**.

1.	On the whole, I am satisfied with myself.	SA	A	D	SD
2.*	At times, I think I am no good at all.	SA	A	D	SD
3.	I feel that I have a number of good qualities.	SA	A	D	SD
4.	I am able to do things as well as most other people.	SA	A	D	SD
5.*	I feel I do not have much to be proud of.	SA	A	D	SD
6.*	I certainly feel useless at times.	SA	A	D	SD
7.	I feel that I'm a person of worth, at least on an equal plane with others.	SA	A	D	SD
8.*	I wish I could have more respect for myself.	SA	A	D	SD
9.*	All in all, I am inclined to feel that I am a failure.	SA	A	D	SD
10.	I take a positive attitude toward myself.	SA	A	D	SD

Scoring: SA = 3, A = 2, D = 1, SD = 0. Items with an asterisk are reverse scored, that is, SA = 0, A = 1, D = 2, SD = 3. Sum the scores for the 10 items. The higher the score, the higher the self-esteem.

Source: Rosenberg, Morris. 1989. Society and the Adolescent Self-Image. Revised edition. Middletown, CT: Wesleyan University Press.

Note. The scale is under public domain but thanks are due to The Morris Rosenberg Foundation c/o Department of Sociology, University of Maryland, 2112 Art/Soc Building, College Park, MD 20742-1315.

Internal Locus of Control, Self-Efficacy, and Satisfaction with Life

An Austrian study that looked at protective factors for suicidal ideation among elderly living in long-term care facilities found that internal locus of control, self-efficacy, and satisfaction with life were important protective determinants (Malfent, Wondrak, Kapusta, & Sonneck, 2009). **Locus of control** is the belief by an individual regarding where the command of happenings in one's life is located. In simple terms it means what or who is responsible for things that happen. There are two broad types of locus of control: internal and external. Internal locus of control is the belief that control of future happenings lies primarily with oneself, whereas external locus of control is the belief that control of future happenings is outside of oneself such as with God, luck, powerful others, and so on.

Self-efficacy refers to the confidence a person has in his or her ability to pursue a behavior. It is behavior specific and is in the present. It is not about past or future. Self-efficacy plays a central role in behavior change and is also related to mental health. Bandura (2004) noted that unless people believe they can produce the changes by their own efforts there will be very little incentive to put in that effort. Some researchers have suggested similarities of this construct with sense of coherence (Posadzki & Glass, 2009). Four strategies can be used in building self-efficacy. First is the breaking down of the complex behavior into practical and doable small steps. The second strategy is to use a demonstration from credible role models. The third strategy to build self-efficacy is by using persuasion and reassurance. If a person has failed in the past to make a behavior change, then those failures can be attributed to external reasons. The fourth strategy in building self-efficacy is to reduce stress. Any behavior change is associated with some amount of negative stress and that hinders the change process. Therefore, reducing stress is an effective means of building self-efficacy.

Satisfaction with life is also associated with good mental health. Some studies have found that satisfaction with life is associated with positive mental health (Abdel-Khalek, 2008; Malfent et al., 2009; Zullig, Valois, Huebner, & Drane, 2005). Low satisfaction with life is associated with decreased mental health (Kamm-Steigelman, Kimble, Dunbar, Sowell, & Bairan, 2006).

Resilience

Resilience is the ability to rebound back in the face of adversity. It is the capacity to recover from extremes of trauma and stress (Atkinson, Martin, & Rankin, 2009). It implies that even when one encounters stress, hardship, adversity, trauma, pain, or tragedy one keeps on functioning, both at the psychological level and the physical level. Resilience helps protect oneself against mental health problems that include depression and anxiety. It also helps offset risk factors for mental illness, such as deficient social support, previous mental trauma, or history of being dominated (Mayo Clinic Staff, 2009). Wagnild and Young (1993) developed a resilience scale that can be used by mental health practitioners that includes some open-ended questions (Wagnild & Collins, 2009).

A study done after Hurricane Katrina found that about one-third of the women studied were resilient from depression and about half were resilient from posttraumatic stress disorder (Harville, Xiong, Buekens, Pridjian, & Elkind-Hirsch, 2010). A study with undiagnosed older African Americans examined the relationship between resilience and willingness of these individuals to seek mental health care for depressive symptoms (Smith, 2009). The study found a direct predictive relationship between resilience and

In order to succeed, people need a sense of self-efficacy, strung together with resilience to meet the inevitable obstacles and inequities of life.

—Albert Bandura (1986)

TABLE 3.3   List of Positive Factors Affecting Mental Health
Hardiness: control, commitment, challenge
Sense of coherence: comprehensibility, manageability, meaningfulness
Acculturation
Social support
Optimism
Self-esteem
Internal locus of control
Self-efficacy
Satisfaction with life
Resilience
Democracy
Social capital
Religiosity

willingness to seek mental health care. Another study on rural older adults in New York State found that resilience was positively correlated with both physical and mental health status (Wells, 2009).

Other Positive Factors

Wise and Sainsbury (2007), using political science literature, traced the development of democracy and studied it in the context of improvements in public health over the past 200 years. They found a link, albeit weak, between democracy and mental health. Safaei (2006) also suggested that democracy has a positive effect on health, including mental health, which is independent of socioeconomic factors.

Another construct related to mental health is **social capital**, defined by Putnam (1996, 2000) as comprising all characteristics of social life such as networks, norms, and trust that enable members to act together in pursuing shared objectives. A Finnish study showed that social capital is linked to mental health (Nyqvist, Finnäs, Jakobsson, & Koskinen, 2008). Another factor related to positive mental health is religiosity (Abdel-Khalek, 2008). **Table 3.3** summarizes positive factors associated with mental health.

NEGATIVE FACTORS AFFECTING MENTAL HEALTH

Several factors hinder mental health, such as poor socioeconomic status, loneliness, negative familial factors, sleep problems, stress-distress, and migration. Each of these factors is discussed below.

Socioeconomic Factors

Socioeconomic factors such as poverty and lack of education have consistently been linked with poorer mental health. A study done in Brazil found that children who were below the poverty line, whose parents had lower levels of education, and lived with single-parent families or those that had stepmother/stepfather exhibited lower social competence and greater number of behavioral problems (Assis, Avanci, & Oliveira Rde, 2009). A study from Australia that looked at links between neighborhood environments and health found that perception of lower levels of neighborhood safety was associated with poorer health (Warr, Feldman, Tacticos, & Kelaher, 2009). A study from India among women found poverty to be independently associated with risk for common mental disorders (Patel, Kirkwood, Pednekar, Weiss, & Mabey, 2006). A study done in Malawi found that poor mental health was related to poverty, inhumane treatment, social isolation, and reduction of hope (Mkandawire-Valhmu, 2010).

Loneliness

Feelings of loneliness are generally associated with poor mental health. A study from Israel among older adults found that loneliness was associated with experiencing more traumatic events, more doctor's visits, and less cognitive vitality (Cohen-Mansfield, Shmotkin, & Goldberg, 2009). Feelings of loneliness are related to physiological stress processes including activity of the hypothalamic-pituitary-adrenal axis and are shown to alter cortisol levels in the body (Doane & Adam, 2009). A study on the elderly population in China found that loneliness was associated with lower mental health (Liu & Guo, 2007). The feeling of being lonely is quite detrimental to mental health and is a negative factor associated with mental health. Loneliness is significantly associated with depression and can be considered as an independent risk factor for depression (Luanaigh & Lawlor, 2008). Besides depression, loneliness is also linked with higher blood pressure, poorer sleep habits, poor immune response, and deterioration in cognition over time (Luanaigh & Lawlor, 2008). In older people loneliness has been found to be the single most important predictor of psychological distress (Paul, Ayis, & Ebrahim, 2006). In another study with older adults a strong association between perceived isolation and mental health was found (Cornwell & Waite, 2009). Loneliness is a problem not only in adults but also in children, where it is a barrier to social development and physical and mental health (Krause-Parello, 2008). Mental health programs must aim at reducing loneliness among people through building social network and social support.

Negative Familial Factors

Several factors associated with dysfunctional families or associated with negative characteristics in families are also detrimental to mental health. A study looked at predictors of emotional problems and physical aggression among immigrant children in Canada (Beiser et al., 2009). Among the significant universal predictors found were depression in parents, dysfunctional family, and parents' lower education status. The study also found migration-specific factors such as country of birth, area of resettlement, resettlement stress, prejudice, and limitations in language fluency. From this study it is evident that negative familial factors such as emotional state of the parents, less education of parents, disharmony in the family, and negative values of the family are important determinants of mental health.

Another study found that parental mental health, number of children, and family structure were consistently associated with health outcomes, again highlighting the role of familial factors (Victorino & Gauthier, 2009). A study done in Greece found that marital status of parents as other than being married, deprived parent–child relationship, and lower levels of subjective maternal mental health were significantly correlated with emotional/behavioral problems in adolescents (Giannakopoulos, Mihas, Dimitrakaki, & Tountas, 2009). The BELLA study from Germany looked at risk and protective factors for mental health among children and found that adverse family climate is a negative contributor to mental health (Ravens-Sieberer, 2008; Wille, Bettge, Ravens-Sieberer, & BELLA Study Group, 2008).

Sleep Problems

Adequate sleep is very important for mental health. The average amount of sleep needed usually varies with age. Newborns and children require more sleep than adults and older adults. Usually, it is recommended that adults sleep for 8 hours every day. About 29% of American adults report sleeping less than 7 hours per night and between 50 and 70 million have chronic sleep disorders (Centers for Disease Control and Prevention [CDC], 2009). Sleep problems or disturbed sleep can lead to poor mental health. A study done with pregnant women to identify determinants of health-related quality of life found that sleep problems were a significant determinant of poorer health-related quality of life in all domains (Da Costa et al., 2009). A study of college students found that students who were poor-quality sleepers reported significantly more problems with physical and mental health as compared with good-quality sleepers (Lund, Reider, Whiting, & Prichard, 2010). A study done in Spain found that extreme sleep durations (≤ 5 hours or ≥ 10 hours) were associated with poorer health-related quality of life (Faubel et al., 2009). A study of children found that shorter sleep duration and sleeping problems were associated with behavioral symptoms (Paavonen, Porkka-Heiskanen, & Lahikainen, 2009). Sleep is also inextricably linked with depression. Depression leads to insomnia, and insomnia is a symptom of depression (Berk, 2009).

Stress-Distress

Stress is defined as the response of the body and mind, including behaviors, as a result of encountering stressors, interpreting them, and making judgments about controlling or influencing the outcomes of these events (Sharma & Romas, 2008). Stress has the potential to produce good effects and is then called as **eustress** (Romas & Sharma, 2010). However, often stress that is not managed effectively can lead to poor mental health and is known as **distress**. (This topic is discussed in depth in Chapter 4.) One stressor is role overload. Role overload is defined as the extent to which a person feels overwhelmed by his or her total responsibilities. A Canadian study done in women found that perceptions of greater role overload were significantly associated with poorer mental health (Glynn, Maclean, Forte, & Cohen, 2009). The study found that women working less than 35 hours per week or 35 to 40 hours per week reported better mental health than nonemployed women. Another study by Bovier, Chamot, and Perneger (2004) found that perceived stress was a risk factor for poor mental health. After exposure to serious stressors such as war, physical abuse, or severe injury one is more prone to developing posttraumatic stress disorder, a mental health disorder discussed in Chapter 6.

Migration

Migration is when individuals move from one country, place, or locality to another. This movement could be in groups or as individuals, unidirectional or bidirectional, and intermittent or continuous (Atri, 2007). The long-term trends of migration can be predicted in terms of the temporal profile of migration, the ethnic groups involved in the process, and the end destinations for the process. The process of migration itself is a complex and heterogeneous one both qualitatively and quantitatively (Mehta, 1998). Bhugra (2004) suggested that the process of migration is not a singular phase but a series of sequential phases each with unique stressors. He divided the process of migration into four phases: (1) premigration experiences, (2) selection for migration, (3) actual process of migration, and (4) postmigration experience.

Higher rates of schizophrenia and other psychotic disorders have consistently been reported in migrant populations (Morgan & Hutchinson, 2009). The very first of these studies explored the linkages of psychosis with the phenomenon of migration. This classic study by Odegaard (1932) reported a higher rate of hospital admission rates for schizophrenia among migrant Norwegians as opposed to their nonmigrant counterparts. Selten and Sijben (1994) also found a positive correlation between schizophrenia and migration. In a meta-analysis of all relevant articles published between 1977 and 2003 Cantor-Graae and Selten (2005) concluded that a personal or family history of migration was an important risk factor for schizophrenia. The evidence linking other mental disorders with migration was, however, equivocal. Some studies have observed a higher rate of psychological distress and mental pathologies among migrant population (Chung & Kagawa-Singer, 1993; Fenta, Hyman, & Noh, 2004; Zilber & Lerner, 1996), whereas others have found no significant increases in the same (Cochrane & Stopes-Roe, 1980). Even if mental disorders do not manifest, the mental health of migrants is often jeopardized due to increased stressors (Anbesse, Hanlon, Alem, Packer, & Whitley, 2009).

> *M* igration is a risk factor for poor mental health.

Other Negative Factors

Limited studies have looked at the relationship of substance use and mental health. Substance use is generally a negative factor that adversely affects mental health. Some studies have found co-occurrence of substance use with mental illness (Rush, Bassani, Urbanoski, & Castel, 2008; Rush et al., 2008; Van Dorn, Williams, Del-Colle, & Hawkins, 2009). A review article found that use of cocaine, amphetamines, cannabis, and alcohol are associated with greater risk for development of psychosis (Thirthalli & Benegal, 2006).

Another factor that has received recent attention is climate change (Berry, Bowen, & Kjellstrom, 2009). There is a direct impact of climate change such as extreme weather events on mental health (Fritze, Blashki, Burke, & Wiseman, 2008). Climate change also impacts the social, economic, and environmental determinants of mental health. Climate change has the potential to produce distress and anxiety.

TABLE 3.4 Negative Factors Affecting Mental Health
Socioeconomic factors, such as poverty and lack of education
Loneliness
Negative familial factors, such as emotional state of the parents, less education of parents, disharmony in the family, negative values of the family
Sleep problems
Stress-distress
Migration
Substance use
Climate change
Physical and sexual abuse
Experiencing physical violence
Suffering from chronic physical illnesses
Work–life imbalance

Studies have also found physical and sexual abuse to be associated with poor mental health, particularly suicidal behavior (Pillai, Andrews, & Patel, 2009). A study among male veterans found that recent physical abuse, recent sexual abuse, and lifetime sexual abuse were significantly related to a higher likelihood of a recent suicide attempt (Tiet, Finney, & Moos, 2006).

Those experiencing physical violence also have poorer mental health. A study done in Brazil with public employees found that after adjusting for age, income, and stressful life events, those exposed to physical violence had a higher risk of manifesting common mental disorders (Lopes, Faerstein, Chor, & Werneck, 2008). A meta-analysis found that exposure to torture and other potentially traumatic events are associated with higher rates of posttraumatic stress disorder and depression (Steel et al., 2009).

Those suffering from chronic physical illnesses also have poorer mental health. A study from India among women found presence of chronic physical illness to be independently associated with risk for common mental disorders (Patel et al., 2006).

Imbalances in work life are also associated with poorer mental health. A Swiss study found that work–life imbalance was a risk factor adversely affecting mental health (Hämmig & Bauer, 2009). The study also found that employees who had work–life conflicts showed a significantly higher relative risk for poor self-rated health. **Table 3.4** summarizes the negative factors affecting mental health.

SKILL-BUILDING ACTIVITY

In this chapter we have been introduced to several factors that either foster mental health or hinder it. In this activity let us choose any one factor such as sense of coherence. Then using that word and "mental health" as key words, conduct a literature search. If you have access to MEDLINE, CINAHL, and ERIC databases usually available through University libraries, then use those databases. If you do not have access to these databases you can search in PubMed (the public version of Medline) at http://www.ncbi.nlm.nih .gov/sites/entrez or Google Scholar at http://scholar.google.com/. Read the abstracts and locate articles that explain the linkage between the factor you have chosen and mental health. If you can locate the full text article, then do so. Prepare a summary and critique of at least one abstract or article.

SUMMARY

Mental health can be measured in several ways, such as the Kessler Psychological Distress Scales K-10 and K-6; the SF-36, which is a short form with 36 questions that also measures physical health; SF-12, a shorter version than SF-36, with just 12 items; and the eight-item Index of Psychological Well-Being, which has also been used for measuring mental health.

Several factors foster mental health, such as hardiness, sense of coherence, acculturation, social support, optimism, self-esteem, internal locus of control, self-efficacy, satisfaction with life, resilience, democracy, social capital, and religiosity. Hardiness is a set of personality traits comprising commitment, control, and challenge that lead to better coping with stressors and improved mental health. Sense of coherence is a theory about a way of seeing the world that enhances mental health and comprises three constructs, namely comprehensibility, manageability, and meaningfulness.

Several factors are detrimental to mental health, such as poor socioeconomic status, loneliness, negative familial factors, sleep problems, stress-distress, migration, substance use, climate change, physical and sexual abuse, experiencing physical violence, suffering from chronic physical illnesses, and work–life imbalance.

REVIEW QUESTIONS

1. How is mental health measured?
2. Define hardiness and its three components. What is its relationship to mental health?
3. Define sense of coherence and its three constructs. How can sense of coherence be built?
4. Describe some factors that promote mental health.
5. Define acculturation and list four modes of acculturation.
6. Describe the stress buffering and main effect model of social support.
7. Define self-esteem. What is its relationship to mental health?
8. List factors that are detrimental to mental health.
9. Discuss the role of migration on mental health.

WEBSITES TO EXPLORE

Aaron Antonovsky (1923–1994)

http://www.angelfire.com/ok/soc/aa.html

This website presents a brief biography of Aaron Antonovsky, the originator of sense of coherence theory. The website also summarizes some of his salient publications.

Read his biography and try to locate one of his publications from the library or the Internet. In two paragraphs summarize the main points from reading this work.

Authentic Happiness

http://www.authentichappiness.sas.upenn.edu/Default.aspx

This website was developed by Dr. Martin Seligman at University of Pennsylvania who coined the concept of learned optimism discussed in this chapter. *You need to register on this website to use all of its resources. The registration is free. After registration take the optimism test and find out your score.*

Duke-UNC Functional Social Support Questionnaire (FSSQ)

http://www.adultmeducation.com/AssessmentTools_4.html

In this chapter we learned about social support. Several scales measure social support. One such scale is the Duke-UNC Functional Social Support Questionnaire (FSSQ), which is presented on this website. *Complete the eight-item questionnaire and find out your score. Is the score good or do you need to improve it?*

More Self-Esteem

http://www.more-selfesteem.com/

This website deals with building self-esteem. Links to topics that include self-esteem, self-confidence, self-help, words of inspiration, mental health, books, and articles have been provided. Also linked are a self-esteem E-book, blog, forum, links, and place for comments. *Follow the link to self-esteem E-book. Read it. Write a reaction of one page.*

Multicultural Center

http://www.multiculturalcenter.org/

This website is linked to Antioch University New England. The mission of the center is to promote multiculturalism within a social justice orientation. It has links to resources, *Journal of Multicultural Counseling and Development*, and disaster services. In this chapter we learned about acculturation and in the resources section under multicultural test titles several scales have been listed. *Choose any one scale and use the reference provided locate that scale. Comment on the strengths and weaknesses of the scale.*

Resilience Scale

http://www.resiliencescale.com

In this chapter we learned about resilience as a positive factor for mental health. This website presents a scale to measure resilience. It has information about its development, how to obtain it for research or other use, information about user's guide, and an online version for finding out your resilience score. *Complete the online resilience scale and find out your score. Possible scores range from 25 to 175. A score below 121 is considered low resilience, 121 to 145 indicates moderate resilience, and scores of 146 and above are considered moderately high to high resilience.*

REFERENCES AND FURTHER READINGS

Abdel-Khalek, A. M. (2008). Religiosity, health, and well-being among Kuwaiti personnel. *Psychological Reports, 102*(1), 181–184.

Anbesse, B., Hanlon, C., Alem, A., Packer, S., & Whitley, R. (2009). Migration and mental health: A study of low-income Ethiopian women working in Middle Eastern countries. *International Journal of Social Psychiatry, 55*(6), 557–568.

Antonovsky, A. (1979). *Health, stress, and coping.* San Francisco: Jossey-Bass.

Antonovsky, A. (1987). *Unraveling the mystery of health: How people manage stress and stay well.* San Francisco: Jossey-Bass.

Assis, S. G., Avanci, J. Q., & Oliveira Rde, V. (2009). Socioeconomic inequalities and child mental health. *Revista de Saude Publica, 43*(Suppl. 1), 92–100.

Atkinson, P. A., Martin, C. R., & Rankin, J. (2009). Resilience revisited. *Journal of Psychiatric and Mental Health Nursing, 16*(2), 137–145.

Atri, A. (2007). Role of social support, hardiness and acculturation as predictors of mental health among the international students of Asian Indian origin in Ohio. (Master's thesis). Available from Ohio Link http://etd.ohiolink.edu.proxy.libraries.uc.edu/view.cgi?acc_num=ucin1178925102

Atri, A., Sharma, M., & Cottrell, R. (2006–2007). Role of social support, hardiness and acculturation as predictors of mental health among the international students of Asian Indian origin. *International Quarterly of Community Health Education, 27*(1), 59–73.

Bandura, A. (1986). *Social foundations of thought and action.* Englewood Cliffs, NJ: Prentice Hall.

Bandura, A. (2004). Health promotion by social cognitive means. *Health Education and Behavior, 31*, 143–164.

Barnett, P., & Gotlib, I. (1988). Psychosocial functioning and depression: Distinguishing among antecedents, concomitants, and consequences. *Psychological Bulletin, 104*(1), 97–126.

Beiser, M., Hamilton, H., Rummens, J. A., Oxman-Martinez, J., Ogilvie, L., Humphrey, C., & Armstrong, R. (2009). Predictors of emotional problems and physical aggression among children of Hong Kong Chinese, Mainland Chinese and Filipino immigrants to Canada. *Social Psychiatry and Psychiatric Epidemiology, 45*(10), 1011–1021.

Ben-Zur, H., Duvdevany, I., & Lury, L. (2005). Associations of social support and hardiness with mental health among mothers of adult children with intellectual disability. *Journal of Intellectual Disability Research, 49*(Pt 1), 54–62.

Berdahl, T. A., & Torres Stone, R. A. (2009). Examining Latino differences in mental healthcare use: The roles of acculturation and attitudes towards healthcare. *Community Mental Health Journal, 45*(5), 393–403.

Berk, M. (2009). Sleep and depression: Theory and practice. *Australian Family Physician, 38*(5), 302–304.

Berkman, P. L. (1971). Measurement of mental health in a general population survey. *American Journal of Epidemiology, 94*(2), 105–111.

Berry, H. L., Bowen, K., & Kjellstrom, T. (2009). Climate change and mental health: A causal pathways framework. *International Journal of Public Health, 55*(2), 123–132.

Berry, J. W. (1997). Immigration, acculturation, and adaptation. *Applied Psychology: An International Review, 46*(1), 5–33.

Bhugra, D. (2004). Migration and mental health. *Acta Psychiatrica Scandinavica, 109*(4), 243–258.

Bíró, E., Balajti, I., Adány, R., & Kósa, K. (2009). Determinants of mental well-being in medical students. *Social Psychiatry & Psychiatric Epidemiology, 45*(2), 253–258.

Blascovich, J., & Tomaka, J. (1991). Measures of self-esteem. In J. P. Robinson, P. R. Shaver, & L. S. Wrightsman (Eds.), *Measures of personality and social psychological attitudes* (Vol. I) (pp. 115–160). San Diego: Academic Press.

Bovier, P. A., Chamot, E., & Perneger, T. V. (2004). Perceived stress, internal resources, and social support as determinants of mental health among young adults. *Quality of Life Research, 13*(1), 161–170.

Burris, J. L., Brechting, E. H., Salsman, J., & Carlson, C. R. (2009). Factors associated with the psychological well-being and distress of university students. *Journal of American College Health, 57*(5), 536–543.

Cantor-Graae, E., & Selten, J. P. (2005). Schizophrenia and migration: A meta-analysis and review. *American Journal of Psychiatry, 162*, 12–24.

Carver, C. S., & Connor-Smith, J. (2010). Personality and coping. *Annual Review of Psychology, 61*, 679–704.

Centers for Disease Control and Prevention. (2009). Perceived insufficient rest or sleep among adults—United States, 2008. *MMWR Morbidity and Mortality Weekly Report, 58*(42), 1175–1179.

Chung, R., & Kagawa-Singer, M. (1993). Predictors of psychological distress among southeast Asian refugees. *Social Science & Medicine, 36*(5), 631–639.

Cochrane, R., & Stopes-Roe, M. (1980). The mental health of immigrants. *New Community, 8*, 123–128.

Cohen, S. (2004). Social relationships and health. *American Psychologist, 59*(8), 676–684.

Cohen, S., & Wills, T. (1985). Stress, social support, and the buffering hypothesis. *Psychological Bulletin, 98*(2), 310–357.

Cohen-Mansfield, J., Shmotkin, D., Goldberg, S. (2009). Loneliness in old age: Longitudinal changes and their determinants in an Israeli sample. *International Psychogeriatrics, 21*(6), 1160–1170.

Cornwell, E. Y., & Waite, L. J. (2009). Social disconnectedness, perceived isolation, and health among older adults. *Journal of Health and Social Behavior, 50*(1), 31–48.

Da Costa, D., Dritsa, M., Verreault, N., Balaa, C., Kudzman, J., & Khalifé, S. (2009). Sleep problems and depressed mood negatively impact health-related quality of life during pregnancy. *Archives of Women's Mental Health, 13*(3), 249–257.

Doane, L. D., & Adam, E. K. (2009). Loneliness and cortisol: Momentary, day-to-day, and trait associations. *Psychoneuroendocrinology, 35*(3), 430–441.

Erikson, M., & Lindstrom, B. (2005). Validity of Antonovsky's sense of coherence scale: A systematic review. *Journal of Epidemiology and Community Health, 59*, 460–466.

Faubel, R., Lopez-Garcia, E., Guallar-Castillón, P., Balboa-Castillo, T., Gutiérrez-Fisac, J. L., Banegas, J. R., & Rodríguez-Artalejo, F. (2009). Sleep duration and health-related quality of life among older adults: A population-based cohort in Spain. *Sleep, 32*(8), 1059–1068.

Fenta, H., Hyman, I., & Noh, S. (2004). Determinants of depression among Ethiopian immigrants and refugees in Toronto. *Journal of Nervous and Mental Disease, 192*(5), 363–372.

Florian, V., Mikulincer, M., & Taubman, O. (1995). Does hardiness contribute to mental health during a stressful real-life situation? The roles of appraisal and coping. *Journal of Personality and Social Psychology, 68*(4), 687–695.

Fritze, J. G., Blashki, G. A., Burke, S., & Wiseman, J. (2008). Hope, despair and transformation: Climate change and the promotion of mental health and wellbeing. *International Journal of Mental Health Systems, 2*(1), 13.

Fox, P. G., Burns, K. R., Popovich, J. M., Belknap, R. A., & Frank-Stromborg, M. (2004). Southeast Asian refugee children: Self-esteem as a predictor of depression and scholastic achievement in the U.S. *International Journal of Psychiatric Nursing Research, 9*(2), 1063–1072.

Furegato, A. R., Santos, J. L., & Silva, E. C. (2008). Depression among nursing students associated to their self-esteem, health perception and interest in mental health. *Revista Latino Americana de Enfermagem, 16*(2), 198–204.

Giannakopoulos, G., Mihas, C., Dimitrakaki, C., & Tountas, Y. (2009). Family correlates of adolescents' emotional/behavioural problems: Evidence from a Greek school-based sample. *Acta Paediatrica, 98*(8), 1319–1323.

Glynn, K., Maclean, H., Forte, T., & Cohen, M. (2009). The association between role overload and women's mental health. *Journal of Women's Health, 18*(2), 217–223.

González, P., & González, G. M. (2008). Acculturation, optimism, and relatively fewer depression symptoms among Mexican immigrants and Mexican Americans. *Psychological Reports, 103*(2), 566–576.

González-Castro, J. L., & Ubillos, S. (2009). Determinants of psychological distress among migrants from Ecuador and Romania in a Spanish city. *International Journal of Social Psychiatry, 57*(1), 30–44.

Gordon, M. (1995). Assimilation in America: Theory and reality. In A. Aguirre & E. Baker (Eds.), *Notable selections in race and ethnicity* (pp. 91–101). Guilford, CT: Dushkin.

Griffiths, C. A. (2009). Sense of coherence and mental health rehabilitation. *Clinical Rehabilitation, 23*(1), 72–78.

Gruber-Baldini, A. L., Ye, J., Anderson, K. E., & Shulman, L. M. (2009). Effects of optimism/pessimism and locus of control on disability and quality of life in Parkinson's disease. *Parkinsonism & Related Disorders, 15*(9), 665–669.

Hämmig, O, & Bauer, G. (2009). Work-life imbalance and mental health among male and female employees in Switzerland. *International Journal of Public Health, 54*(2), 88–95.

Harville, E. W., Xiong, X., Buekens, P., Pridjian, G., & Elkind-Hirsch, K. (2010). Resilience after Hurricane Katrina among pregnant and postpartum women. *Women's Health Issues, 20*(1), 20–27.

Heaney, C. A., & Israel, B. A. (2008). Social networks and social support. In K. Glanz, B. K. Rimer, & K. Viswanath (Eds.), *Health behavior and health education: Theory, research and practice* (4th ed., pp. 189–210). San Francisco: Jossey-Bass.

House, J. S. (1981). *Work stress and social support.* Reading, MA: Addison-Wesley.

Johnson, E., Kamilaris, T., Chrousos, G., & Gold, P. (1992). Mechanisms of stress: A dynamic overview of hormonal and behavioral homeostasis. *Neuroscience & Biobehavioral Reviews, 16*(2), 115–130.

Kamm-Steigelman, L., Kimble, L. P., Dunbar, S., Sowell, R. L., & Bairan, A. (2006). Religion, relationships and mental health in midlife women following acute myocardial infarction. *Issues in Mental Health Nursing, 27*(2), 141–159.

Kawachi, I., & Berkman, L. (2001). Social ties and mental health. *Journal of Urban Health, 78*(3), 458–467.

Kessler, R. C., Andrews, G., Colpe, L. J., Hiripi, E., Mroczek, D. K., Normand, S. L.T., & Zaslavsky, A. (2002). Short screening scales to monitor population prevalences and trends in nonspecific psychological distress. *Psychological Medicine, 32*(6), 959–976.

Kessler, R. C., Barker, P. R., Colpe, L. J., Epstein, J. F., Gfroerer, J. C., Hiripi, E., & Zaslavsky, A. M. (2003). Screening for serious mental illness in the general population *Archives of General Psychiatry, 60*(2), 184–189.

Kidd, S., & Shahar, G. (2008). Resilience in homeless youth: The key role of self-esteem. *American Journal of Orthopsychiatry, 78*(2), 163–172.

Kim, Y. H. (2003). Correlation of mental health problems with psychological constructs in adolescence: Final results from a 2-year study. *International Journal of Nursing Studies, 40*(2), 115–124.

Kobasa, S. C. (1979a). Personality and resistance to illness. *American Journal of Community Psychology, 7*, 413–423.

Kobasa, S. C. (1979b). Stressful life events, personality, and health: An inquiry into hardiness. *Journal of Personality and Social Psychology, 37*, 1–11.

Kobasa, S. C. (1985). Stressful life events, personality, and health: An inquiry into hardiness. In A. Monat & R. S. Lazarus (Eds.), *Stress and coping: An anthology* (pp. 174–188). New York: Columbia University Press.

Krause-Parello, C. A. (2008). Loneliness in the school setting. *Journal of School Nursing, 24*(2), 66–70.

Lambert, V. A., Lambert, C. E., Petrini, M., Li, X. M., & Zhang, Y. J. (2007). Workplace and personal factors associated with physical and mental health in hospital nurses in China. *Nursing & Health Sciences, 9*(2), 120–126.

LaRocco, J., House, J., & French, J. R. (1980). Social support, occupational stress, and health. *Journal of Health and Social Behavior, 21*(3), 202–218.

Liu, L. J., & Guo, Q. (2007). Loneliness and health-related quality of life for the empty nest elderly in the rural area of a mountainous county in China. *Quality of Life Research, 16*(8), 1275–1280.

Lopes, C. S., Faerstein, E., Chor, D., & Werneck, G. L. (2008). Higher risk of common mental disorders after experiencing physical violence in Rio de Janeiro, Brazil: The Pró-Saúde Study. *International Journal of Social Psychiatry, 54*(2), 112–117.

Luanaigh, C. O., & Lawlor, B. A. (2008). Loneliness and the health of older people. *International Journal of Geriatric Psychiatry, 23*(12), 1213–1221.

Lund, H. G., Reider, B. D., Whiting, A. B., & Prichard, J. R. (2010). Sleep patterns and predictors of disturbed sleep in a large population of college students. *Journal of Adolescent Health, 46*(2), 124–132.

Maddi, S. R., & Khoshaba, D. M. (1994). Hardiness and mental health. *Journal of Personality Assessment, 63*(2), 265–274.

Malfent, D., Wondrak, T., Kapusta, N. D., & Sonneck, G. (2009). Suicidal ideation and its correlates among elderly in residential care homes. *International Journal of Geriatric Psychiatry, 25*(8), 843–849.

Malinauskiene, V., Leisyte, P., & Malinauskas, R. (2009). Psychosocial job characteristics, social support, and sense of coherence as determinants of mental health among nurses. *Medicina (Kaunas), 45*(11), 910–917.

Mann, G. S., & Gamba, R. J. (1996). A new measurement of acculturation for Hispanics: The Biodimensional Acculturation Scale for Hispanics (BAS). *Hispanic Journal of Behavioral Sciences, 18*(3), 297–316.

Mann, M., Hosman, C. M., Schaalma, H. P., & de Vries, N. K. (2004). Self-esteem in a broad-spectrum approach for mental health promotion. *Health Education Research, 19*(4), 357–372.

Mayo Clinic Staff (2009). Resilience: Build skills to endure hardship. Retrieved from http://www.mayoclinic.com/health/resilience/MH00078.

Mehta, S. (1998). Relationship between acculturation and mental health for Asian Indian immigrants in the United States. *Genetic, Social, and General Psychology Monographs, 124*(1), 61–78.

Mkandawire-Valhmu, L. (2010). "Suffering in thought": An analysis of the mental health needs of female domestic workers living with violence in Malawi. *Issues in Mental Health Nursing, 31*(2), 112–118.

Morgan, C., & Hutchinson, G. (2009). The social determinants of psychosis in migrant and ethnic minority populations: A public health tragedy. *Psychological Medicine, 40*(5), 705–709.

Mosing, M. A., Zietsch, B. P., Shekar, S. N., Wright, M. J., & Martin, N. G. (2009). Genetic and environmental influences on optimism and its relationship to mental and self-rated health: A study of aging twins. *Behavior Genetics, 39*(6), 597–604.

Neria, Y., Guttmann-Steinmetz, S., Koenen, K., Levinovsky, L., Zakin, G., & Dekel, R. (2001). Do attachment and hardiness relate to each other and to mental health in real-life stress? *Journal of Social & Personal Relationships, 18*(6), 844–858.

Norekvål, T. M., Fridlund, B., Moons, P., Nordrehaug, J. E., Sævareid, H. I., Wentzel- Larsen, T., & Hanestad, B. R. (2009). Sense of coherence-a determinant of quality of life over time in older female acute myocardial infarction survivors. *Journal of Clinical Nursing, 19*(5–6), 820–831.

Nyqvist, F., Finnäs, F., Jakobsson, G., & Koskinen, S. (2008). The effect of social capital on health: The case of two language groups in Finland. *Health and Place, 14*(2), 347–360.

Odegaard, O. (1932). *Emigration and insanity: A study of mental disease among the Norwegian-born population of Minnesota.* Oppenhagen, Norway: Levib & Munksgaard.

Paavonen, E. J., Porkka-Heiskanen, T., & Lahikainen, A. R. (2009). Sleep quality, duration and behavioral symptoms among 5–6-year-old children. *European Child & Adolescent Psychiatry, 18*(12), 747–754.

Patel, V., Kirkwood, B. R., Pednekar, S., Weiss, H., & Mabey, D. (2006). Risk factors for common mental disorders in women. Population-based longitudinal study. *British Journal of Psychiatry, 189*, 547–555.

Paul, C., Ayis, S., & Ebrahim, S. (2006). Psychological distress, loneliness and disability in old age. *Psychology Health & Medicine, 11*(2), 221–232.

Pillai, A., Andrews, T., & Patel, V. (2009). Violence, psychological distress and the risk of suicidal behaviour in young people in India. *International Journal of Epidemiology, 38*(2), 459–469.

Posadzki, P., & Glass, N. (2009). Self-efficacy and the sense of coherence: Narrative review and a conceptual synthesis. *Scientific World Journal, 9*, 924–933.

Putnam, R. D. (1996, Winter). The strange disappearance of civic America. *American Prospect, 7*(24).

Putnam, R.D. (2000). *Bowling alone. The collapse and revival of American community.* New York: Simon & Schuster.

Ramanaiah, N. V., Sharpe, J. P., & Byravan, A. (1999). Hardiness and major personality factors. *Psychological Reports, 84*(2), 497–500.

Ravens-Sieberer U. (2008). The contribution of the BELLA study in filling the gap of knowledge on mental health and well-being in children and adolescents in Germany. *European Child and Adolescent Psychiatry, 17*(Suppl. 1), 5–9.

Redfield, R., Linton, R., & Herskovits, M. J. (1936). Memorandum for the study of acculturation. *American Anthropologist, 38*, 149–152.

Rogler, L., Cortes, D., & Malgady, R. (1991). Acculturation and mental health status among Hispanics. Convergence and new directions for research. *American Psychologist, 46*(6), 585–597.

Romas, J. A., & Sharma, M. (2010). *Practical stress management. A comprehensive workbook for managing change and promoting health* (5th ed.). San Francisco: Benjamin Cummings.

Rosenberg, M. (1965). *Society and the adolescent self-image*. Princeton, NJ: Princeton University Press.

Rosenberg, M. (1989). *Society and the adolescent self-image* (revised edition). Middletown, CT: Wesleyan University Press.

Rush, B. R., Bassani, D. G., Urbanoski, K. A., & Castel, S. (2008). Influence of co-occurring mental and substance use disorders on the prevalence of problem gambling in Canada. *Addiction, 103*(11), 1847–1856.

Rush, B., Urbanoski, K., Bassani, D., Castel, S., Wild, T. C., Strike, C., & Somers, J. (2008). Prevalence of co-occurring substance use and other mental disorders in the Canadian population. *Canadian Journal of Psychiatry, 53*(12), 800–809.

Ryder, A. G., Alden, L. E., & Paulhus, D. L. (2000). Is acculturation unidimensional or bidimensional? Ahead to head comparison in the prediction of personality, self-identity, and adjustment. *Journal of Personality and Social Psychology, 79*(1), 77–88.

Safaei, J. (2006). Is democracy good for health? *International Journal of Health Services: Planning, Administration, Evaluation, 36*(4), 767–786.

Scheier, M. F., & Carver, C. S. (1985). Optimism, coping, and health: Assessment and implications of generalized outcome expectancies. *Health Psychology, 4*, 219–247.

Scheier, M. F., Carver, C. S., & Bridges, M. W. (1994). Distinguishing optimism from neuroticism (and trait anxiety, self-mastery, and self-esteem): A reevaluation of the Life Orientation Test. *Journal of Personality and Social Psychology, 67*, 1063–1078.

Segerstrom, S. C. (2007). Optimism and resources: Effects on each other and on health over 10 years. *Journal of Research in Personality, 41*(4), 772–786.

Seligman, M. E. P. (1990). *Learned optimism*. New York: Pocket Books.

Seligman, M. E. P. (1994). *What you can change and what you can't: The complete guide to self-improvement*. New York: Alfred A. Knopf.

Selten, J., & Sijben, N. (1994). First admission rates for schizophrenia in immigrants to The Netherlands. The Dutch National Register. *Social Psychiatry and Psychiatric Epidemiology, 29*(2), 71–77.

Sharaf, A. Y., Thompson, E. A., Walsh, E. (2009). Protective effects of self-esteem and family support on suicide risk behaviors among at-risk adolescents. *Journal of Child and Adolescent Psychiatric Nursing, 22*(3), 160–168.

Sharma, M., & Romas, J. A. (2008). *Theoretical foundations of health education and health promotion*. Sudbury, MA: Jones and Bartlett.

Sheard, M. (2009). A cross-national analysis of mental toughness and hardiness in elite university rugby league teams. *Perceptual and Motor Skills, 109*(1), 213–223.

Shen, B., & Takeuchi, D. (2001). A structural model of acculturation and mental health status among Chinese Americans. *American Journal of Community Psychology, 29*(3), 387–418.

Smith, P. R. (2009). Resilience: Resistance factor for depressive symptom. *Journal of Psychiatric and Mental Health Nursing, 16*(9), 829–837.

Steel, Z., Chey, T., Silove, D., Marnane, C., Bryant, R. A., & van Ommeren, M. (2009). Association of torture and other potentially traumatic events with mental health outcomes among populations exposed to mass conflict and displacement: A systematic review and meta-analysis. *Journal of the American Medical Association, 302*(5), 537–549.

Taylor, S. E., & Aspinwall, L. G. (1996). Mediating and moderating processes in psychosocial stress. Appraisal, coping, resistance, and vulnerability. In H. B Kaplan (Ed.), *Psychosocial stress: Perspectives on structure, theory, life course and methods* (pp. 71–110). San Diego: Academic Press.

Thirthalli, J., & Benegal, V. (2006). Psychosis among substance users. *Current Opinion in Psychiatry, 19*(3), 239–245.

Tiet, Q. Q., Finney, J. W., & Moos, R. H. (2006). Recent sexual abuse, physical abuse, and suicide attempts among male veterans seeking psychiatric treatment. *Psychiatric Services, 57*(1), 107–113.

Urakawa, K., & Yokoyama, K. (2009). Sense of coherence (SOC) may reduce the effects of occupational stress on mental health status among Japanese factory workers. *Industrial Health, 47*(5), 503–508.

Van Dorn, R. A., Williams, J. H., Del-Colle, M., & Hawkins, J. D. (2009). Substance use, mental illness and violence: The co-occurrence of problem behaviors among young adults. *The Journal of Behavioral Health Services and Research, 36*(4), 465–477.

Veselska, Z., Madarasova Geckova, A., Gajdosova, B., Orosova, O., van Dijk, J. P., & Reijneveld, S. A. (2009). Socio-economic differences in self-esteem of adolescents influenced by personality, mental health and social support. *European Journal of Public Health, 20*(6), 647–652.

Victorino, C. C., & Gauthier, A. H. (2009). The social determinants of child health: Variations across health outcomes—a population-based cross-sectional analysis. *BMC Pediatrics, 9,* 53.

Wagnild, G. M., & Collins, J. A. (2009). Assessing resilience. *Journal of Psychosocial Nursing and Mental Health Services, 47*(12), 28–33.

Wagnild, G. M., & Young, H. M. (1993). Development and psychometric evaluation of the Resilience Scale. *Journal of Nursing Measurement, 1,* 165–178.

Ware, J. E. (n.d.). SF-36® health survey update. Retrieved from http://www.sf-36.org/tools/SF36.shtml

Ware, J. E., Gandek, B., & the IQOLA Project Group. (1994). The SF-36® health survey: Development and use in mental health research and the IQOLA Project. *International Journal of Mental Health, 23*(2), 49–73.

Ware, J. E., Kosinski, M., & Keller, S. D. (1994). *SF-36® physical and mental health summary scales: A user's manual.* Boston: The Health Institute.

Ware, J. E., Kosinski, M., & Keller, S. D. (1995). *SF-12®: How to score the SF-12® physical and mental health summary scales* (2nd ed.). Boston: The Health Institute.

Warr, D., Feldman, P., Tacticos, T., & Kelaher, M. (2009). Sources of stress in impoverished neighbourhoods: Insights into links between neighbourhood environments and health. *Australian and New Zealand Journal of Public Health, 33*(1), 25–33.

Webster, C., & Austin, W. (1999). Health-related hardiness and the effect of a psycho-educational group on clients' symptoms. *Journal of Psychiatric and Mental Health Nursing, 6*(3), 241–247.

Wells, M. (2009). Resilience in rural community-dwelling older adults. *Journal of Rural Health, 25*(4), 415–419.

Wille, N., Bettge, S., Ravens-Sieberer, U., & BELLA study group. (2008). Risk and protective factors for children's and adolescents' mental health: Results of the BELLA study. *European Child and Adolescent Psychiatry, 17*(Suppl. 1), 133–147.

Wise, M., & Sainsbury, P. (2007). Democracy: The forgotten determinant of mental health. *Health Promotion Journal of Australia, 18*(3), 177–183.

Zilber, N., & Lerner, Y. (1996). Psychological distress among recent immigrants from the former Soviet Union to Israel, I. Correlates of level of distress. *Psychological Medicine, 26*(3), 493–501.

Zullig, K. J., Valois, R. F., Huebner, E. S., & Drane, J. W. (2005). Adolescent health-related quality of life and perceived satisfaction with life. *Quality of Life Research, 14*(6), 1573–1584.

CHAPTER 4

Stress and Coping

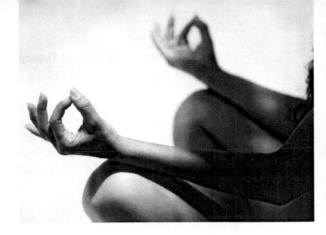

CHAPTER OBJECTIVES

After reading this chapter you should be able to
- Describe the historical genesis of theories of stress and coping
- List the constructs of the expanded transactional model
- Summarize the applications of theories of stress and coping in health education and health promotion
- Identify educational methods and match these to modify each construct from theories of stress and coping
- Apply the theories of stress and coping to reduce stress

This chapter discusses the concepts of stress and coping. Understanding stress is an integral part of understanding mental health. Stress and stressors are inevitable parts of living. Stress can be produced by a variety of external and internal events, such as acquiring a new behavior or changing an existing one. As we have seen in Chapter 3 sometimes this stress is harmful and causes negative sequelae known as distress. Sometimes this stress is helpful and leads to positive outcomes known as eustress.

Various theories, models, and constructs have been developed to explain the stress process. Some of these theories and models focus on the effects of stress, some on the causes of stress, others on personality characteristics, and some on coping responses. This chapter integrates the understanding of stress across these various models and theories. In health education and health promotion we are interested in understanding the stress process and in finding ways to reduce negative stress, so the emphasis is on the modifiability of constructs that can be altered.

I t is not the stressor but your perception of the stress that is important.

—Romas and Sharma (2010, p. 1)

In this chapter we begin by describing the historical aspects of the genesis of these theories. Next, we describe the various constructs that make up these theories and discuss the applications of theories of stress and coping in health education and health promotion. We then explore the limitations of the theories of stress and coping and present a skill-building application.

HISTORICAL PERSPECTIVES

The concept of **stress** in physiology and psychology was not known before 1932. Before that time the term was used mainly in physical sciences to denote cracks in the structure of buildings caused by pressure. Walter Cannon (1932), a physiologist, first defined stress as a "fight or flight" syndrome. He stated that when an organism is presented with a stressful stimulus, it responds by either fighting with it or running away from it. This was the origin of **response-based models** of stress.

The response-based concept was further elaborated by the work of Swedish physiologist Hans Selye (1936, 1974a, 1974b, 1982, 1985), who described the **general adaptation syndrome**. While trying to isolate a new sex hormone in rats, Selye observed that exposing rats to events such as cold, heat, injury, infection, loss of blood, pain, and other noxious stimuli resulted in their adrenal glands secreting corticoid hormones (a steroid) and their bodies going through three stages he called the general adaptation syndrome (**Figure 4.1**). He labeled the first stage the *alarm reaction*, in which a living organism's homeostasis, or balance, is disrupted by the noxious stimuli. In this phase the endocrine glands (ductless glands that pour their secretions directly into the blood), especially the adrenal glands, start secreting their hormones (corticosteroids), which help to supply more energy to the body. This is accompanied by a shrinkage of lymphatic structures, decrease in blood volume, and development of ulcers in the stomach. The second stage is *resistance*, in which the body tries to resist the noxious stimuli. In this stage the adaptation energy continues to get depleted. The third and final stage of the general adaptation syndrome is *exhaustion*. Exhaustion causes permanent damage to the system; if the noxious agent is not removed, the organism's energy becomes depleted, and death may ensue.

The response-based modeling of stress, which originated from the work of physiologists and discussed hormonal and physiological responses, remained the major model of stress until the 1960s, when event-based models and the concept of coping became understood in psychology. Thomas Holmes and Richard Rahe (1967) developed the Social Readjustment Rating Scale, which listed 43 life events, each with a predetermined weight, and asked a person to identify events he or she had experienced in the past year. They empirically found that the higher a person's score on the scale, the greater the chances

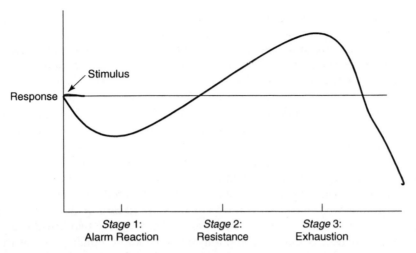

FIGURE 4.1 Stages of general adaptation syndrome

Source: Sharma, M., & Romas, J. A. (2012). *Theoretical foundations of health education and health promotion* (2nd ed., p. 148). Sudbury, MA: Jones and Bartlett. Reprinted with permission from Jones and Bartlett.

of that individual developing sickness in the subsequent year. The **event-based models** changed the paradigm from the effect (response) to the cause (stressor).

Alongside the event-based models the concept of **coping** was also developed, which led to the establishment of the transactional model of coping. The term *coping* can be traced back to the concept of **defense mechanisms** described in the psychoanalytical model by the famous Austrian neurologist Sigmund Freud (1923). In the 1920s Freud described the mechanisms of defense that a person's mind uses to protect itself. These include methods such as introjection, isolation, projection reversal, reaction formation, regression, repression, sublimation, turning against the self, and undoing. According to Freud, defense mechanisms were the devices the mind used to alter the individual's perception of situations that disturbed the internal milieu or mental balance. He applied the concept in identifying sources of anxiety through the free association technique on patients.

In the 1930s one of Freud's associates, Austrian-born physician Alfred Adler, differed from Freud and argued that defense mechanisms were protective against external threats or challenges (Sharma, 2003). Sigmund Freud's daughter and renowned psychologist, Anna Freud (1937), included both these viewpoints and underscored the role of defense mechanisms as being protective against both internal and external threats. She also extended the repertoire of defense mechanisms to include denial, intellectualization, ego restriction, and identifying with the aggressor. Therefore, it appears the concept of defense mechanisms is very similar to that of coping, which it preceded. However, in the 1970s psychologist Norma Haan (1977) distinguished defense mechanisms from coping. She explained that coping is purposive and involves choices, whereas defense mechanisms are rigid and set. Coping, according to Haan, is focused on the present, whereas defense mechanisms are premised on the past and distort the present.

Using the concept of coping, Richard Lazarus (1966, 1984), a professor of psychology at the University of California–Berkley, came up with the **transactional model**. According to this model all stressful experiences, including chronic illnesses, are perceived as person–environment transactions. In these transactions the person undertakes a four-stage assessment known as *appraisal* (Lazarus & Folkman, 1984). When confronted with any stressor the first stage is the *primary appraisal* of the event. In this stage the person internally determines the severity of the stressor and whether he or she is in trouble. If the stressor is perceived to be severe or threatening, has caused harm or loss in the past, or has affected someone known to the person, then the stage of secondary appraisal occurs. If, on the other hand, the stressor is judged to be irrelevant or poses minimal threat, then stress does not develop any further, and no further coping occurs. The *secondary appraisal* determines how much control the person has over the stressor. Based on this understanding the individual ascertains what means of control are available to him or her. This is the stage known as *coping*. According to the transactional model there are two broad categories of coping: problem-focused coping and emotion-focused coping. Finally, the fourth stage is *reappraisal*, during which the person determines whether the effects of the stressor have been effectively negated.

In the 1970s Suzanne Kobasa (1979a, 1979b) conducted an 8-year study of executives undergoing the major stress of losing their jobs or being reassigned and found that individuals who displayed a certain set of personality characteristics remained healthier and happier during the crisis. She labeled such personality traits *hardiness* (discussed in Chapter 3). Friedman and Rosenman (1974) classified people into type A and type B personalities. The **type A personality** was characterized by hurrying, exercising control over people and things, a sense of urgency, and a challenging nature. The **type B personality**

> *The nature and severity of the stress disorder could depend on at least three factors: (1) the formal characteristics of the environmental demands, (2) the quality of the emotional response generated by the demands, or in particular individuals facing these demands, and (3) the process of coping mobilized by the stressful commerce.*
>
> –Lazarus (1974, p. 327)

was more laid back and had a more relaxed disposition. It was found that type B personalities had less stress and type A had more stress. In the late 1970s and 1980s a medical sociologist, Aaron Antonovsky (1979, 1987), proposed the theory of sense of coherence (discussed in Chapter 3), which postulated that people who possess a higher sense of coherence tend to cope with life better. In the 1980s another construct that moderates the influence of stressors was discovered, namely, social support (discussed in Chapter 3). Scheier and Carver (1985) also suggested the construct of optimism as having a beneficial effect on coping (discussed in Chapter 3).

CONSTRUCTS OF THEORIES OF STRESS AND COPING

The primary construct of theories of stress and coping is **stressors**, which are demands from the internal or external environment an individual perceives as being harmful or threatening (Lazarus & Folkman, 1984). These are divided into three general classes: discrete, major life events; ongoing, everyday chronic stressors; and the absence of major happenings, or nonevents (Romas & Sharma, 2010).

Life events, or **life change events**, are discrete, observable, and objectively reportable events that require some social or psychological adjustment, or both, on the part of the individual (Wheaton, 1994). Examples of such events are the death of a family member, starting a new job, and buying a new home. If these happened in the recent past (within the last year), they are called **recent life events**; if they occurred further in the past (such as childhood events) and are bothersome as memories, they are called **remote life events.**

McLean and Link (1994) classified **chronic stressors** into five types:

1. *Persistent life difficulties:* These are life events that last longer than 6 months, such as long-term disability.
2. *Role strains:* These comprise of strain from either performing a specific role (such as parenting, working, or being in a relationship) or performing a multiplicity of roles at the same time.
3. *Chronic strains:* These are due to responses of one social group to another, such as overt or covert, intentional or unintentional discriminatory behavior due to race, ethnicity, minority status, and so on.
4. *Daily hassles:* These are everyday problems, such as getting stuck in traffic or waiting in a line.
5. *Community-wide strains:* These are stressors that operate at an ecological level, such as residing in a high-crime neighborhood.

Nonevents are classified as three types: (1) when desired or anticipated events do not occur (e.g., wanting to graduate but not having enough credits), (2) when desired events do not occur even though their occurrence is normative for people of a certain group (e.g., a person does not get married when most people of his or her age are married), and (3) not having anything to do (e.g., being bored).

Most of the time stressors cannot be modified and have to be endured. However, what can be changed in these cases is a person's perception of the stressors. Some stressors can be changed by modification of the environment. For example, if one is stressed about taking a class from a certain instructor and that class is being offered by another instructor, then making a change to the second instructor can alleviate the stress.

The second construct of the theories of stress and coping is that of primary appraisal, in which the person determines the severity of the stressor and makes an assessment regarding whether he or she is in trouble. To modify this construct in an educational program, participants could be asked to keep a stress diary, or they could participate in a brainstorming session to identify the stressors that are affecting them at any given time, or they could discuss the stressors and their severity.

In secondary appraisal the person determines how much control he or she has over the stressor. If control is high, then no stress develops; if control is low, then stress develops. To modify secondary appraisal in an educational program, stress diaries, brainstorming, or discussion can be helpful.

The construct of **problem-focused coping** is based on a person's capability to think and to alter the environmental event or situation. Examples of this strategy at the thought process level include utilization of problem-solving skills, interpersonal conflict resolution, advice seeking, time management, goal setting, and gathering more information about what is causing the stress. Problem solving requires thinking through various alternatives, evaluating the pros and cons of different solutions, and then implementing a solution that seems most advantageous to reduce the stress. Examples of this strategy at the behavioral or action level include activities such as joining a smoking cessation program, compliance with a prescribed medical treatment, adherence to a diabetic diet plan, and scheduling and prioritizing tasks for managing time.

In the construct of **emotion-focused coping**, the focus is on altering the way one thinks or feels about a situation or an event. Examples of this strategy at the thought process level include denying the existence of the stressful situation, freely expressing emotions, avoiding the stressful situation, making social comparisons, and looking at the bright side of things. Examples of this strategy at the behavioral or action level include seeking social support to negate the influence of the stressful situation; use of exercise, relaxation, or meditation; joining support groups; and practicing religious rituals. Negative examples include escaping through the use of alcohol and drugs.

The final construct of theories of stress and coping is **reappraisal**, which is the feedback loop by which the person determines whether the effects of the stressor have been effectively negated. To modify this construct techniques such as stress diaries, brainstorming, or discussion can again be helpful. **Table 4.1** summarizes the constructs.

TABLE 4.1 **Key Constructs from Theories of Stress and Coping**		
Construct	**Definition**	**How to Modify?**
Stressors	Demands from the internal or external environment that one perceives as being harmful or threatening. There are three kinds: life events, chronic stressors, and nonevents.	Most stressors cannot be modified and must be endured. What can be modified is the perception toward stressors. Some stressors can be modified by environmental engineering.
Primary appraisal	Person determines the severity of the stressor and makes an assessment whether he or she is in trouble.	• Stress diary • Brainstorming • Discussion
Secondary appraisal	Person determines how much control he or she has over the stressor.	• Stress diary • Brainstorming • Discussion
Problem-focused coping	Method of dealing with a given stressor by one's ability to think and alter the environmental event or situation.	• Problem-solving skills • Interpersonal conflict resolution • Advice seeking • Time management • Goal setting • Discussion to gather more information about what is causing one stress
Emotion-focused coping	Method of dealing with a stressor where the focus is inward on altering the way one thinks or feels about a situation or an event.	• Use of exercise • Relaxation • Meditation • Joining support groups
Reappraisal	Feedback loop where the person determines whether the effects of stressor have been effectively negated or not.	• Stress diary • Brainstorming • Discussion

APPLICATIONS OF THE THEORIES OF STRESS AND COPING

Theories of stress and coping have been used in a variety of health education and promotion applications, such as for cardiac rehabilitation after myocardial infarction (Macinnes, 2005), coping after traumatic brain injury (Anson & Ponsford, 2006; Strom & Kosciulek, 2007), coping in breast cancer survivors (Lebel, Rosberger, Edgar, & Devins, 2008; Wonghongkul, Dechaprom, Phumivichuvate, & Losawatkul, 2006), coping in the elderly (Poderico, Ruggiero, Iachini, & Iavarone, 2006), coping in the elderly with arthritis (Tak, 2006), coping in head and neck cancer patients (Vidhubala, Latha, Ravikannan, Mani, & Karthikesh, 2006), coping in newly incarcerated adolescents (Brown & Ireland, 2006), coping in old-age psychosis (Berry, Barrowclough, Byrne, & Purandare, 2006), coping in siblings with sickle cell disease (Gold, Treadwell, Weissman, & Vichinsky, 2008), coping in survivors of domestic violence (Lewis et al., 2006; Watlington & Murphy, 2006), coping with diabetes mellitus (Samuel-Hodge, Watkins, Rowell, & Hooten, 2008), coping with exacerbation of psoriasis and eczema (Wahl, Mork, Hanestad, & Helland, 2006), prevention of atherosclerosis (Jedryka-Goral et al., 2006), prevention of recurrent depression (Bockting et al., 2006), quality of life assessment for stroke caregivers (Van Puymbroeck & Rittman, 2005), smoking cessation (Friis, Forouzesh, Chhim, Monga, & Sze, 2006), and worksite stress management programs (Shimazu, Umanodan, & Schaufeli, 2006). **Table 4.2** summarizes these applications.

> *E*ach person must find a way to relieve his pent-up energy without creating conflicts with his fellow men. Such an approach not only insures peace of mind but also earns goodwill, respect, and even love of our neighbors, the highest degree of security and the noblest status symbol to which the human being can aspire.
>
> —Selye (1985, p. 28)

TABLE 4.2   Examples of Applications of Theories of Stress and Coping in Health Education and Health Promotion

Cardiac rehabilitation after myocardial infarction

Coping after traumatic brain injury

Coping in breast cancer survivors

Coping in elderly

Coping in elderly with arthritis

Coping in head and neck cancer patients

Coping in newly incarcerated adolescents

Coping in old-age psychosis

Coping in siblings with sickle cell disease

Coping in survivors of domestic violence

Coping with exacerbation in psoriasis and eczema

Prevention of atherosclerosis

Prevention in recurrent depression

Quality of life assessment for stroke caregivers

Smoking cessation

Worksite stress management program

FOCUS FEATURE 4.1 RELAXATION TECHNIQUES

Relaxation techniques are the core of stress management programs. Through relaxation we restore and consolidate energy that has been lost in everyday activities. Several techniques can be used for relaxation:

1. *Progressive muscle relaxation:* This technique was first described by Edmund Jacobson (1938, 1977) and entails systematic contraction and relaxation of various skeletal muscles in the body. It requires a person to lie down and then starting from feet, going to legs, abdomen, chest, upper limbs, neck and head region contract and relax various muscle groups. It is a mind–body technique that relaxes the system.

2. *Autogenic training:* This technique was first described by Johannes Schultz (1932) and entails a self-hypnotic procedure in which the mind focuses on heaviness and warmth sensations in different parts of the body. It is a mind–body technique that relaxes the system.

3. *Visual imagery:* This technique entails mental visualization with the help of imagination and is similar to dreaming (Romas & Sharma, 2010). One can focus on a past event that caused happiness and relaxation, or focus on the present with the help of music or some other soothing sounds, or focus on a future event that might bring happiness. Visualization of these events brings about relaxation. It is mind–body technique that relaxes the system.

4. *Yoga and meditation:* Practicing yogic breathing techniques (*pranayama*) and performing low-physical-impact postures (*asanas*) and meditation (*dhyana*) are also useful relaxation techniques. In *pranayama* inhalation pausing or holding the breath and exhalation are done in a ratio of 1:4:2. *Asanas* involve holding the body in various postures that provide relaxation to the system. One of the *asanas* is *shava asana* or the corpse pose in which one lies down and totally relaxes the mind and body. In meditation (*dhyana*) one concentrates on breathing or various endocrine glands or a *mantra* (a Sanskrit phrase) or on inner life force and in the process the mind gets subtler and subtler. In meditation based on electroencephalographic recordings, the mind starts from beta waves (14–40 cycles per second) and then goes to alpha (8–13 cycles per second) to theta waves (4–7 cycles per second) to delta waves (1 cycle per second).

5. *Biofeedback:* This technique entails use of instruments to comprehend physiological processes that one is not normally aware of but that may be brought under voluntary control. Usually, physiological processes such as blood pressure, heart rhythm, and muscle tension are recorded and feedback given to participants. This is a mind–body technique that relaxes the system.

LIMITATIONS OF THE THEORIES OF STRESS AND COPING

As discussed, there are three major theories of stress and coping. The strength of response-based models is that they explicate the physiological relationships involved in stress, but some of the limitations of this model are the nonspecificity of stimuli, the lack of accounting for individual variations, the lack of accounting for differences in stressors, and lack of attention to cognitive processing of stressors. Event-based models are strong in terms of clarifying stressors, introducing the notion of coping, and explaining the differences in stressors, but the limitations are not covering physiological mechanisms and not distinguishing between cause and effect (e.g., disease is an event that produces stress as well as an outcome of stress).

The strengths of the transactional model of stress are that it explains coping in steps; underscores the importance of thinking, perception, and determination of controllability; emphasizes the role of chronic stressors or daily hassles as being more important than occasional life events; takes into account the interaction between individual and environment;

TABLE 4.3 Comparison of Response-Based, Event-Based, and Transactional Models of Stress and Coping

Model	Strengths	Weaknesses
Response based	Explicates the physiological mechanisms	Nonspecificity of stimuli/stressors
		Does not account for individual variations
		Multiplicity of stressors not addressed
		No attention to the cognitive processing of the stressor(s)
Event based	Clarifies stressors	Does not cover physiological mechanisms
	Introduces the notion of coping (or dealing with environmental events)	Does not distinguish between cause and effect, for example, disease is an event that produces stress and it is considered an outcome of stress
	Explains multiplicity of stressors	
Transactional	Explains coping in steps	Lack of objective measurement of coping
	Underscores the importance of thinking, perception, and determination of controllability	Does not consider personality characteristics
	Emphasizes the role of chronic stressors or daily hassles as being more important than occasional life events	Does not cover physiological mechanisms
	Takes into account the communication process or interaction between individual and environment including other people	
	Feedback mechanism or "closed loop" system in this model (Reappraisal)	

and has a feedback mechanism or "closed-loop" system in the form of reappraisal. The chief limitations of this model are that coping is not measured objectively, it does not cover personality characteristics, and it does not cover physiological mechanisms. **Table 4.3** summarizes the strengths and weaknesses of the major models of stress and coping.

SKILL-BUILDING ACTIVITY

Let us see how we can apply the transactional model of stress and coping for developing healthy coping behavior in a group of college students. **Figure 4.2** depicts each of the constructs of the transactional model of coping and links these with the educational processes and behavioral objectives in this example.

The health education intervention starts with the construct of primary appraisal, or stressor identification. This can be done by keeping a stress diary. Secondary appraisal can be modified through a brainstorming session. Problem-focused coping can be used to build problem-solving skills in the students. A demonstration of how to apply the steps of problem solving to help participants think through many solutions and identify the pros and cons of each solution before choosing one solution will be used as an educational method.

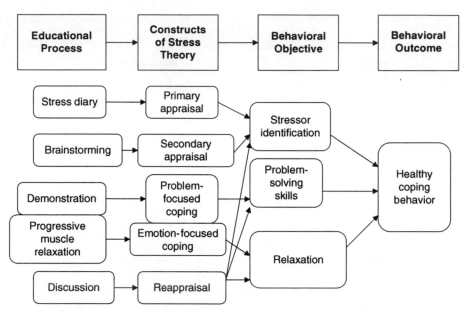

FIGURE 4.2   How the transactional model can be used to modify healthy coping.

Emotion-focused coping involves teaching the behavioral skill of relaxation to the students. The technique of progressive muscle relaxation can be taught in this regard. The final construct, reappraisal, can be facilitated through a discussion in which the participants think about how successful they have been with identifying stressors, using problem-solving skills, and learning relaxation. Using this approach, you can plan a coping intervention either as a standalone as shown in this example or as an adjuvant to another behavior change program. **Table 4.4** provides a set of questions.

TABLE 4.4   Choosing the Educational Method for Health Education Program Planning Using the Transactional Theory of Stress and Coping
What is the best method to facilitate *primary appraisal*?
☐ Stress diary
☐ Brainstorming
☐ Discussion
☐ Other
What is the best educational method to facilitate *secondary appraisal*?
☐ Stress diary
☐ Brainstorming
☐ Discussion
☐ Other

TABLE 4.4 Choosing the Educational Method for Health Education Program Planning Using the Transactional Theory of Stress and Coping (*Continued*)

What is the best educational method to facilitate *problem-focused coping*?

- ☐ Demonstration of problem-solving skills
- ☐ Interpersonal conflict resolution
- ☐ Advice seeking
- ☐ Time management
- ☐ Goal setting
- ☐ Discussion
- ☐ Other

What is the best educational method to facilitate *emotion-focused coping*?

- ☐ Exercise
- ☐ Relaxation
- ☐ Meditation
- ☐ Support groups
- ☐ Other

What is the best educational method to facilitate *reappraisal*?

- ☐ Stress diary
- ☐ Brainstorming
- ☐ Discussion
- ☐ Other

SUMMARY

In physiology and psychology the concept of stress originated in the 1930s with the response-based models based on the work of Walter Cannon and Hans Selye. These models looked at a myriad of physiological effects of stress on the body. This conceptualization was followed by the event-based models, which looked at the role of life events or discrete stressors in the causation of stress. Between the 1960s and 1980s Richard Lazarus proposed the transactional model of stress, in which a person interacts with the environment while going through four stages: primary appraisal, secondary appraisal, coping, and reappraisal. Coping is of two types: problem focused and emotion focused.

Stressors are divided into three general classes: discrete, major life events; ongoing, everyday chronic stressors; and the absence of major happenings, or nonevents. Life events are of two types: recent and remote. Chronic stressors are of five types: persistent life difficulties, role strains, chronic strains, daily hassles, and community-wide strains.

REVIEW QUESTIONS

1. Differentiate between response-based and event-based models.
2. Describe the transactional model.
3. Discuss the general adaptation syndrome.
4. Define stressors. Provide a classification of stressors.

5. Differentiate between problem-focused and emotion-focused coping.
6. Apply the transactional model of stress and coping for developing healthy coping behavior in a group of college students.

WEBSITES TO EXPLORE

American Institute of Stress

http://www.stress.org/

This website provides information about the American Institute of Stress, a not-for-profit organization established in 1978 to serve as a clearinghouse for information on stress-related issues. *Use this website to explore the contributions of some of the well-known personalities in the stress field.*

International Stress Management Association

http://www.isma.org.uk/

This is the website of a multidisciplinary professional membership organization based in the United Kingdom and the Republic of Ireland. This organization sets standards for stress management professionals and organizes conferences and other events. *Explore this website to learn about stress and this organization. Find out about the annual ISMA conference.*

Stress and Disease: Contributions of Hans Selye

http://home.cc.umanitoba.ca/~berczii/page2.htm

This website at University of Manitoba summarizes the contributions of Hans Selye. The website provides links to the Canadian Institute of Stress and several books and sites related to neuroimmunobiology. *Review this website and summarize the contributions of Hans Selye to stress field.*

Stress Free Net

http://www.stressfree.com/

Visit this website and review the graphic model of stress provided as a link on this website. *Check the featured item and write a brief summary of what was on the featured item.*

Transactional Model of Stress and Coping: University of Twente

http://www.tcw.utwente.nl/theorieenoverzicht/Theory%20clusters/Health%20Communication/transactional_model_of_stress_and_coping.doc/

This website at University of Twente, Netherlands summarizes the transactional model of stress and coping. Its history, assumptions, conceptual model, favorite methods, scope and application, and example are presented. *Review the website and determine which constructs were discussed in the chapter and which were new.*

REFERENCES AND FURTHER READINGS

Anson, K., & Ponsford, J. (2006). Coping and emotional adjustment following traumatic brain injury. *Journal of Head Trauma Rehabilitation, 21*(3), 248–259.

Antonovsky, A. (1979). *Health, stress, and coping.* San Francisco: Jossey-Bass.

Antonovsky, A. (1987). *Unraveling the mystery of health: How people manage stress and stay well.* San Francisco: Jossey-Bass.

Berry, K., Barrowclough, C., Byrne, J., & Purandare, N. (2006). Coping strategies and social support in old age psychosis. *Social Psychiatry and Psychiatric Epidemiology, 41*(4), 280–284.

Bockting, C. L., Spinhoven, P., Koeter, M. W., Wouters, L. F., Visser, I., & Schene, A. H. (2006). Differential predictors of response to preventive cognitive therapy in recurrent depression: A 2-year prospective study. *Psychotherapy and Psychosomatics, 75*(4), 229–236.

Brown, S. L., & Ireland, C. A. (2006). Coping style and distress in newly incarcerated male adolescents. *Journal of Adolescent Health, 38*(6), 656–661.

Cannon, W. B. (1932). *The wisdom of the body.* New York: Norton.

Freud, A. (1937). *The ego and mechanism of defense.* London: Hogarth Press.

Freud, S. (1923). *The ego and the id.* New York: Norton.

Friedman, M., & Rosenman, R. H. (1974). *Type A behavior and your heart.* New York: Fawcett Crest.

Friis, R. H., Forouzesh, M., Chhim, H. S., Monga, S., & Sze, D. (2006). Sociocultural determinants of tobacco use among Cambodian Americans. *Health Education Research, 21*(3), 355–365.

Gold, J. I., Treadwell, M., Weissman, L., & Vichinsky, E. (2008). An expanded transactional stress and coping model for siblings of children with sickle cell disease: Family functioning and sibling coping, self-efficacy and perceived social support. *Child: Care, Health, & Development, 34*(4), 491–502.

Haan, N. (1977). *Coping and defending: Processes of self-environment organization.* New York: Academic Press.

Holmes, T. H., & Rahe, R. H. (1967). The social readjustment rating scale. *Journal of Psychosomatic Research, 11,* 213–218.

Jacobson, E. (1938). *Progressive relaxation* (2nd ed.). Chicago: University of Chicago.

Jacobson, E. (1977). The origins and developments of progressive relaxation. *Journal of Behavior Therapy and Experimental Psychiatry, 8,* 119–123.

Jedryka-Goral, A., Pasierski, T., Zabek, J., Widerszal-Bazyl, M., Radkiewicz, P., Szulczyk, G. A., ... Bugajska, J. (2006). Risk factors for atherosclerosis in healthy employees—a multidisciplinary approach. *European Journal of Internal Medicine, 17*(4), 247–253.

Kobasa, S. C. (1979a). Personality and resistance to illness. *American Journal of Community Psychology, 7,* 413–423.

Kobasa, S. C. (1979b). Stressful life events, personality, and health: An inquiry into hardiness. *Journal of Personality and Social Psychology, 37,* 1–11.

Lazarus, R. S. (1966). *Psychological stress and the coping process.* New York: McGraw-Hill.

Lazarus, R. S. (1974). Psychological stress and the coping in adaptation and illness. *International Journal of Psychiatry in Medicine, 5,* 321–333.

Lazarus, R. S. (1984). Puzzles in the study of daily hassles. *Journal of Behavioral Medicine, 7,* 375–389.

Lazarus, R. S., & Folkman, S. (1984). *Stress, appraisal, and coping.* New York: Springer.

Lebel, S., Rosberger, Z., Edgar, L., & Devins, G. M. (2008). Predicting stress-related problems in long-term breast cancer survivors. *Journal of Psychosomatic Research, 65*(6), 513–523.

Lewis, C. S., Griffing, S., Chu, M., Jospitre, T., Sage, R. E., Madry, L., & Primm, B. J. (2006). Coping and violence exposure as predictors of psychological functioning in domestic violence survivors. *Violence Against Women, 12*(4), 340–354.

Macinnes, J. D. (2005). The illness perceptions of women following acute myocardial infarction: Implications for behaviour change and attendance at cardiac rehabilitation. *Women and Health, 42*(4), 105–121.

McLean, D. E., & Link, B. G. (1994). Unraveling complexity: Strategies to refine concepts, measures, and research designs in the study of life events and mental health. In W. R. Avison & I. H. Gotlib (Eds.), *Stress and mental health: Contemporary issues and prospects for the future* (pp. 15–42). New York: Plenum Press.

Poderico, C., Ruggiero, G., Iachini, T., & Iavarone, A. (2006). Coping strategies and cognitive functioning in elderly people from a rural community in Italy. *Psychological Reports, 98*(1), 159–168.

Romas, J. A., & Sharma, M. (2010). *Practical stress management. A comprehensive workbook for managing change and promoting health* (5th ed.). San Francisco: Benjamin Cummings.

Samuel-Hodge, C. D., Watkins, D. C., Rowell, K. L., & Hooten, E. G. (2008). Coping styles, well-being, and self-care behaviors among African Americans with type 2 diabetes. *Diabetes Educator, 34*(3), 501–510.

Scheier, M. F., & Carver, C. S. (1985). Optimism, coping, and health: Assessment and implications of generalized outcome expectancies. *Health Psychology, 4,* 219–247.

Schultz, J. H. (1932). *Das Autogene Training-Konzentrative Selbstentspannung.* Leipzig, Germany: Thieme.

Selye, H. (1936). A syndrome produced by diverse nocuous agents. *Nature, 138,* 32.

Selye, H. (1974a). *Stress without distress.* Philadelphia: Lippincott.

Selye, H. (1974b). *The stress of life.* New York: McGraw Hill.

Selye, H. (1982). History and present status of stress concept. In L. Goldberger & S. Breznitz (Eds.), *Handbook of stress: Theoretical and clinical aspects* (pp. 7–17). New York: Free Press.

Selye, H. (1985). History and present status of the stress concept. In A. Monat & R. S. Lazarus (Eds.), *Stress and coping: An anthology* (pp. 17–29). New York: Columbia University Press.

Sharma, M. (2003). Coping: Strategies. In N. A. Pitrowski (Ed.), *Magill's encyclopedia of social science: Psychology* (pp. 442–446). Pasadena, CA: Salem Press.

Shimazu, A., Umanodan, R., & Schaufeli, W. B. (2006). Effects of a brief worksite stress management program on coping skills, psychological distress and physical complaints: A controlled trial. *International Archives of Occupational and Environmental Health, 80*(1), 60–69.

Strom, T. Q., & Kosciulek, J. (2007). Stress, appraisal and coping following mild traumatic brain injury. *Brain Injury, 21*(11), 1137–1145.

Tak, S. H. (2006). An insider perspective of daily stress and coping in elders with arthritis. *Orthopaedic Nursing, 25*(2), 127–132.

Van Puymbroeck, M., & Rittman, M. R. (2005). Quality-of-life predictors for caregivers at 1 and 6 months poststroke: Results of path analyses. *Journal of Rehabilitation Research and Development, 42*(6), 747–760.

Vidhubala, E., Latha, Ravikannan, R., Mani, C. S., & Karthikesh, M. (2006). Coping preferences of head and neck cancer patients—Indian context. *Indian Journal of Cancer, 43*(1), 6–11.

Wahl, A. K., Mork, C., Hanestad, B. R., & Helland, S. (2006). Coping with exacerbation in psoriasis and eczema prior to admission in a dermatological ward. *European Journal of Dermatology, 16*(3), 271–275.

Watlington, C. G., & Murphy, C. M. (2006). The roles of religion and spirituality among African American survivors of domestic violence. *Journal of Clinical Psychology, 62*(7), 837–857.

Wheaton, B. (1994). Sampling the stress universe. In W. R. Avison & I. H. Gotlib (Eds.), *Stress and mental health: Contemporary issues and prospects for the future* (pp. 15–42). New York: Plenum Press.

Wonghongkul, T., Dechaprom, N., Phumivichuvate, L., & Losawatkul, S. (2006). Uncertainty appraisal coping and quality of life in breast cancer survivors. *Cancer Nursing, 29*(3), 250–257.

CHAPTER 5

Understanding Major Psychotic Disorders

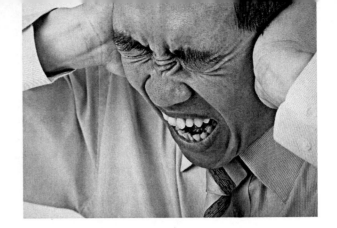

CHAPTER OBJECTIVES

After reading this chapter you should be able to
- Describe the salient clinical features of a psychotic disorder
- Define the major types of psychotic disorders
- Discuss the epidemiology, course, and burden of illness for schizophrenia
- Identify the preventative and treatment strategies available for psychotic disorders
- Delineate the important features of psychosocial models developed for schizophrenia and related illnesses
- Discuss the assertive community treatment model

In this chapter we discuss psychotic disorders and the treatments and interventions available to treat or remedy those disorders. Psychotic conditions such as schizophrenia are, undoubtedly, the most disabling of all mental illnesses. No text on mental health can be complete without an elaborate focus on psychotic disorders.

We begin with an introduction into psychosis and cover some basic concepts and definitions that serve as a background for the remaining text. We then discuss the epidemiology, risk factors, diagnostic criteria, course, and prognosis and consequences of schizophrenia and other psychotic disorders. In the last section we discuss how the prevention and treatment approaches have evolved in the past few decades.

PSYCHOTIC DISORDERS: AN INTRODUCTION

The latest version of the *Diagnostic and Statistical Manual of Mental Disorders* offers multiple definitions for the term **psychosis** (Ivleva & Tamminga, 2007). One of the many definitions restricts psychosis to "delusions and prominent hallucinations, with the hallucinations occurring in the absence of insight into their pathological nature" (American Psychiatric Association, 2000, p. 297). By this definition an individual hearing one or more voices that are not present would not be considered psychotic as long as he or she realizes the voices are imaginary. A less restrictive definition describes it as "prominent hallucinations that the individual realizes are hallucinatory experiences" (American Psychiatric Association, 2000, p. 297). This second definition accepts **insight** toward one's symptoms as spectrum, which hugely varies in different psychotic disorders and among different individuals. Somewhat more encompassing than the first definition, this second characterization of psychosis allows for the fact that a huge proportion of individuals with psychosis have some insight into their condition. It is the very few and perhaps sickest individuals who are truly completely oblivious to the nature of their symptoms. Perhaps the best definition of the term is to describe it as "a gross impairment of reality testing." **Table 5.1** lists some of the basic terms that are helpful during a formal discussion of psychosis.

> *Normality is an ideal fiction.*
>
> —Sigmund Freud

TABLE 5.1	Basic Definitions
Term	**Definition**
Delusion	A false belief based on incorrect inferences about reality at odds with the person's social and cultural background.
Hallucination	A false sensory perception occurring in the absence of any relevant external stimulation of the sensory modality involved.
Insight	A conscious recognition of one's own condition. In psychiatry it refers to the conscious awareness and understanding of one's own symptoms of maladaptive behavior; highly important in effecting changes in the personality and behavior of a person.
Disorganized speech	Loss of the orderliness of one's speech characterized by impairments in speech production, the tempo, lucidity, and content.
Cognition	Mental process of knowing and becoming aware; function is closely associated with judgment.
Reality testing	The ability to differentiate between the external world and the internal world and to accurately judge the relation between the self and the environment.

Delusions, hallucinations, problems in **reality testing**, **disorganized speech**, and disorganized behavior are the hallmark symptoms of **schizophrenia** or any other psychotic disorder. Depending on the etiology of a particular psychosis, these symptoms may present in isolation or in different combinations. Psychosis presents in its greatest severity in schizophrenia. Bizarre delusions and **hallucinations** may lead to dramatic and often frightening behavioral manifestations. Patients with schizophrenia may endorse hearing multiple voices conversing among themselves, commenting on the patient's life or behavior, or talking to the patient directly.

SCHIZOPHRENIA

Epidemiology

Undoubtedly, schizophrenia remains the most chronic and debilitating of all psychiatric disorders. Descriptions closely mimicking the symptoms of schizophrenia are found in literature from earliest documented history. At various times in human history, individuals with schizophrenia-like symptoms have either been exalted as seers and prophets or condemned as witches and devils. A scientific understanding of schizophrenia as a human brain disease started developing around the 19th century. Then, the **humane treatment** often prescribed for "insanity" was a method that advocated care, protection, and human understanding for those afflicted (Tamminga, 2007).

Two million Americans are presently diagnosed with schizophrenia. Interestingly, the incidence rates per year of schizophrenia in adults fall within a narrow range between 0.1 and 0.4 per 1,000 population across the globe. It was around the middle of the 20th century that antipsychotic drug treatments became widely available. Presently, there are two generations of antipsychotic medications, multiple psychotherapeutic techniques that have been found to help alleviate some of the symptoms, several known risk genes, and an evolving understanding of the anatomy of schizophrenia. With an emergence of a fundamental understanding in the brain sciences, it is fairly rational to predict that rational treatments for the condition may be developed within the next few decades.

Risk factors for schizophrenia have been grouped under three headings (Cooper, 1978):

1. Sociodemographic characteristics
2. Predisposing factors
3. Precipitating factors

Among the sociodemographic factors, social class and marital status are important predictors of schizophrenia. Epidemiological studies have consistently maintained an association between lower social class and schizophrenia in urban areas of developed countries. Marital status also seems to have a strong association with the risk ratio for unmarried individuals in comparison with their married counterparts calculated to be around 4 (Eaton, Day, & Kramer, 1988).

Genetic determinants seem to be the most important predisposing factor. Concordance rates of less than 50% in monozygotic twins and lifetime risk of about 45% in children of two schizophrenic parents leave ample room for environmental influences. It is believed that given the heterogeneous nature of schizophrenic disorders, it is also possible that both genetic and nongenetic forms of the disorder exist.

A variety of interpersonal, social, and cultural variables have been proposed as potential precipitating factors. Of these, family environment remains the best studied. Family interaction patterns characterized by unclear or fragmented communication, negative affective style, criticism, hostility, and over-involvement are strong predictors of relapse in schizophrenia, but their influence on the onset of the disorder remains limited (Miklowitz, 1994).

Diagnostic Criteria

Schizophrenia has been defined as a disturbance lasting at least 6 months (if untreated) not due to substance use or a general medical condition such as a brain tumor and in which two or more of the following symptoms are present for at least 1 month (American Psychiatric Association, 2000):

1. Delusions or hallucinations
2. Disorganized speech
3. Disorganized or catatonic behavior
4. Negative symptoms (described below)

The symptoms of schizophrenia have been divided into positive, negative, and cognitive. When a symptom involves an addition to an individual's normal experiences, it is said to be a **positive symptom**. Examples include auditory and visual hallucinations (hearing voices and seeing things), **thought broadcasting** or the feeling that one's thoughts are being broadcast into the environment, and delusions. **Negative symptoms** refer to affects and behaviors that are lacking in persons with schizophrenia and include a **flat or blunted affect** (reduction in the normal range of facial expressions), **thought blocking** (inability to completely articulate a thought), poverty of speech, and social withdrawal.

Cognitive symptoms may include memory and attention deficits, language difficulties, and problems with executive functioning. Patients with schizophrenia may have problems with executive functioning as evidenced by difficulties in ordering sequential behaviors, establishing goal-directed plans, maintaining tasks when interrupted, monitoring personal behavior, and associating knowledge with required responses (Beebe, 2003).

"Voices" are the most common type of hallucination in schizophrenia.

Course and Prognosis

Schizophrenia is usually first diagnosed in adolescence or early adulthood. A **prodromal period** (defined as the early symptoms and signs of an illness that pave the way for the characteristic manifestations of the acute, fully developed illness) usually precedes the actual disorder and may be characterized by peculiar behaviors, unusual speech, bizarre ideas, and strange perceptions. For example, individuals in the prodromal phase may claim to have special powers, such as the ability to communicate with inanimate objects. In its most classic form the disorder is characterized by episodes of symptom exacerbations and remissions. Within 5 to 10 years of diagnosis the positive symptoms appear to level out, whereas the negative symptoms become more evident (Beebe, 2003).

Individuals with schizophrenia become increasingly socially disabled over time. Prominent negative symptoms, a lack of social support, and social withdrawal are predictors of a poor outcome. Also, cognitive deficits (memory and attention problems, language difficulties, etc.) are correlated with poor community functioning to a greater extent than symptom levels (Beebe, 2003).

Consequences

Schizophrenia is a devastating illness in many ways. The consequences of this disorder can be grave, with implications both for the patient and their social network. The consequences can best be studied by dividing them under five broad headings (World Health Organization [WHO], 1998):

1. Mortality and morbidity
2. Social disability
3. Social stigma
4. Impact on caregivers
5. Social costs

In addition to psychotic symptoms, cognitive deficits, and social impairments, persons with schizophrenia are faced with multiple barriers to optimal health. Medical comorbidities are fairly common in schizophrenia, composed mainly of common diseases that affect schizophrenic patients more frequently than attributable to chance, as well as certain rare conditions or abnormalities that tend to co-occur with the disorder (Tamminga, 2007). Comorbid diseases in schizophrenic patients tend to be seriously undetected and underdiagnosed. Persons with schizophrenia have a mortality rate approximately 1.6 to 2.6 times higher and a life expectancy 20% shorter than those of the general population (Harris & Barraclough, 1998). They have significantly higher death rates from obesity-related diseases, diabetes, and respiratory and cardiovascular diseases.

Disability arising in the aftermath of schizophrenia can impair social functioning in many different ways (Janca et al., 1996). Self-care, in the form of personal hygiene, dressing, and feeding, may be impaired. Occupational performance or performance at the workplace may be hampered. An individual's functioning with respect to the family and household members may be affected. Finally, in a broader sense, socially appropriate interaction with community members and participation in leisure and other social activities may be curtailed.

Social stigma has been defined as a set of "deeply discrediting attributes, related to negative attitudes and beliefs towards a group of people, likely to affect a person's identity and thus leading to a damaged sense of self through social rejection, discrimination and social isolation" (Goffman, 1963, p. 116). The label of mentally ill is closely associated with stigma and is often unrelated to the actual symptoms, characteristics, or behaviors of those who are stigmatized. Social stigma can obstruct an optimal integration of patients with schizophrenia (and other mental health disorders) into the community, can be a strong barrier to treatment (both because of a fear of being labeled "mentally ill" and because health care providers may harbor negative attitudes toward patients), and may even lead to negative self-perceptions in those stigmatized and loss of self-esteem (WHO, 1998).

The enormous burden schizophrenia often places on families and others in close contact with a mentally ill person has only recently been explored. Caregiver burden may present in multiple forms, such as the economic costs associated with the need to support the patient and the loss of productivity of the family unit, emotional reactions (such as guilt and denial) in response to the family member's illness, concerns about the future, the stress of coping with disturbed behavior, disruption of a regular household routine, problems coping with social withdrawal or awkward interpersonal behavior, and curtailment of social activities of the caregiver.

Schizophrenia comes with profound social costs. The measure of disability-adjusted life years is often used as a health status indicator. Disability-adjusted life years can be used to compare different diseases and disorders in terms of their contribution to the overall burden. Schizophrenia is ranked 26th in the list of the diseases, arranged according to their contribution to the overall burden in terms of disability-adjusted life years. The indirect costs have not been reliably measured but are considered to be fairly sizeable.

OTHER PSYCHOTIC DISORDERS

There are many other psychiatric disorders that can have partial or even complete symptomatic overlap with schizophrenia. Many of these disorders share many of the risk factors with schizophrenia, and often the management for either disorder is the same. These disorders include **schizophreniform disorder, schizoaffective disorder, delusional disorder, shared psychotic disorder (folie à deux), brief psychotic disorder, substance-induced psychotic disorder**, and **psychotic disorder due to a medical condition**. Some of the salient features of these disorders are discussed in **Table 5.2**.

TABLE 5.2   Other Psychotic Disorders

Disorder	Diagnostic Clues
Schizophreniform disorder	An episode of schizophrenia lasting more than 1 but less than 6 months
Schizoaffective disorder	A combination of schizo (psychotic) + affective (mood) symptoms
Delusional disorder	Nonbizarre delusion of at least 1 month duration
Shared psychotic disorder (folie à deux)	A delusion develops in an individual in the context of a close relationship with another person(s), who has an already established delusion
Brief psychotic disorder	Combination of psychotic symptoms for more than 1 day but less than a month
Substance-induced psychotic disorder	Prominent hallucinations or delusions
	Evidence that the above developed within 1 month of substance abuse or withdrawal
Psychotic disorder due to a medical condition	Delusions/hallucinations occurring as the direct consequence of a general medical condition

Prevention, Treatment, and Care

We discuss the prevention, treatment, and care for patients with schizophrenia under the following five headings:

1. Preventive interventions
2. Medications
3. Family interventions
4. Other psychosocial interventions
5. Models of service delivery

Some of these sections are also dealt with elsewhere in this book. For instance, in the section on medications we only focus here on the points most relevant to the diagnosis of schizophrenia and psychotic disorders. The medications themselves are covered in more detail in other chapters.

Preventive Interventions

Primary prevention seeks to avoid the development of a disease in individuals who are as yet unaffected with that disease. Interventions that seek to reduce the incidence of a disease in a given population are included under **primary prevention** efforts. The two broad preventive strategies used in a public health context are illness prevention and health promotion (Eisenberg, 1993). The former, illness prevention, seeks to modify one or more risk factors thereby establishing specific interventions for specific disorders. Health promotion, on the other hand, aims to enhance health-promoting behaviors in a given community to foster well-being and prevent the onset of a wider group of disorders.

Secondary prevention attempts to identify individuals afflicted with a disease at an early stage (sometimes called the prodromal stage) and seeks to reduce morbidity through prompt treatment. When the onset of a disease or condition is unavoidable, preventive strategies conceptually shift from primary to secondary (Eaton, Badawi, & Melton, 1995). For a proper differentiation between primary and secondary prevention efforts, accurate knowledge of the natural history of an illness, risk factors, and whether the disease is amenable to preventive strategies should be known.

For most, if not all, psychiatric disorders risk factors and prodromal symptoms have a low specificity. Further, reliable methods to assess and predict the vulnerability to the disorder are almost nonexistent. Also, the early course of most such disorders is highly variable among individuals. Finally, most psychiatric disorders are thought to be multifactorial in origin. All these factors significantly limit the development of targeted preventive interventions (WHO, 1998).

For instance, although the role of genetic transmission in increasing the likelihood of developing schizophrenia has been well documented, the probable existence of nongenetic forms of the disorder and the absence of genetic markers make genetic risk prediction highly imprecise. The fact that only a small minority of individuals with schizophrenia come from families with a relative who is also affected further makes the use of genetic markers quite inaccurate. Because of the above considerations, genetic counseling cannot be offered to an individual "at risk" for developing the disorder.

Preventative strategies for schizophrenia have been advocated with the help of models using a psychosocial approach (Laporta & Falloon, 1992; Birchwood, McGorry, & Jackson, 1997; WHO, 1998). It is important to focus on preventive strategies given that treatment lag in first-episode schizophrenia has been estimated at 1 or more years (Birchwood et al., 1997). Such models involve some combination of the following strategies:

- Community education programs about psychotic disorders.
- Integrating mental health services into primary care.
- Detection of early warning signs by primary care practitioners and other communal agencies. Some research has been done into the early warning or prodromal signs of psychotic disorders, but due to the imprecise nature of such research it is not widely disseminated or known.
- Rigorous home-based assessment and interventions targeting at-risk individuals and key persons in their social networks to enhance stress management strategies and problem-solving skills.

The models that advocate a psychosocial approach are based on the underlying assumption that the development of health-promoting coping attitudes in individuals showing at-risk mental states and in their social environment could prevent the onset or retard the progression of overt psychotic disorders, even through nonspecific interventions. Also, by intercepting at-risk individuals before a frank psychotic episode, the prospects of starting active treatment at the right time increase.

The above approach is also worth mentioning because by attempting to integrate mental health interventions with primary care it seeks to reduce the stigma associated with psychiatric services thereby facilitating access to early treatment. However, its value as a truly preventive strategy remains uncertain.

Medications

Antipsychotic medications provide symptomatic improvement in schizophrenia and other psychotic disorders. These medications have been used in the treatment of psychotic conditions for more than four decades. Psychopharmacology in general and antipsychotic medications are discussed in more detail in Chapter 8. However, here we highlight the most important principles:

- Most antipsychotic medications work better for positive symptoms, whereas their effect on negative symptoms is less clear-cut.
- Therapy with medications can help delay but not avoid the risk of future relapses. The risk of relapse during the first year after an acute episode in patients on antipsychotic medications is reduced to about 20% compared with about 60% on placebo (Dixon, Lehman, & Levine, 1995).
- For first-episode (also called first break psychosis) patients who achieve full remission, some clinicians suggest that the medication should be tapered or discontinued within a period of 6 months to 2 years (Dixon et al., 1995). However, with

multiple episodes or in individuals who have an incomplete or partial remission the guidelines are not clear. In such cases medication-related decisions should be made on an individual basis, balancing the costs and benefits of treatment.

- All antipsychotic medications induce distressing and occasionally hazardous side effects, some of which can even mimic certain symptoms of psychiatric diseases. Any dose adjustment should be done in close cooperation with the patient. Some of the potential side effects can be minimized with the use of the newer or "atypical" antipsychotic medications sometimes labeled "second-generation antipsychotics."
- As is the case for most psychiatric illnesses, treatment adherence remains a major factor limiting therapeutic success.

Family Interventions

Early social theories of schizophrenia during the 1950s and the late 1970s focused determinedly on the possible causal role of dysfunctional child-rearing patterns and disturbed family communications. Such theories were widely popular among mental health professionals both in the United States and other Western countries and unfortunately contributed to negative attitudes toward patients' relatives and occasionally adversarial relationships between professionals and families. The **double bind theory of schizophrenia**, which gained widespread recognition, described the "double bind" situation in which no matter what an individual did, they "could not win." It was hypothesized that a person caught in the double bind could develop schizophrenic symptoms (Bateson, Jackson, Haley, & Weakland, 1956).

Eventually, research moved away from overambitious causal explanations to more pragmatic antecedents within the framework of studies of expressed emotion, factors related to family interaction and family members' beliefs and expectations that were likely to influence the course of schizophrenia, and other mental and physical disorders (Leff & Vaughn, 1985; WHO, 1998).

Family-based interventions developed as an outcome of the above mentioned paradigm shift. Such interventions sought to enhance the resources of the family unit in its caring function, mitigate family burden, and temper family interactions and attitudes that were predictive of relapse. Such interventions were variously labeled **"psychoeducational,"** "supportive," or "behavioral" and had some common constituents (Goldman, 1988; Goldstein, 1995):

- Early engagement of the family in the treatment process
- Education about schizophrenia (risk factors, prognostic variability, available treatments and rationale for them, suggestions for coping with the disorder)
- Communication training attempting to improve the clarity of communication within the family unit
- Problem-solving training aimed at improving ways of managing everyday problems, coping with stressful life events, and planning to deal with anticipated stressors by generalizing problem-solving skills
- Crisis intervention at times of extreme stress or when signs of relapse are evident

Strong research supports culturally sensitive family interventions in the comprehensive care of people with schizophrenia. Such interventions have consistently been found to reduce the risk of relapse and increase patients' and family members' satisfaction with service. With the identification and acceptance of family interventions as a vital component of community care of patients with schizophrenia, such interventions should now be seen as a long-term support rather than as a short time-limited treatment (Dixon & Lehman, 1995).

Other Psychosocial Interventions

The different psychotherapeutic approaches are covered in detail in Chapter 8. Here we briefly discuss other psychosocial interventions currently available for the treatment of schizophrenia. Long-term psychodynamic psychotherapy that originated from the psychoanalytic tradition remained the single most important psychological approach to the treatment of schizophrenia for many decades both in America and in Europe. Because of its high status this model deeply influenced the training and professional attitudes of many clinicians. However, over the past several decades several drawbacks were recognized. Absence of empirical testing through clinical trials, prohibitive costs, and limited adaptability to community settings led to the search for alternative models of psychotherapy more suited to the current times (Mueser and Berenbaum, 1990).

The cognitive approach focuses on an individuals' subjective response to dysfunctional thoughts or perceptions. The central notion of **cognitive behavioral therapy** (CBT) is that the way in which people make sense of their environment (including psychotic experiences) influences their affect and behavior (Turkington, Dudley, Warman, & Beck, 2004). Central to the CBT approach with schizophrenia is the importance of linking thoughts and feelings about current symptoms and then reevaluating these thoughts in relation to these symptoms. However, the crucial element in CBT for schizophrenia is the formation of a trusting therapeutic alliance. A focus on engaging the psychotic patient is maintained in every session. The patient's model of symptom initiation and maintenance is always carefully explored before other explanations are considered. It attempts to modify beliefs associated with delusions and ways of coping with auditory hallucinations. The strength of the CBT model lies in the fact that it attempts to build on natural coping strategies already used by people with schizophrenia when faced with positive symptoms, thereby linking professional intervention with self-help efforts. Moreover, it places psychotic symptoms within the context of a stress vulnerability model emphasizing that we all have the capacity of developing such symptoms if placed under sufficient stress. By highlighting that psychotic symptoms lie on a spectrum of differences in thought or behavior and are not an outcome of fundamentally different psychological processes, CBT-based approaches challenge long-held beliefs about the discontinuity between schizophrenia and ordinary experience (Chadwick, Birchwood, & Trower, 1996; Turkington et al., 2004).

Other interventions usually included under psychosocial rehabilitation are social skills training. Social skills training refers to a group of interventions that aim to teach the perceptual, motor, and interpersonal skills vital to achieving community survival, independence, and socially rewarding relationships. As part of these interventions, complex behaviors are evaluated and broken down into smaller components. Various behavioral techniques such as problem specification, instruction, modeling, role playing, behavioral rehearsal, coaching, reinforcement, structured feedback, and homework assignment are then used to teach those behaviors piece by piece (WHO, 1998). Despite the improvement evident for specific behavioral performances, it remains unclear whether the learning transfers from the training environment to everyday life. Vocational training linked to supported employment (Lehman, 1995) is another promising development.

Models of Service Delivery

Any health care intervention occurs within the larger context of a health care system. One of the many components of a health care system is the model or models of service delivery used to impart health care. For psychiatric disorders like schizophrenia ways of providing care, treatment settings, and service organization are critical as outcome determinants, more so than any single treatment modality. This is partly because unlike many other medical disorders, complete symptomatic remission is often an exception rather than the rule for psychiatric illnesses, especially psychotic disorders like schizophrenia.

Several decades ago care for schizophrenia was delivered almost exclusively at large institutions where many patients spent years. The deleterious effect of such an environment, particularly on social outcomes, has been well documented over many years. Despite being unavoidable for many patients, custodial care is increasingly being seen as a short-term and often secondary alternative to **community-based care**, the hallmark feature of which is provision of services in the users' own social environments. Community-based care services are currently adjudged to be the best context for service delivery to people with schizophrenia (Santos, Henggeler, Burns, Arana, & Meisler, 1995).

Advanced models of community care have been described and implemented in many countries around the world (Santos et al., 1995; WHO, 1998). A growing body of evidence from all over the globe supports both the viability and the benefits of comprehensive community care for people with schizophrenia and other severe mental disorders (Santos et al., 1995). All models of community care have certain common features:

- Services are offered to the entire population in a well-defined catchment area.
- Community care services attempt to provide individualized treatment aimed at empowering users and building on their assets and strengths.
- Services are primarily targeted at the seriously ill and most disabled patients.
- Continuity of care across treatment settings and over time is attempted.
- Services are provided preferably in the users' social environment.
- An attempt is made to offer services in the least restrictive setting.
- Long-term hospitalization is discouraged and recommended only in the extreme cases.
- Services are linked closely with primary health care.
- Social and vocational rehabilitation is provided in a natural environment.
- Users and their caregivers are involved in planning, implementing, and evaluating services.

FOCUS FEATURE 5.1 ASSERTIVE COMMUNITY TREATMENT

Assertive community treatment (ACT) is a service-delivery model that provides comprehensive, locally based treatment to people with serious mental illnesses. It provides highly individualized services directly to consumers. The ACT approach takes the multidisciplinary, round-the-clock staffing of a psychiatric unit directly to patients within the comfort of their home and community. For delivering such a comprehensive level of care, ACT members are trained in the disciples of psychiatry, social work, nursing, substance abuse, and vocational rehabilitation. The ACT team provides these necessary services 24 hours a day, 7 days a week, and 365 days a year.

The ACT model was developed in the late 1960s from work led by Arnold Marx, MD, Leonard Stein, MD, and Mary Ann Test, PhD, on an inpatient research unit of Mendota State Hospital, Madison, Wisconsin. These researchers noted that the gains made by patients in the hospital were often lost when they moved back into the community. It was hypothesized that the hospital's round-the-clock care helped alleviate clients' symptoms and that ongoing support and treatment were very important after discharge.

ACT seeks to reduce or eliminate the incapacitating symptoms of mental illness and to minimize or avoid recurrent acute episodes of the illness, to meet basic needs and enhance quality of life of the clients, to improve functioning in adult social and employment roles, to enhance an individual's ability to live independently in his or her own community, and to lessen the family's burden of providing care.

Treatment, rehabilitation, and support services are the three arms of the ACT model. Treatment includes psychopharmacological treatment, individual supportive therapy, mobile crisis intervention, hospitalization substance abuse treatment, and group therapy (for clients with a dual diagnosis of substance abuse and mental illness). Rehabilitation includes behaviorally oriented skill teaching, including structuring time and handling activities of daily living; supported employment, both paid and volunteer work; and support for resuming education. Support services include collaboration with families and assistance to clients with children; support, education, and skill-teaching to family members; and direct support to help clients obtain legal and advocacy services, financial support, supported housing, money-management services, and transportation.

The ACT model helps and supports individuals across all age groups who have a severe and persistent mental illness causing symptoms and impairments that produce distress and major disability in adult functioning (e.g., employment, self-care, and social and interpersonal relationships). Participants are usually individuals with schizophrenia and other disabling psychiatric disorders who have not been helped by traditional outpatient models for a multitude of reasons (difficulty getting to appointments, bad experiences in the traditional system, or a limited comprehension of their need for help).

ACT clients spend significantly less time in hospitals and more time in independent living situations, have less time unemployed, earn more income from competitive employment, experience more positive social relationships, express greater satisfaction with life, and are less symptomatic.

Unfortunately, despite the documented treatment success of ACT, only a small percentage of those with the greatest needs have access to this uniquely effective program. In the United States adults with severe and persistent mental illnesses constitute 0.5% to 1% of the adult population. Estimates suggest that 20% to 40% of this population could be helped by the ACT model if it were available.

Source: National Alliance on Mental Illness (NAMI). Treatment and Services. (2010). Available at: http://www.nami .org/Template.cfm?Section=About_Treatments_and_Supports&template=/ContentManagement/ContentDisplay .cfm&ContentID=8075. Accessed August 10, 2011.

SKILL-BUILDING ACTIVITY

In this chapter we discussed some of the major clinical features of psychotic illnesses. Watch the movie "A Beautiful Mind" and compile a list of the symptoms you were able to recognize. How different is the management of psychotic illnesses now from what it was several decades ago? Did any part of the movie surprise you? Compile a reflection paper discussing your feelings toward the male lead in the movie, John Nash.

SUMMARY

Psychosis is defined as a "gross impairment of reality testing, which is the ability to differentiate the external world and the internal world and to accurately judge the relations between the self and the environment" (American Psychiatric Association, 2000, p. 297). Delusions, hallucinations, problems in reality testing, disorganized speech, and disorganized behavior are the hallmark symptoms of schizophrenia or any other psychotic disorder.

Schizophrenia remains the most chronic and debilitating of all psychiatric disorders. An improved fundamental understanding in the brain sciences has raised hopes that rational treatments for the condition may be developed within the next few decades. Risk factors for schizophrenia are grouped under sociodemographic characteristics, predisposing factors, and precipitating factors. The symptoms of schizophrenia are divided into positive, negative, and cognitive types.

Schizophrenia is usually first diagnosed in adolescence or early adulthood. In its most classic form the disorder is characterized by episodes of symptom exacerbations and remissions. Schizophrenia is a devastating illness with manifold consequences, not just for the patient but also for the family and the society at large. Many other psychiatric disorders can have partial or even complete symptomatic overlap with schizophrenia.

Primary prevention seeks to avoid the development of a disease in individuals who are as yet unaffected with that disease, whereas secondary prevention attempts to identify individuals afflicted with a disease at an early stage (sometimes called the prodromal stage) and seeks to reduce morbidity through prompt treatment. Preventative strategies for schizophrenia that use a psychosocial model involve some combination of community education programs, integration of mental health services into primary care, detection of early warning signs by primary care practitioners, and rigorous home-based assessment and interventions targeting at-risk individuals and key persons in their social networks to enhance stress management strategies and problem-solving skills.

Antipsychotic medications provide symptomatic improvement in schizophrenia and other psychotic disorders. They are one of the cornerstones in the management of psychotic illnesses. They have been used in the treatment of psychotic conditions for more than four decades and have evolved with the introduction of newer agents.

Family-based interventions help enhance the resources of the family unit in its caring function, mitigate family burden, and temper family interactions and attitudes that are predictive of relapse.

Other psychosocial interventions currently available for the treatment of schizophrenia and other psychoses include long-term psychodynamic psychotherapy, the more prevalent and widely accepted CBT approach, and social skills training. Central to the CBT approach with schizophrenia is the importance of linking thoughts and feelings about current symptoms and then reevaluating these thoughts in relation to these symptoms. Social skills training are a group of interventions that aim to teach the perceptual, motor, and interpersonal skills vital to achieving community survival, independence, and socially rewarding relationships.

Any health care intervention occurs within the larger context of a health care system. One of the many components of a health care system is the model or models of service delivery used to impart health care. For psychiatric disorders like schizophrenia ways of providing care, treatment settings, and service organization are more critical as outcome determinants than any single treatment modality. Custodial care for the mentally ill is increasingly being seen as a short-term and less preferable alternative to community-based care. Community-based care services are currently adjudged to be the best context for service delivery to people with schizophrenia, and advanced models of community care have been described and implemented in many countries around the world. ACT is a service-delivery model that provides comprehensive, locally based treatment to people with serious mental illnesses.

REVIEW QUESTIONS

1. Define psychosis. What is the major difference between schizophrenia and schizophreniform disorder?
2. Enumerate the major diagnostic criteria for schizophrenia.
3. Discuss the social consequences of schizophrenia.
4. Differentiate between primary and secondary prevention.
5. Define community-based care. Discuss the major features of assertive community treatment.

WEBSITES TO EXPLORE

National Alliance for Research on Schizophrenia and Depression (NARSAD)

http://www.narsad.org/index.php

NARSAD is one of the most important private funders of psychiatric disorders. It came into being in 1981 as the American Schizophrenia Foundation and was formed by three leading national mental health organizations: National Alliance for the Mentally Ill, National Mental Health Association, and National Depressive and Manic Depressive Association. NARSAD raises money from donors around the world and invests it directly in the most promising research projects in mental health. *Explore the "Research News" section of the NARSAD website and compile a broad list of the major areas on which current research in schizophrenia is focused.*

Schizophrenia and Related Disorders Alliance of America (SARDAA)

http://www.sardaa.org/about_sardaa.html

SARDAA is a not-for-profit organization formed in February 2008 and dedicated to the support of persons who live with schizophrenia and related disorders. The organization focuses on providing materials and information to assist people in their own personal journey in living with their illness. *Download a copy of "Minds Unleashed—A Collection of Poetry by People with a Mental Illness" available on this website. Compile a reflection of your feelings and reactions as you read some of the poems.*

National Alliance on Mental Illness (NAMI)

http://www.nami.org/

Founded in 1979 NAMI is a grassroots mental health advocacy organization in North America. Through the efforts of grassroots leaders, NAMI focuses on three cornerstones of activity that offer hope, reform, and health: support, education, and advocacy. *Browse the website and explore the NAMI WALKS program.*

Mental Health America (MHA)

http://www.mentalhealthamerica.net/go/programs

Formerly known as the National Mental Health Association (NMHA), Mental Health America is a nonprofit organization that aims at promoting mental health and preventing mental disorders through advocacy, education, research, and services. *Use this website to locate a local support group for schizophrenia and related disorders.*

REFERENCES AND FURTHER READINGS

American Psychiatric Association. (2000). *Diagnostic and statistical manual of mental disorders* (4th ed., text revision). Washington, DC: Author.

Bateson, G., Jackson, D. D., Haley, J., & Weakland, J. (1956). Toward a theory of schizophrenia. *Behavioral Science, 1*, 251–264.

Beebe, L. H. (2003). Health promotion in persons with schizophrenia: Atypical medications. *Journal of the American Psychiatric Nurses Association, 9*, 115–122.

Birchwood, M., McGorry, P., & Jackson, H. (1997). Early intervention in schizophrenia. *British Journal of Psychiatry, 170*(1), 2–5.

Chadwick, P., Birchwood, M., & Trower, P. (1996). *Cognitive therapy for delusions, voices and paranoia.* Chichester, UK: Wiley.

Cooper, B. (1978). Epidemiology. In J. K. Wing (Ed.), *Schizophrenia: Towards a new synthesis.* New York: Grune & Stratton.

Dixon, L.B., & Lehman A.F. (1995). Family interventions for schizophrenia. *Schizophrenia Bulletin, 21*, 631–643.

Dixon, L. B., Lehman, A. F., & Levine, J. (1995). Conventional antipsychotic medications for schizophrenia. *Schizophrenia Bulletin, 21*, 567–577.

Eaton, W. W., Badawi, M., & Melton, B. (1995). Prodromes and precursors: Epidemiological data for primary prevention of disorders with slow onset. *American Journal of Psychiatry, 152,* 967–972.

Eaton, W. W., Day, R. & Kramer, M. (1988). The use of epidemiology for risk factor research in schizophrenia: An overview and methodological critique. In M.T. Tsuang & J. C. Simpson (Eds.), *Handbook of schizophrenia. Vol. 3: Nosology, epidemiology and genetics.* Amsterdam: Elsevier.

Eisenberg, L. (1993). Relation between treatment and prevention policies. In N. Sartorius, G. de Girolamo, G. Andrews, & L. Eisenberg (Eds.), *Treatment of mental disorders: A review of effectiveness.* Washington, DC: American Psychiatric Press.

Goffman, E. (1963). *Stigma. The negated identity.* Englewood Cliffs, NJ: Prentice-Hall.

Goldman, C. R. (1988). Toward a definition of psychoeducation. *Hosp Community Psychiatry, 29,* 666–668.

Goldstein, M. J. (1995). Psychoeducation and relapse prevention. *International Clinical Psychopharmacology, 9*(Suppl. 5), 59–69.

Harris, E. C., & Barraclough, B. (1998). Lifetime risk of suicide for affective disorder, alcoholism and schizophrenia. *British Journal of Psychiatry, 173,* 11–53.

Ivleva, E. I., & Tamminga, C. A. (2007). Psychosis as a defining dimension in schizophrenia. In B. J. Sadock, V. A. Sadock, & P. Ruiz (Eds.), *Kaplan and Sadock's comprehensive textbook of psychiatry* (pp. 1594–1595). Philadelphia: Lippincott Williams & Wilkins.

Janca A., Kastrup M., Katschnig, H., Lopez Ibor J. J., Jr., Mezzich, J. E., & Sartorius, N. (1996). The World Health Organization Short Disability Assessment Schedule (WHO DAS-S): A tool for the assessment of difficulties in selected areas of functioning of patients with mental disorders. *Social Psychiatry and Psychiatric Epidemiology, 31,* 349–354.

Laporta, M., & Falloon, I. (1992). Preventive interventions in the community. In D. J. Kavanagh (Ed.), *Schizophrenia: An overview and practical handbook.* London: Chapman and Hall.

Leff, J., & Vaughn, C. (1985). *Expressed emotion in families.* New York: Guilford Press.

Lehman, A. F. (1995). Vocational rehabilitation in schizophrenia. *Schizophrenia Bulletin, 21,* 645–656.

Miklowitz, D. J. (1994). Family risk indicators in schizophrenia. *Schizophrenia Bulletin, 20,* 137–149.

Mueser, K. T., & Berenbaum, H. (1990). Psychodynamic treatment of schizophrenia: Is there a future? *Psychological Medicine, 2,* 253–262.

National Alliance on Mental Illness. (2010). *Assertive Community Treatment.* Retrieved from http://www.nami.org/Template.cfm?Section=About_Treatments_and_Supports&template=/ContentManagement/ContentDisplay.cfm&ContentID=8075.

Santos, A. B., Henggeler, S. W., Burns, B. J., Arana, G. W., & Meisler, N. (1995). Research on field based services: Models for reform in the delivery of mental health care to populations with complex clinical problems. *American Journal of Psychiatry, 152,* 1111–1123.

Tamminga, C. A. (2007). Schizophrenia and other psychotic disorders. In B. J. Sadock, V. A. Sadock, & P. Ruiz (Eds.), *Kaplan and Sadock's comprehensive textbook of psychiatry* (pp. 1432–1462). Philadelphia: Lippincott Williams & Wilkins.

Turkington, D., Dudley, R., Warman, D. M., & Beck, A. T. (2004). Cognitive-behavioral therapy for schizophrenia: A review. *Journal of Psychiatric practice, 10*(1), 5–16.

World Health Organization (WHO). (1998). *Schizophrenia and public health.* Retrieved from http://www.who.int/mental_health/media/en/55.pdf.

CHAPTER 6

Understanding Mood, Anxiety, and Personality Disorders

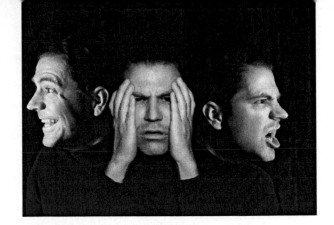

CHAPTER OBJECTIVES

After reading this chapter you should be able to
- Discuss the epidemiological impact and the main features of depression and bipolar disorder
- Describe the risk factors for suicide and be able to discuss suicide prevention
- Enumerate the main features of different anxiety disorders

- Define culture-bound syndromes and be able to discuss one or more of the syndromes described in this text
- Define personality disorders and be able to identify the salient features of different kinds of personality disorders

In this chapter we provide an overview of mood, anxiety, and personality disorders. There is a significant overlap between mood and anxiety disorders, with patients diagnosed with one often meeting the diagnostic criteria for another group of disorders. We begin with a discussion of depression and bipolar disorder and then explore anxiety and personality disorders.

DEPRESSION AND SUICIDE

Clinical Symptoms and Diagnostic Criteria of Depression

Depression is a common mental disorder that presents with depressed mood, loss of interest or pleasure, feelings of guilt or low self-worth, disturbed sleep or appetite, low energy, and poor concentration. These problems may become chronic, leading to substantial impairments in an individual's ability to take care of his or her everyday responsibilities. The worst possible outcome of depression is suicide, a tragedy associated with the loss of about 850,000 lives every year (World Health Organization [WHO], 2010). Depressive disorders are strongly associated with limitations in well-being and daily functioning that are equal to or greater than those of several chronic medical conditions.

Depression is the leading cause of disability and the fourth leading contributor to the global burden of disease (disability-adjusted life years, or DALYs) in 2000. By the year 2020 depression is projected to reach second place in the ranking of DALYs calculated for all ages and both genders. Today, depression is already the second contributor to DALYs in the age category 15 to 44 years for both genders combined (WHO, 2010).

Epidemiology

Two large studies, the Epidemiological Catchment Area Study and the National Comorbidity Survey, found the lifetime rates of major depressive disorders to be 4.9% and 17.1% respectively. The 1-year prevalence rates in these studies of major depressive disorder were 2.7% and 10.3%, respectively. More recent estimates have pegged the prevalence rates for major depression as intermediate between the Epidemiological Catchment Area Study and National Comorbidity Survey estimates (Rihmer & Angst, 2007).

The factors that predispose an individual to depression can be broken down into demographic, social, psychosocial, and seasonal, geographical, and dietary factors. We discuss each of these factors in some detail.

Demographic (Gender, Age, Race, and Ethnicity) Factors

Depression has been found to be approximately twice as common among women than men in almost all epidemiological studies on the prevalence and incidence of unipolar major depression. This gender difference unravels in early adulthood, becomes most pronounced in people between the ages of 30 and 45, and continues to persist in the elderly population. Among people younger than 45 years depressive disorders show much higher lifetime prevalence. However, the age at onset differs between familial and nonfamilial cases.

The average age at onset of recurrent unipolar major depressive episode falls between the ages of 30 and 35 years, whereas single-episode major depression that often lacks family history of mood disorders usually begins some years later. Because it is a frequent and highly recurrent illness, the probability of recurrence of major depressive disorder does not decrease with age.

It is well accepted that cultural differences may color the clinical presentation of depression, often leading to unreliable statistics in prevalence studies performed by standard methodology. Recent research (Alegria et al., 2008) has found that, after controlling for demographic factors, Asian Americans and Hispanic Americans have a significantly lower lifetime prevalence of unipolar depressive disorders.

Social Factors

Marital status and mood disorders have a very complicated relationship. For instance, being single, divorced, or separated can be both a risk factor for depression and the outcome of undesirable life events set into motion by depressive disorders. Major depressive disorders are most frequent among divorced, separated, or widowed individuals. Single women have lower rates of depression than married women, but for men the opposite holds true. The risk of a major depressive episode is quite high among recently widowed individuals across all ages but particularly so for the elderly.

Socioeconomic Factors

Despite being well documented, the relationship between depressive symptoms and low social class is only supported by a weak correlation. Individuals with lower socioeconomic status consistently have lower levels of education, income, and living conditions, coupled with higher rates of unemployment. Just as in the case of marital status and mood disorder, there is a possibility that cause and effect may be reversed here. Mood disorder could easily lead to unemployment, divorce, or low income, resulting in a downward slide on the social ladder.

Psychosocial Factors

Social stressors and social support are two of the most important psychosocial factors that can have a major role in influencing and precipitating depressive episodes. Social stressors have been well documented as risk factors for mood disorders. The type of stressor (acute vs. chronic, positive life event vs. negative life event, etc.) can play an important role in influencing and precipitating depressive disorders. In the genesis of mood disorders, chronic stressors (e.g., physical disability or difficult marital situation) play a more significant role than acute stressors. That said, the strongest predisposing factor is an accumulation of stressful negative life events. More important than the event is the subjective perception of that individual of the event. Acute positive events can also precipitate major depression.

Social support can help improve coping and temper the occurrence of psychosocial stressors or their unpleasant outcomes. Research has consistently shown that living alone, having low socioeconomic status, and being unemployed are important risk factors for mood disorders. A weak or nonexistent social support can also be considered a major risk factor.

Depression can be seen across all age groups and in all populations. However, certain population groups deserve special mention, either because the manifestations of depressive illnesses in these populations have unique features or because the prognosis of depression in those groups is more guarded. These special groups include pregnant females and children.

Seasonal Depression

Many functions of the human body, such as sleeping and temperature regulation, depend on biological cycles called circadian rhythms. These biological rhythms depend on the season and length of the day. **Seasonal depression** is the name given to the specific kind of depression precipitated by the disruption of these rhythms during the winter months (WHO, 2006). Excessive lethargy, excessive sleep, and overeating are symptoms somewhat specific to this form of depression, in addition to the usual symptoms elucidated above. Research suggests that seasonal depression may be related to light deprivation. Apart from standard drug therapy, phototherapy (exposing the depressed person to bright lights for predetermined lengths of time) may be effective in improving depression in such patients.

Postpartum Depression

The postpartum period immediately follows childbirth. The risk of depression in women is increased in the postpartum period, and approximately 10% of women develop **postpartum depression**, an incapacitating illness with devastating effects on the patient and her family if not recognized and treated in a timely fashion. Women with personal or family history of depression or other mood disorders are particularly at high risk (WHO, 2006). Even though the symptoms of postpartum depression are generally the same as other forms of depression, maternal guilt is an important part of the presentation because mothers may feel especially guilty about not being able to fully respond to the needs of their newborn infant.

Depression in Children

Earlier beliefs maintained that children and young adolescents were incapable of experiencing depressive symptoms and consequently could not suffer from depression. Research has revealed, however, that depression is quite common during childhood and adolescence (WHO, 2006).

Suicide

Suicide is undoubtedly one of the most tragic outcomes of any mental illness. Completed suicide is a relatively uncommon phenomenon, and this makes the precise prediction of suicidal attempts very difficult if not impossible. There are approximately 30,000 suicidal deaths annually in the United States (more than 80 per day) and at least 7 to 10 times this number of attempts. In 2007 suicide was the third leading cause of death in young people ages 15 to 24. Adolescent suicide accounted for 4,140 deaths (12%) of the total 34,598 suicide deaths in that year (National Institute of Mental Health [NIMH], 2010; Sudak, 2007).

Estimates put the number of suicide attempts at a staggering 10 times that of completed attempts. Despite remarkable increases in the suicide death rates for certain subpopulations during the last century (for instance, increased adolescent and decreased elderly rates), the overall rate of approximately 20 suicidal deaths per 100,000 persons has remained stable.

Gender Differences

Irrespective of race, males in the United States have suicide completion rates roughly three times that of females. However, females attempt suicide approximately three times as often as males. The discrepancy is not entirely understood but has been explained in different ways.

First, it is explained as an outcome of the methodology of suicide preferred by the two genders. For instance, females usually choose less lethal methods, those causing less disfigurement, and those that would be comparably less painful, such as pills. This choice leads to a greater margin of safety after an attempted suicide for females compared with males, who are more likely to select more lethal methods such as guns.

Another theory links the lower rate of alcohol abuse or dependence in females as a likely contributor to this differential. When studies control for this difference in alcohol abuse or dependence, completed suicide rates are more comparable between the two genders.

Another explanation is the fact that women are more likely to seek medical help when they are depressed or have another mental problem than men. The "sick role" is less uncomfortable and more socioculturally acceptable for women, whereas many men may feel compelled to "tough it out."

Age Differences

Suicide is rare before puberty across all races. For White males rates then increase in nearly direct proportion to age. African American male rates are comparable with White male rates up to age 25 to 30 but then decrease rather than increase with increased age.

From 1950 (19 per 100,000) to 1980 (20 per 100,000) the overall rate of suicide remained stable. However, during the same time adolescent rates tripled, but elderly (55+) rates dropped enough to balance out the adolescent increase.

Racial Differences

White male and female rates are approximately two to three times as high as African American male and female rates across the life cycle. The suicide rates in 2007 across the major ethnic/racial groups were as follows (Centers for Disease Control and Prevention, 2005):

- Highest rates
  - Native American and Alaska Natives: 14.3 per 100,000
  - Non-Hispanic Whites: 13.5 per 100,000
- Lowest rates:
  - Hispanics: 6.0 per 100,000
  - Non-Hispanic Blacks: 5.1 per 100,000
  - Asian and Pacific Islanders: 6.2 per 100,000

Miscellaneous Group Differences

As mentioned above, Native Americans have the highest rates in the United States. This is attributed partially or entirely to their high rates of substance abuse, high poverty, and gun availability. The rates for Protestants and Jews are slightly higher than Catholics. Rates for first-generation Americans parallel those of the countries from which their parents emigrated but over succeeding generations these rates approach U.S. rates. Homosexual men and women appear to have higher rates of suicide than matched heterosexuals.

Etiology of Suicide

Suicide is usually a multifactorial phenomenon with biological, psychological, and social factors acting together and culminating in the final, drastic outcome of suicide. The following have been documented as risk factors for suicide:

- Depression and other mental disorders or a substance-abuse disorder (often in combination with other mental disorders). More than 90% of people who die by suicide have the above-mentioned risk factors (Moscicki, 2001).
- Previous suicide attempt
- Family history of mental disorder or substance abuse
- Family history of suicide
- Family violence, including physical and/or sexual abuse
- Firearms in the home (Miller, Azrael, Hepburn, Hemenway, & Lippmann, 2006)
- Incarceration
- Exposure to the suicidal behavior of others, such as family members, peers, or media figures (Arango, Huang, Underwood, & Mann, 2002)

Prevention

Because suicide is a relatively uncommon phenomenon, positive predictions of suicide are uncommon. This difficulty in prediction holds true even for subgroups with very high rates (e.g., young adult, male, and Native Americans).

It is neither feasible nor possible to prevent all suicides. Interventions also cannot be expected to absolutely protect a given individual from suicide. However, the likelihood of suicide can certainly be reduced at both the population and individual level (Sudak, 2007).

Suicide prevention can also be targeted at different levels of prevention. Primary prevention attempts to eliminate diseases before they start. Primary preventative efforts include genetic counseling, gene manipulation, improved quality of life for all, and smoking cessation. Secondary prevention seeks to minimize the effects of the disease and could be conceived as better therapy for depression and prevention of suicide attempts in depression. Finally, tertiary prevention attempts to minimize the morbidity and mortality once a suicide attempt has occurred. Counseling after suicide could be seen as one instance of tertiary prevention.

The Centers for Disease Control and Prevention survey (Centers for Disease Control and Prevention, 2005) estimates that approximately 75% or more of suicide completers saw a primary care physician in the month before their deaths. Consequently, a natural prevention strategy is to educate primary care physicians to enhance their recognition and treatment of depression and suicide.

Research into suicide has facilitated the understanding of modifiable risk factors and interventions appropriate for specific population groups. Before being implemented, prevention programs should be tested through research to determine their safety and effectiveness (Gould, Greenberg, Velting, & Shaffer, 2003). For instance, because research has shown that mental and substance-abuse disorders are major risk factors for suicide, many interventions focus on treating these disorders as well as addressing suicide risk directly.

Suicide brings up ethical constraints for researchers who cannot randomly divide apparently suicidal patients into treated versus untreated arms. Consequently, the number of programs and practices identified that can be truly called "evidence based" in terms of suicide prediction or treatment is scant. The Best Practice Registry (a joint project of the American Foundation for Suicide Prevention and the Suicide Prevention Resource Center) seeks to enumerate programs and practices that appear to be both safe and clinically useful, even if they do not completely qualify as being evidence based (American Foundation for Suicide Prevention, 2010).

A specific kind of psychotherapy called cognitive therapy has been identified to reduce the rate of repeated suicide attempts by 50% during 1 year of follow-up. A previous suicide attempt is known to be among the strongest predictors of subsequent suicide. Cognitive therapy helps suicide attempters contemplate alternative actions when thoughts of self-harm surface (Brown et al., 2005). Specific kinds of psychotherapy may be helpful for specific groups of people. For example, a treatment called dialectical behavior therapy reduces suicide attempts by half, compared with other kinds of therapy, in people with borderline personality disorder (Linehan et al., 2006).

The U.S. Food and Drug Administration has approved the medication clozapine for suicide prevention in people with schizophrenia (Meltzer et al., 2003). Other potential medications and psychosocial treatments for suicidal people are being tested.

Because research shows that older adults and women who die by suicide are likely to have seen a primary care provider in the year before death, improving primary care providers' ability to recognize and treat risk factors may help prevent suicide among these groups (Luoma, Pearson, & Martin, 2002). Improving outreach to men at risk is a major challenge in need of investigation.

BIPOLAR DISORDER

Bipolar disorder (also called manic-depressive illness) is a brain disorder associated with abnormal shifts in mood, energy, activity levels, and the ability to carry out daily activities. Bipolar disorder has severe symptoms that are qualitatively different from the normal ups and downs people usually go through from time to time. Bipolar disorder symptoms can result in damaged relationships, poor job or school performance, and even suicide. Bipolar disorder can be treated, however, and people with this illness can lead full and productive lives (NIMH, 2008).

Bipolar disorder often develops in a person's late teens or early adult years. At least half of all cases start before age 25 (Kessler et al., 2005). Although some individuals develop their first symptoms in childhood, others may develop symptoms later on in their lives. The condition is difficult to diagnose, and there may be a lag time of years before people suffering from bipolar disorder are properly diagnosed and treated.

Symptoms

Individuals with bipolar disorder experience intense emotional states in distinct periods called "**mood episodes.**" A euphoric, overexcited state is termed a **manic episode**, whereas a sad and hopeless state is called a **depressive episode**. A mood episode may have symptoms of both depression and mania and is then called a "**mixed state.**" Irritability may also be a common symptom of bipolar disorder. During a mixed state symptoms often include agitation, trouble sleeping, major changes in appetite, and suicidal thinking. People in a mixed state may feel extremely sad and hopeless but at the same time also feel highly energized. Intense changes in energy, activity, sleep, and behavior often accompany these changes in mood. In place of discrete episodes of depression or mania, a person with bipolar disorder may experience chronically unstable moods (NIMH, 2008). Symptoms of a depressive episode are similar to those discussed above for depression. The major symptoms of a manic episode are as follows:

- A long period of feeling elated or excessively happy or outgoing mood
- Extreme irritability, agitation
- Talking rapidly, jumping from one idea to another, or having racing thoughts
- Being easily distractible
- Increasing goal-directed activities, such as taking on new projects
- Being restless
- Sleeping less than usual
- Having an unrealistic belief in one's abilities
- Impulsive and reckless behavior such as spending sprees, impulsive sex, and impulsive business investments

Sometimes a person with severe episodes of mania or depression may also have psychotic symptoms such as hallucinations or delusions. (Psychotic symptoms were discussed in detail in Chapter 5.) Psychotic symptoms tend to reflect the person's extreme mood, for instance, a person may believe he or she is renowned, has a lot of money, or has special powers. In the same way a person with a depressive episode may believe he or she is ruined and destitute or has committed a crime. As a result people with bipolar disorder who have psychotic symptoms are sometimes wrongly diagnosed as having schizophrenia, a psychotic disorder (discussed in Chapter 5) that also manifests hallucinations and delusions. Finally, individuals diagnosed with bipolar disorder may also develop behavioral problems such as alcohol and substance abuse and may experience poor performance at work or school and relationship problems.

Longitudinal Course of Bipolar Disorder

Bipolar disorder is generally a chronic and lifelong illness. Episodes of mania and depression usually come back over time. Between episodes some individuals may be completely free of symptoms, whereas others may have some residual or lingering symptoms (NIMH, 2008).

The *Diagnostic and Statistical Manual of Mental Disorders*, fourth edition, revised (DSM-IV-TR; American Psychiatric Association, 2000) divides bipolar disorder into four subtypes:

1. *Bipolar I Disorder*. The hallmark is manic or mixed episodes that last at least 7 days or manic symptoms that are so intense the individual requires immediate hospital care. Usually, the person also has depressive episodes, typically lasting at least 2 weeks. The symptoms of mania or depression must be a major change from the person's normal behavior and must not be due to substance abuse.

2. *Bipolar II Disorder*. The hallmark is an episodic shift between depressive and hypo-manic episodes, without full-blown manic or mixed episodes.

3. *Bipolar Disorder Not Otherwise Specified*. Diagnosed when an individual has symptoms of the illness that do not meet diagnostic criteria for either of the above two categories. The symptoms may be less intense or less frequent or less in number to be diagnosed with bipolar I or II. However, the symptoms are clearly out of the individual's normal range of behavior.

4. *Cyclothymic Disorder (Cyclothymia)*. **Cyclothymia** is a milder form of bipolar disorder where episodes of hypomania shift back and forth with mild depression for at least 2 years. However, the symptoms fail to meet the diagnostic requirements for any other type of bipolar disorder.

Without treatment, bipolar disorder worsens with time. Successive mood episodes may be both more frequent and more severe than the first episode (Goodwin & Jamison, 2007). Also, delays in getting the correct diagnosis and treatment make a person more likely to experience personal, social, and work-related problems (National Depressive and Manic-Depressive Association, 2001).

Coexisting Illnesses

Substance abuse is quite common among people with bipolar disorder, but the reasons remain unclear (Bizzarri et al., 2007). Some people with bipolar disorder may attempt to self-medicate with alcohol or drugs. However, substance abuse may also precipitate or prolong bipolar symptoms. Finally, the behavioral control problems associated with mania can result in a person consuming too much alcohol.

Anxiety disorders, such as posttraumatic stress disorder (PTSD) and social phobia, frequently co-occur among people with bipolar disorder (Krishnan, 2005; Mueser et al., 1998; Strakowski et al., 1998). Attention deficit hyperactivity disorder also frequently co-occurs with bipolar disorder, and there is some overlap in the symptoms between the two such as feeling restless and being easily distracted.

Bipolar disorder is also associated with a higher risk of thyroid disease, migraine headaches, heart disease, diabetes, obesity, and other physical illnesses (Krishnan, 2005; Kupfer, 2005). These illnesses can precipitate symptoms of mania or depression. Alternatively, they may also result from treatment of bipolar disorder.

Risk Factors

Because bipolar disorder tends to run in families, contemporary research focuses on identifying genes that may increase a person's likelihood of developing the illness. Genes are contained inside a person's cells that are passed down from parents to children. Children with a parent or sibling diagnosed with bipolar disorder are four to six times more likely to develop the illness compared with those who do not have a family history of bipolar disorder (Nurnberger & Foroud, 2000).

Technological research has helped advance genetic research on bipolar disorder. The launch of the Bipolar Disorder Phenome Database, funded in part by NIMH (2008), has helped facilitate the linking of visible signs of the disorder with the genes that may influence them. So far, researchers (Potash et al., 2007) using this database discovered that most people with bipolar disorder had

- Missed work because of their illness
- Other illnesses at the same time, especially alcohol and/or substance abuse and panic disorders
- Been treated or hospitalized for bipolar disorder

The researchers (Potash et al., 2007) also identified certain traits that appeared to run in families:

- History of psychiatric hospitalization
- Co-occurring obsessive-compulsive disorder (OCD)
- Age at first manic episode
- Number and frequency of manic episodes

Diagnosis

Like most psychiatric disorders there are no physical or laboratory tests currently available to make a diagnosis of bipolar disorder. However, tests may help rule out other possibilities or co-occurring conditions. The doctor or mental health professional should conduct a complete diagnostic evaluation. A complete history should also focus on family history. An attempt should be made to contact the individual's close relatives or spouse and note how they describe the person's symptoms and family medical history.

People with bipolar disorder are more likely to seek help when they are depressed than when experiencing mania or hypomania (Hirschfeld, 2008). Because the manic episodes are not seen, a thorough medical history is needed to ensure that bipolar disorder is not mistakenly diagnosed simply as major depressive disorder.

Treatment

Although there is no cure for bipolar disorder, proper treatment can still help most people gain better control of their mood swings and symptoms. This applies to the most severe form of the illness as well (Huxley, Parikh, & Baldessarini, 2000; Sachs, Printz, Kahn, Carpenter, & Docherty, 2000; Sachs & Thase, 2000).

Because of its chronic nature, people with bipolar disorder require long-term treatment to maintain control of bipolar symptoms. An effective maintenance treatment plan includes medication (psychopharmacological) and psychotherapy (commonly referred to as "talk therapy") with a goal of preventing future relapses and reducing symptom severity (Miklowitz, 2006). Usually, bipolar medications are prescribed by a physician. However, in some states clinical psychologists, psychiatric nurse practitioners, and advanced psychiatric nurse specialists can also legally prescribe medications. Three broad classes of medications are used to treat symptoms of bipolar disorder: mood-stabilizing medications, antipsychotic medications, and antidepressant medications.

Psychopharmacological

Mood-stabilizing medications are usually the first line of treatment for bipolar disorder and help control the abnormal mood episodes. Usually, treatment with mood stabilizers is continued for many years. Some of these medications are also used in the treatment of seizures and are therefore also called "anticonvulsants." Commonly used mood stabilizers are lithium, valproic acid, and lamotrigine. (More details on drug treatment can be found in Chapter 8).

   Antipsychotic medications are mainly used to target symptoms of psychotic conditions such as hallucinations and delusions but are occasionally used to treat symptoms of bipolar disorder. Such medications are divided into two groups: typical and atypical. Atypical antipsychotic medications (also called second-generation antipsychotics) are called "atypical" to set them apart from earlier medications, which are called "conventional" or "first-generation" antipsychotics (NIMH, 2008).

   Antidepressant medications are commonly used in the treatment of depression and help improve the mood and other symptoms of depression like low energy, poor appetite, and insomnia. However, individuals with bipolar disorder usually take antidepressants only in combination with either mood stabilizers of antipsychotic medications, because using only an antidepressant can increase a person's risk of switching to mania or hypomania or of developing rapid cycling symptoms (Thase & Sachs, 2000).

Psychotherapy

Psychotherapy is an effective tool in that it helps provide support, education, and guidance to individuals with bipolar disorder and their families. The following psychotherapy treatments are used to treat bipolar disorder (NIMH, 2008):

- **Cognitive behavioral therapy** helps people with bipolar disorder learn to change harmful or negative thought patterns and behaviors (also called **cognitive distortions**).
- **Family-focused therapy** involves the entire family unit and assists in developing and enhancing coping strategies, such as early recognition of new mood episodes. It also helps improve communication between family members.
- **Interpersonal and social rhythm therapy** helps people with bipolar disorder improve their relationships with others and manage their daily routines. Regular daily routines and sleep schedules may help protect against manic episodes.
- **Psychoeducation** teaches about bipolar disorder and its treatment both to the individual and the family. This approach helps people identify early signs of relapse so they can seek treatment early and perhaps avert a full-blown mood episode. It can be delivered in group or individual settings and may also prove helpful for family members and caregivers.

Licensed psychologists, social workers, or counselors usually provide the above-mentioned therapies. The number, frequency, and type of therapy sessions should be based on the individual treatment needs of each person. For individuals with a better awareness of the disease process, cognitive behavioral approach might be preferable to other approaches. For individuals with dysfunctional families and family dynamics that may obstruct treatment, a psychoeducational model might be preferable.

ANXIETY DISORDERS

Research focused on the constellation of mental conditions labeled *anxiety disorders* has expanded dramatically since the 1970s. In the clinical sense **anxiety** refers to the presence of fear or apprehension that is out of proportion to the context of the life situation (McClure-Tone & Pine, 2007; Pine, 2007). Therefore, extreme apprehension is considered clinically relevant anxiety if it is inappropriate to an individual's life circumstances (e.g., unremitting worries by a millionaire banker regarding his future financial well-being). We briefly discuss the most important symptoms of the major types of anxiety disorders, which are broadly divided into five major types:

1. Panic disorder and agoraphobia
2. Phobias
3. OCD
4. PTSD and acute stress disorders
5. Generalized anxiety disorder

Panic Disorder and Agoraphobia

Recurrent **"panic attacks"** represent the main feature of panic disorder. A panic attack is described as a discrete period of intense fear or discomfort that develops abruptly and peaks within 10 minutes. It is characterized by anxiety-based symptoms such as subjective feeling of one's heart beating, an increase in the heart rate, sweating, shaking, shortness of breath, chest pain, a fear of either losing control or of dying, feelings of unreality (**derealization**) or feelings of being detached from oneself (**depersonalization**), sensation of tingling, pricking, or numbness of a person's skin collectively called **paresthesias** and dizziness (American Psychiatric Association, 2000). For being diagnosed with panic disorder, a person should also have anticipatory anxiety associated with the fear of having more panic attacks, in addition to the attacks themselves (American Psychiatric Association, 2000).

Agoraphobia is the feeling of intense anxiety about being in places or situations from which escape might be difficult (or embarrassing) or in which help may not be available in the event of having an unexpected panic attack or panic-like symptoms. Agoraphobic fears typically involve characteristic clusters of situations that include being outside the home alone, being in a crowd or standing in a line, being on a bridge, and traveling in a bus, train, or automobile. Panic disorder can occur by itself or often in association with agoraphobia (McClure-Tone & Pine, 2007; Pine, 2007).

Phobias

A **phobia** is an excessive fear of a specific object, circumstance, or situation. Phobias are classified based on the nature of the feared object or situation, and the DSM-IV-TR recognizes three distinct classes of phobia: agoraphobia (considered to relate closely to panic disorder), **specific phobia**, and **social phobia**.

There are two important features of specific phobia (American Psychiatric Association, 2000):

1. Marked and persistent fear that is excessive or unreasonable, cued by the presence or anticipation of a specific object or situation (e.g., flying, heights, animals, receiving an injection, seeing blood)
2. Exposure to the phobic stimulus almost invariably provokes an immediate anxiety response

The four primary subtypes of specific phobias are animal type, natural environment type, blood-injury type, and situational type, along with a residual category for phobias that do not clearly fit any of these four categories.

Claustrophobia: fear of confined spaces
Autophobia: fear of being alone

Social phobia, on the other hand, includes a marked or persistent fear of one or more social or performance situations in which the person is exposed to unfamiliar people or to possible scrutiny by others. The individual is afraid of acting in a manner (or exhibiting anxiety symptoms) that will be humiliating or embarrassing.

Obsessive-Compulsive Disorder

Obsessive-compulsive disorder is another important anxiety disorder. The characteristic features of OCD are obsessions and compulsions. Obsessions provoke anxiety, and therefore the condition is classified as an anxiety disorder. **Obsessions** are defined as "persistent ideas, thoughts, impulses, or images that are experienced as intrusive and inappropriate" (American Psychiatric Association, 2000, p. 457). The obsession should be more than simply excessive worrying about everyday life situations. A common obsession is one of contamination where the individual has intrusive thoughts that he or she may be dirty or unclean.

Compulsions are defined as "repetitive acts, behaviors, or thoughts that are designed to counteract the anxiety associated with an obsession." (American Psychiatric Association, 2000, p. 457). The main feature of a compulsion is that it lessens the anxiety associated with the obsession. The compulsive ritual of hand washing may be used by an individual obsessed with contamination. Compulsions can also manifest as thoughts. For example, an individual obsessed with having sinned may chose to lessen his or her anxiety by compulsively repeating a prayer.

In the 1997 romantic comedy "As Good as It Gets," actor Jack Nicholson plays the character of Melvin Udall, a grouchy novelist who suffers from obsessive-compulsive disorder and takes his own silverware to the same restaurant every day because of his obsessions with cleanliness and/or possible contamination.

Posttraumatic Stress Disorder

As the name suggests, **posttraumatic stress disorder** is characterized by the onset of psychiatric symptoms immediately after exposure to a traumatic event. The DSM-IV-TR necessitates that to be able to cause PTSD, the traumatic event must include experiencing or witnessing events that involve actual or threatened death or injury or threats to the physical integrity of oneself or others. It also states that the individual's response to the traumatic event must involve intense fear or horror (American Psychiatric Association, 2000; McClure-Tone & Pine, 2007).

Such traumatic experiences could include physical assault, a violent accident or crime, natural disasters, military combat, being abducted, being diagnosed with a life-threatening illness, or experiencing systematic physical or sexual abuse. There is some evidence for a "dose–response relationship" between the intensity of trauma and the likelihood of developing symptoms. The higher the proximity and the greater the intensity of the trauma, the greater the likelihood that an individual will develop symptoms. PTSD symptoms are typically characterized into three areas:

*M*rs. Z sought help for symptoms she developed after an assault that occurred approximately 10 weeks before her evaluation at a mental health clinic. While leaving work late one evening, Mrs. M was attacked by a group of males in the parking lot next to the mall at which she worked. She was raped and violently assaulted, leading to multiple fractures and lacerations. However, eventually she was able to escape and call for help. On her initial evaluation Mrs. Z reported frequent invasive thoughts about the assault. She also had daily nightmares about the event and recurrent visions of her assailants. She reported that she now took a longer detour and parked in an alternative lot to avoid the attack scene. She also experienced some difficulty in dealing with males, particularly those who resembled her attackers. She reported being "very jumpy" and being startled very easily even by moderate noises. Mrs. Z described difficulty staying asleep at night, inability to focus, feeling irritable all the time, and an overall increased focus on her environment, particularly after dark.

1. *Reexperiencing the trauma.* **Flashbacks** are psychological phenomena in which an individual has a sudden, usually powerful, reexperiencing of a past experience or elements of a past experience. Reexperiencing can manifest in other ways, such as distressing recollections or dreams and either physiological or psychological stress reactions on exposure to stimuli that are linked to the trauma.
2. *Avoiding stimuli associated with the trauma.* Symptoms of avoidance associated with PTSD include efforts to avoid thoughts or activities related to the trauma, inability to remember all or part of the details related to the trauma, feelings of detachment or derealization, and a sense of a foreshortened future.
3. *Experiencing symptoms of increased autonomic arousal.* Symptoms of increased arousal include insomnia, irritability, hypervigilance, and exaggerated startle.

Finally, the diagnosis of PTSD is only made when symptoms persist for at least 1 month. In the absence of this last requirement, the diagnosis of **acute stress disorder** is usually applied. Acute stress disorder is characterized by reexperiencing, avoidance, and increased arousal, much like PTSD.

Generalized Anxiety Disorder

Generalized anxiety disorder is characterized by frequent and lasting worry and anxiety inconsistent with the actual events or circumstances on which the anxiety is focused.

For instance, even though a certain degree of concern regarding one's financial health is needed, worrying about an impending financial disaster all the time despite having good financial support may signal an underlying generalized anxiety disorder.

Individuals with generalized anxiety disorder are distressed by the degree of their anxiety even though they may not necessarily acknowledge the excessive nature of their anxiety. Also, the excessive worrying should have continued for most days of the week during at least a 6-month period. The condition is often associated with other somatic (concerning the body) or cognitive (pertaining to thinking) symptoms:

- Restlessness or feeling keyed up or on edge
- Easily fatigued
- Difficulty concentrating
- Irritability
- Muscle tension
- Sleep disturbance (difficulty falling or staying asleep or restless, unsatisfying sleep)

Worry is a common characteristic of a variety of anxiety disorders: Patients with panic disorder worry about having future panic attacks, patients with social phobia worry about their social interactions and the potential embarrassment that might ensue from an interaction gone wrong, and patients with OCD worry about their obsessions. For an individual to be diagnosed with generalized anxiety disorder his or her worries must surpass in breadth or scope the worries that characterize these other anxiety disorders.

CULTURE-BOUND SYNDROMES

Culture-bound syndromes have been discussed under a variety of names and have been defined as "episodic and dramatic reactions specific to a particular community locally defined as discrete patterns of behavior" (Littlewood & Lipsedge, 1985, p. 109). However, there is no clear consensus on what label should be used for a culture-bound syndrome. The term is contested both because of difficulties inherent in discussions of these experiences and in relating such phenomena to psychiatric diagnostic categories (Lewis-Fernández, Guarnaccia, & Ruiz, 2007).

The DSM-IV-TR contains symptomatic descriptions of 25 culture-bound syndromes and defines it as follows (American Psychiatric Association, 2000, p. 898):

> The term culture-bound syndrome denotes recurrent, locality-specific patterns of aberrant behavior and troubling experience that may or may not be linked to a particular DSM-IV diagnostic category. Many of these patterns are indigenously considered to be illnesses, or at least afflictions and most have local names. Culture-bound syndromes are generally limited to specific societies or culture areas and are localized, folk, diagnostic categories that frame coherent meanings for certain repetitive, patterned and troubling sets of experiences and observations.

Many culture-bound syndromes are currently recognized. Eating disorders are considered by many experts to be culture-bound syndromes. However, for sake of simplicity we limit our discussion to only three: amok, dhat, and ataque de nervios.

Amok

The DSM-IV-TR glossary of culture-bound syndromes contains the following definition of **amok** (American Psychiatric Association, 2000, p. 665):

> A dissociative episode characterized by a period of brooding followed by an outburst of violent, aggressive, or homicidal behavior directed at people and objects. The episode tends to be precipitated by a perceived slight or insult and seems to be prevalent only among males. The episode is often accompanied by persecutory ideas, automatism, amnesia, exhaustion, and a return to premorbid state following the episode. Some instances of amok may occur during a brief psychotic episode or constitute the onset or an exacerbation of a chronic psychotic process.

Similar behavior patterns have been reported from Laos, Philippines, Puerto Rico, India, Israel, Kenya, and North America. Similar reaction patterns exhibiting symptoms closely resembling amok have been found in other cultures, and controversy remains as to whether all these patterns should be labeled similarly and analyzed together (Lewis-Fernández et al., 2007).

Dhat

Dhat derives from the Sanskrit word *dhatu* meaning "metal" or "constituent part of the body." It was first mentioned in contemporary Western psychiatric texts as early as the 1960s by Wig (1960).

The symptoms of dhat include vague somatic complaints of fatigue, weakness, anxiety, appetite loss, guilt, and sexual dysfunction attributed by the patient to loss of semen in nocturnal emissions, through urine, and/or masturbation. Such symptoms have been well described in historical writings in India. In ancient Ayurvedic texts dating between the 5th millennium BC and the 7th century AD the process of semen production is described as a cyclical one where food is converted to blood, blood is converted to flesh, and flesh is converted to marrow, which is eventually converted to semen. It is said that it takes 40 days for 40 drops of food to be converted to 1 drop of blood, 40 drops of blood to 1 drop of flesh, and so on (Bhugra & Buchanan, 1989).

Such ideas can easily intimidate the individual into developing a sense of impending doom if a single drop of semen is lost, the anxiety culminating in a series of somatic symptoms (Chadha & Ahuja, 1990). These notions of semen loss and consequent anxiety have been reported from Sri Lanka and other parts of the subcontinent as well.

Ataque de Nervios

Ataque de nervios is a culture-bound syndrome mainly reported from the Latino population from the Caribbean but recognized among many other Latin American countries. Ataques de nervios frequently occur as a direct outcome of a life stressor pertaining to the family (e.g., death or injury to a close relative, divorce or spousal conflicts, or witnessing an accident involving a family member).

Individuals may experience amnesia for the entire duration of the ataque de nervios but otherwise return rapidly to their usual premorbid level of functioning. A common characteristic of an ataque de nervios is a feeling of being out of control. Other symptoms include uncontrollable shouting, paroxysms of crying, trembling, heat rising from the chest into the head, and verbal or physical aggression. Dissociative experiences, seizure-like or fainting episodes, and suicidal gestures are prominent in some but absent in other attacks (Lewis-Fernández et al., 2007).

Even though descriptions of some ataques de nervios may closely fit the DSM-IV-TR description of panic attacks, the association of most episodes with a precipitating event and the usual absence of the hallmark symptom of acute fear or apprehension helps distinguish them from panic disorder.

PERSONALITY DISORDERS

Personality disorders are usually defined by first delineating the concept of normal personality. This normality is usually defined either directly using criteria of health ideals or indirectly as opposite that of deviant personality. The distinction between "normal" and "abnormal" personality is, however, relative and subjective mainly because it relies on arbitrary cutoff points on the continuum between two extremes (very low and very high) of any behavior. The distinction is also context dependent because the same behavior, manifested in different situations, could be viewed as normal or as maladaptive (e.g., invariant cautiousness when danger is unlikely and the same trait when danger is likely).

The American Psychiatric Association (2000) has defined personality disorder as "an enduring pattern of inner experience and behavior that deviates markedly from the expectations of the individual's culture" (p. 685). Further, the above-mentioned pattern should be visible in two (or more) of the following areas:

1. Cognition (i.e., ways of perceiving and interpreting self, other people, and events)
2. **Affectivity** (i.e., the range, intensity, responsiveness, and appropriateness of emotional response)
3. Interpersonal functioning
4. Impulse control

The pattern is stable and of long duration, and its onset can be traced back at least to adolescence or early adulthood. It is inflexible and pervasive across a broad range of personal and social situations and leads to clinically significant distress or impairment in social, occupational, or other important areas of functioning. Personality disorders have been grouped into three clusters, shown in **Table 6.1**, based on common themes/characteristics.

Paranoid Personality Disorder

The hallmarks of paranoid personality disorder are excessive suspiciousness and distrust of others expressed as a pervasive tendency to interpret actions of others as deliberately demeaning, malevolent, threatening, exploiting, or deceiving. Individuals with paranoid personality disorder may exhibit an unusual hypersensitivity to and unforgiveness of insults, slights, and rebuffs; an unjustifiable tendency to question the loyalty of friends or the fidelity of spouse or sexual partners; and a reluctance to confide in others because

TABLE 6.1	Personality Disorders
Cluster	**Characteristics**
Cluster A	1. Paranoid personality disorder
	2. Schizoid personality disorder
	3. Schizotypal personality disorder
Cluster B	1. Antisocial personality disorder
	2. Narcissistic personality disorder
	3. Histrionic personality disorder
	4. Borderline personality disorder
Cluster C	1. Avoidant personality disorder
	2. Dependent personality disorder

of unwarranted fear that the information will be used against him or her (Cloninger & Svrakic, 2007).

Schizoid Personality Disorder

Schizoid personality disorder manifests as a pervasive pattern of social detachment and a restricted range of expressed emotions in interpersonal settings beginning by early adulthood and present in a variety of contexts signaled by

- Indifference to praise and criticism
- Preference for solitary activities and fantasy ("loner")
- Lack of interest in sexual interactions
- Lack of desire for or pleasure in close relationships
- Emotional coldness, detachment, or flattened affectivity
- No close friends or confidants other than family members
- Pleasure experienced in few, if any, activities

Schizotypal Personality Disorder

Schizotypal personality disorder is characterized by social and interpersonal deficits as indicated by pervasive discomfort with reduced capacity for close relationships as well as cognitive and perceptual distortions and eccentric and peculiar behavior such as odd beliefs and magical thinking (superstitious beliefs, beliefs in clairvoyance, telepathy, "sixth sense"; in children and adolescents bizarre fantasies or preoccupation), and lack of close friends, except family members (American Psychiatric Association, 2000; Cloninger & Svrakic, 2007).

Antisocial Personality Disorder

Antisocial personality disorder manifests as a pervasive disregard for and violation of the rights of others occurring since the age of 15 years and continuing into adulthood. Other clinical features are failure to conform to social norms (resulting in frequent arrests); deceitfulness, including lying and conning others for personal profit or pleasure; impulsivity or failure to plan ahead; irritability and aggressiveness, including repeated physical fights or assaults; recklessness, with disregard for the safety of self and others; irresponsibility, indicated by the failure to honor financial obligations or to sustain consistent work behavior; and lack of remorse, indicated by indifference or rationalizing having hurt, mistreated, or stolen from others.

Narcissistic Personality Disorder

The hallmarks of narcissistic personality disorder are a pervasive sense of grandiosity (in fantasy or in behavior), need for admiration, lack of empathy, and chronic intense envy. Other characteristics include a grandiose sense of self-importance and specialness; preoccupation with fantasies of unlimited success, power, brilliance, beauty, or ideal love; sense of entitlement; interpersonal exploitativeness, such as taking advantage of others to achieve own needs; lack of empathy; excessive need for admiration and acclaim; and an arrogant and haughty attitude.

Histrionic Personality Disorder

The hallmarks of histrionic personality disorder are pervasive and excessive self-dramatization, excessive emotionality, and attention seeking. Other features can include an inappropriate sexual seductiveness or provocativeness and an excessive need to be at the center of attention.

Borderline Personality Disorder

A pervasive and excessive instability of self-image and interpersonal relationships is the hallmark of this disorder. It also includes marked impulsivity. Diagnostic features may also include frantic efforts to avoid real or imagined abandonment, unstable and intense interpersonal relationships, markedly and persistently unstable self-image or sense of self, and recurrent suicidal behavior, gestures, threats, or self-mutilating behaviors.

Avoidant Personality Disorder

The hallmarks of avoidant personality disorder are pervasive and excessive hypersensitivity to negative evaluation, social inhibition, and feelings of inadequacy. It also includes an avoidance of occupational activities that involve significant interpersonal contact because of fears of criticism, rejection, or disapproval; an unwillingness to be involved with others unless certain of being liked; restraint in intimate relationships because of the fear of being shamed or ridiculed; and a preoccupation of being criticized or rejected in social situations.

Dependent Personality Disorder

The hallmarks of dependent personality disorder are pervasive and excessive need to be taken care of that leads to clinging behavior, submissiveness, fear of separation, and interpersonal dependency. Other features may include difficulty in making everyday decisions without excessive reassurance and advice from others, a need for others to assume responsibility for major areas of the individual's life, and difficulties in expressing disagreement with others because of fear of loss of support or approval.

FOCUS FEATURE 6.1 CASE HISTORY OF A PATIENT WITH PARANOID PERSONALITY DISORDER

Marc is a 25-year-old White man in his senior year of college. On the surface he appears to be a regular college student with the usual stressors that come with college. However, he was recently referred for psychological evaluation after he created a scene at the college cafeteria and accused a peer of following him around. This episode was only the most recent in a series of instances where Marc got into heated arguments with peers or authority figures. Marc was referred to the university psychologist.

During the first encounter Marc often made snide remarks insinuating the likelihood that the psychologist was a part of an elaborate scheme involving the peers he argued with and refused to accept any explanation as to his true role. He also refused any note taking or recording during the session. He revealed he was sick of having his phones tapped, his mail intercepted and inspected, and his place being wrecked days after he had an argument with a senior law enforcement officer. Per Marc, this senior officer had been parked in front of his apartment for a "suspiciously long time" for no obvious reasons.

During the next several evaluations a pattern emerged of an individual who was extremely hypersensitive to insults, slights, and rebuffs even from close friends. Despite an initial reluctance to trust the therapist to any degree, with the course of time Marc somewhat opened up. He admitted to the therapist that as long as he could remember, he had always been extremely reluctant to confide in others. This was because of a deep rooted fear that people, even friends, would use that information against him. Marc had few close friends, and his friendships and past intimate relationships had often been destroyed because of his constant questioning of the loyalty of his friends and the fidelity of his partners. Marc narrated all of this with little insight into the fact that his behaviors had been the cause of all the trouble. He had sued three of his previous employers on claims of discrimination. Marc had grown increasingly distant from his family after moving to college and would sometimes wonder if "they were all a part of it as well." After a thorough evaluation Marc was diagnosed with paranoid personality disorder.

SKILL-BUILDING ACTIVITY

Let's consider a hypothetical scenario. One of your close friends calls you at 8 p.m. and shocks you by making the revelation that he or she is contemplating suicide, that they have been depressed for quite some time now and have failed to get any help. Compile a list of five steps you would take, given the severity of the situation, to ensure your friend's safety. Feel free to consult any resources (including scholarly journals, websites, books, and so on). Compose a one- to two-page paper listing those steps and the rationale for such a plan. Share your paper with another peer and compare your choices with that of your peer.

SUMMARY

Depression is a common mental disorder that presents with depressed mood, loss of interest or pleasure, feelings of guilt or low self-worth, disturbed sleep or appetite, low energy, and poor concentration. These problems may become chronic, leading to substantial impairments in an individual's ability to take care of his or her everyday responsibilities. The worst possible outcome of depression is suicide, a tragedy associated with the loss of about 850,000 lives every year. Depression is the leading cause of disability and the fourth leading contributor to the global burden of disease (DALYs) in 2000. The factors that predispose an individual to depression can be broken down into demographic, social, psychosocial, and seasonal, geographic and dietary factors.

Suicide is undoubtedly one of the most tragic outcomes of any mental illness. Completed suicide is a relatively uncommon phenomenon, and this makes the precise prediction of suicidal attempts very difficult if not impossible. There are approximately 30,000 suicidal deaths annually in the United States (more than 80 per day) and at least 7 to 10 times this number of attempts. In 2007 suicide was the third leading cause of death for young people ages 15 to 24. Gender, age, racial, and miscellaneous group differences seem to exist in suicide completion rates across different groups. Native American and Alaska Natives have the highest rates, whereas Asian and Pacific Islanders have the lowest rates of suicide. Suicide is a multifactorial phenomenon with biological, psychological, and social factors acting together and culminating in the final, drastic outcome of suicide. The Best Practice Registry (a joint project of the American Foundation for Suicide Prevention and the Suicide Prevention Resource Center) seeks to enumerate programs and practices that appear to be both safe and clinically useful, even if they do not completely qualify as being evidence based.

Bipolar disorder (also called manic-depressive illness) is a brain disorder associated with abnormal shifts in mood, energy, activity levels, and the ability to carry out daily activities. Bipolar disorder has severe symptoms that are qualitatively different from the normal ups and downs people usually experience from time to time. Bipolar disorder symptoms can result in damaged relationships, poor job or school performance, and even suicide.

Bipolar disorder is generally a chronic and lifelong illness. Episodes of mania and depression usually come back over time. Like most psychiatric conditions, the treatment of bipolar disorder can be divided into two approaches: psychopharmacological (treatment with drugs) and psychotherapeutic (commonly referred to as "talk therapy"). Usually, bipolar medications are prescribed by a physician. However, in some states clinical psychologists, psychiatric nurse practitioners, and advanced psychiatric nurse specialists can also legally prescribe medications. The three broad classes of medications used to treat symptoms of bipolar disorder are mood-stabilizing medications, antipsychotic medications, and antidepressant medications.

Research focused on the constellation of mental conditions labeled "anxiety disorders" has expanded dramatically since the 1970s. In the clinical sense anxiety refers to the presence of fear or apprehension that is out of proportion to the context of the life situation. Therefore, extreme apprehension is considered clinically relevant anxiety if it is inappropriate to an individual's life circumstances (e.g., unremitting worries by a millionaire banker regarding his future financial well-being). Anxiety disorders are broadly divided into five major types: panic disorder and agoraphobia, phobias, OCD, PTSD and acute stress disorders, and generalized anxiety disorder.

Culture-bound syndromes have been defined as "episodic and dramatic reactions specific to a particular community locally defined as discrete patterns of behavior" (American

Psychiatric Association, 2000, p. 898). The currently recognized culture-bound syndromes are amok, dhat, and ataque de nervios.

The American Psychiatric Association and other authorities have defined personality disorders as "an enduring pattern of inner experience and behavior that deviates markedly from the expectations of the individual's culture." (American Psychiatric Association, 2000, p. 685). The pattern is stable and of long duration and its onset can be traced back at least to adolescence or early adulthood. It is inflexible and pervasive across a broad range of personal and social situations and leads to clinically significant distress or impairment in social, occupational, or other important areas of functioning. Personality disorders have been grouped into clusters A, B, and C based on common themes/characteristics.

REVIEW QUESTIONS

1. Define depression. Discuss the predisposing factors for depression.
2. Enumerate the risk factors for suicide.
3. Discuss suicide prevention.
4. Differentiate between bipolar I disorder and cyclothymia.
5. How can you differentiate an anxiety disorder from normal day to day anxiety?
6. What is a culture-bound syndrome?

WEBSITES TO EXPLORE

American Foundation for Suicide Prevention

http://www.afsp.org/

This website provides information about the American Foundation for Suicide Prevention (AFSP), a national not-for-profit organization established in 1987 that seeks to understand and prevent suicide through research, education, and advocacy and to reach out to people with mental disorders and those impacted by suicide. Visit the above website and browse to the section on "Best Practices Registry for Suicide Prevention," a collaborative effort of the AFSP and the Suicide Prevention Resource Center to develop and maintain an online registry of best practices for suicide prevention. *Compile a list of five evidence-based programs that hold promise for suicide prevention efforts.*

National Institute of Mental Health

http://www.nimh.nih.gov/health/publications

The National Institute of Mental Health (NIMH) is the largest research organization in the world specializing in mental illness. It is a part of the federal government of the United States. The stated mission of NIMH is to reduce the burden of mental illness and behavioral disorders through ("biomedical") research on mind, brain, and behavior. *Visit the above website and compile a one-page paper on a mental illness not discussed in this text.*

Suicide.org

http://www.suicide.org/about-suicide-org.html

Suicide.org is nonprofit organization with the following mission: "Our mission is to prevent suicides, support suicide survivors, and educate the public about suicide." *Check out the Suicide Myths section and compile a list of myths you thought were true before checking out this site.*

National Association of Cognitive-Behavioral Therapists

http://www.nacbt.org/whatiscbt.htm

The National Association of Cognitive-Behavioral Therapists (NACBT) is dedicated exclusively to supporting, promoting, teaching, and developing cognitive behavioral therapy and its practitioners. Cognitive behavioral therapy has often been claimed to be superior to other therapeutic approaches because it is "evidence based." *Explore the website and compile the reasons why CBT is called evidence based.*

REFERENCES AND FURTHER READINGS

Alegria, M., Canino, G., Shrout, P. E., Woo, M., Duan, N., Vila, D., Torres, M., Chen, C. N., Meng, X. L. (2008). *Prevalence of mental illness in immigrant and non-immigrant U.S. Latino groups, 165*(3), 359–369.

American Foundation for Suicide Prevention. (2010). Best Practices Registry (BPR) for suicide prevention. Retrieved from http://www2.sprc.org/bpr/section-i-evidence-based-programs.

American Psychiatric Association. (2000). *Diagnostic and statistical manual of mental disorders* (4th ed., text revision). Washington, DC: Author.

Arango, V., Huang, Y. Y., Underwood, M. D., & Mann, J. J. (2003). Genetics of the serotonergic system in suicidal behavior. *Journal of Psychiatric Research, 37*, 375–386.

Berrios, G. E. (1993). European views on personality disorders: A conceptual history. *Comprehensive Psychiatry, 34*(1), 14–30.

Bhugra, D., & Buchanan, A. (1989). Impotence in ancient Indian texts. *Sexual and Marital Therapy, 4*, 87–92.

Bizzarri, J. V., Sbrana, A., Rucci, P., Ravani, L., Massei, G. J., Gonnelli, C., Spagnolli, S., Doria, M. R., Raimondi, F., Endicott, J., Dell'Osso, L., Cassano, G. B. (2007). The spectrum of substance abuse in bipolar disorder: reasons for use, sensation seeking and substance sensitivity. *Bipolar disorders, 9*(3), 213–220.

Brown, G. K., Ten Have, T., Henriques, G. R., Xie, S. X., Hollander, J. E., & Beck, A. T. (2005). Cognitive therapy for the prevention of suicide attempts: a randomized controlled trial. *Journal of the American Medical Association, 294*(5), 563–570.

Centers for Disease Control and Prevention, National Center for Injury Prevention and Control. (2005). Web-based Injury Statistics Query and Reporting System (WISQARS). Retrieved January 31, 2007, from http://www.cdc.gov/injury/wisqars/index.html.

Chadha, C., & Ahuja, N. (1990). Dhat syndrome. A sex neurosis of the Indian subcontinent. *British Journal of Psychiatry, 156*, 577–579.

Cloninger, C. R., & Svrakic, D. M. (2007). Personality disorders. In B. J. Sadock, V. A. Sadock, & P. Ruiz (Eds.), *Kaplan & Sadock's comprehensive textbook of psychiatry* (pp. 2197–2240). Philadelphia: Lippincott Williams & Wilkins.

Goodwin, F. K., & Jamison, K. R. (2007). *Manic-depressive illness: Bipolar disorders and recurrent depression* (2nd ed.). New York: Oxford University Press.

Gould, M. S., Greenberg, T., Velting, D. M., & Shaffer, D. (2003). Youth suicide risk and preventive interventions: A review of the past 10 years. *Journal of the American Academy of Child and Adolescent Psychiatry, 42*(4), 386–405.

Hirschfeld, R. M. (2008). Psychiatric management. In Guideline watch: Practice guideline for the treatment of patients with bipolar disorder (2nd ed.). Retrieved from http://www.psychiatryonline.com/content.aspx?aID=148440.

Huxley, N. A., Parikh, S. V., & Baldessarini, R. J. (2000). Effectiveness of psychosocial treatments in bipolar disorder: state of the evidence. *Harvard Review of Psychiatry, 8*, 126–140.

Kessler, R. C., Berglund, P., Demler, O., Jin, R., Merikangas, K. R., & Walters, E. E. (2005). Lifetime prevalence and age-of-onset distributions of DSM-IV disorders in the National Comorbidity Survey Replication. *Archives of General Psychiatry, 62*(6), 593–602.

Krishnan, K. R. (2005). Psychiatric and medical comorbidities of bipolar disorder. *Psychosomatic Medicine, 67*(1), 1–8.

Kupfer, D. J. (2005). The increasing medical burden in bipolar disorder. *Journal of American Medical Association, 293*, 2528–2530.

Lewis-Fernández, R., Guarnaccia, P. J., & Ruiz, P. (2007). Culture-bound syndromes. In B. J. Sadock, V. A. Sadock, & P. Ruiz (Eds.), *Kaplan & Sadock's comprehensive textbook of psychiatry* (pp. 2520–2538). Philadelphia: Lippincott Williams & Wilkins.

Linehan, M. M., Comtois, K. A., Murray, A. M., Brown, M. Z., Gallop, R. J., Heard, H. L. et al. (2006). Two-year randomized controlled trial and follow-up of dialectical behavior therapy vs therapy by experts for suicidal behaviors and borderline personality disorder. *Archives of General Psychiatry, 63*(7), 757–766.

Littlewood, R., & Lipsedge, M. (1985). Culture bound syndromes. In K. Granville-Grossman (Ed.), *Recent advances in clinical psychiatry* (pp.105–142). Edinburgh, UK: Churchill Livingstone.

Luoma, J. B., Pearson, J. L., & Martin, C. E. (2002). Contact with mental health and primary care prior to suicide: A review of the evidence. *American Journal of Psychiatry, 159*, 909–916.

McClure-Tone, E., B., & Pine, D. S. (2007). Clinical features of the anxiety disorders. In B. J. Sadock, V. A. Sadock, & P. Ruiz (Eds.), *Kaplan & Sadock's comprehensive textbook of psychiatry* (pp. 1845–1856). Philadelphia: Lippincott Williams & Wilkins.

Meltzer, H. Y., Alphs, L., Green, A. I., Altamura, A. C., Anand, R., Bertoldi, A. et al. (2003). International Suicide Prevention Trial Study Group. Clozapine treatment for suicidality in schizophrenia: International Suicide Prevention Trial (InterSePT). *Archives of General Psychiatry, 60*(1), 82–91.

Miklowitz, D. J. (2006). A review of evidence-based psychosocial interventions for bipolar disorder. *Journal of Consulting & Clinical Psychology, 67*(Suppl. 11), 28–33.

Miller, M., Azrael, D., Hepburn, L., Hemenway, D., & Lippman, S. J. (2006). The association between changes in household firearm ownership and rates of suicide in the United States, 1981–2002. *Injury Prevention, 12*, 178–182.

Moscicki, E. K. (2001). Epidemiology of completed and attempted suicide: Toward a framework for prevention. *Clinical Neuroscience Research, 1*, 310–323.

Mueser, K. T., Goodman, L. B., Trumbetta, S. L., Rosenberg, S. D., Osher, C., Vidaver, C. et al. (1998). Trauma and posttraumatic stress disorder in severe mental illness. *Journal of Consulting & Clinical Psychology, 66*(3), 493–499.

National Depressive and Manic-Depressive Association (NMDA). (2001). *Constituency survey: living with bipolar disorder: how far have we really come?* Retrieved from http://www.dbsalliance.org/pdfs/bphowfar1.pdf.

National Institute of Mental Health (NIMH). (2008). Bipolar disorder. Retrieved from http://www.nimh.nih.gov/health/publications/bipolar-disorder/complete-index.shtml.

National Institute of Mental Health (NIMH). (2010). Suicide: A major, preventable mental health problem   Retrieved   from   http://www.nimh.nih.gov/health/publications/suicide-a-major-preventable-mental-health-problem-fact-sheet/suicide-a-major-preventable-mental-health-problem.shtml.

Nurnberger, J. I., & Foroud, T. (2000). Genetics of bipolar affective disorder. *Current Psychiatric Reports, 2*(2), 147–157.

Pine, D. S. (2007). Anxiety disorders: Introduction and overview. In B. J. Sadock, V. A. Sadock, & P. Ruiz (Eds.), *Kaplan & Sadock's comprehensive textbook of psychiatry* (pp. 1839–1844). Philadelphia: Lippincott Williams & Wilkins.

Potash, J. B., Toolan, J., Steele, J., Miller, E. B., Pearl, J., Zandi, P. P. et al. (2007). The Bipolar Disorder Phenome Database: A resource for genetic studies. *American Journal of Psychiatry, 164*(8), 1229–1237.

Rihmer, Z., & Angst, J. (2007). Mood disorders: Epidemiology. In B. J. Sadock, V. A. Sadock, & P. Ruiz (Eds.), *Kaplan and Sadock's comprehensive textbook of psychiatry* (pp. 1646–1647). Philadelphia: Lippincott Williams & Wilkins.

Sachs, G. S., Printz, D. J., Kahn, D. A., Carpenter, D., & Docherty, J. P. (2000). The Expert Consensus Guideline Series: Medication treatment of bipolar disorder 2000. *Postgraduate Medicine, 1*, 1–104.

Sachs, G. S., & Thase, M. E. (2000). Bipolar disorder therapeutics: Maintenance treatment. *Biological Psychiatry, 48*(6), 573–581.

Strakowski, S. M., Sax, K. W., McElroy, S. L., Keck, P. E., Jr., Hawkins, J. M., & West, S. A. (1998). Course of psychiatric and substance abuse syndromes co-occurring with bipolar disorder after a first psychiatric hospitalization. *Journal of Consulting & Clinical Psychology, 59*, 465–471.

Sudak, H. S. (2007). Psychiatric emergencies. In B. J. Sadock, V. A. Sadock, & P. Ruiz (Eds.), *Kaplan & Sadock's comprehensive textbook of psychiatry* (pp. 2717–2731). Philadelphia: Lippincott Williams & Wilkins.

Thase, M. E., & Sachs, G. S. (2000). Bipolar depression: Pharmacotherapy and related therapeutic strategies. *Biological Psychiatry, 48*(6), 558–572.

Wig, N. N. (1960). Problems of the mental health in India. *Journal of Clinical and Social Psychiatry, 17*, 48–53.

World Health Organization (WHO). (2006). Mental health and substance abuse. Retrieved from http://www.searo.who.int/EN/Section1174/Section1199/Section1567/Section1826_8109.htm.

World Health Organization (WHO). (2010). Depression. Retrieved from http://www.who.int/mental_health/management/depression/definition/en/index.html.

CHAPTER 7

Alcohol Dependence, Tobacco Use, and Substance Abuse

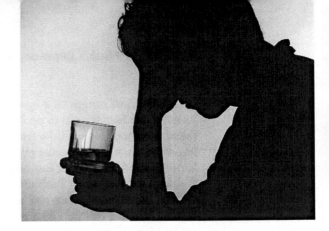

KEY CONCEPTS

- alcohol
- alcohol use
- alcoholism (alcohol dependence)
- amphetamines
- cocaine
- delirium tremens
- depressants
- drug abuse (substance abuse)
- drug dependence (substance dependence)
- drug misuse
- hallucinogens
- marijuana
- opioids
- stimulants
- tobacco use

CHAPTER OBJECTIVES

After reading this chapter you should be able to
- Describe the effects of alcohol
- Discuss the problem of alcohol abuse and alcoholism
- Discuss strategies for prevention and control of alcohol abuse
- Describe strategies for prevention and control of tobacco use
- Define drug abuse and misuse
- Identify commonly abused psychoactive drugs
- Discuss strategies for prevention and control of substance abuse

ALCOHOL

Alcohol as a beverage has been used by humankind since time immemorial, as records show alcohol use in all ancient civilizations. **Alcohol use** commonly involves the drinking of beer, wine, or spirits. In some parts of the world local home-brewed alcoholic beverages are also drunk, such as *burukutu* in Nigeria or *desi sharab* in India. Today, alcohol and tobacco are considered gateway drugs, meaning the use of these drugs leads one to experiment with other psychoactive drugs.

Saitz (2005) suggests a spectrum of alcohol use starting from abstinence (no use) to low risk use to risky use to problem drinking to harmful use (alcohol abuse) to alcoholism (alcohol dependence). Risky use for women and persons older than 65 years entails drinking more than seven drinks per week or more than three drinks per occasion. Risky use for men aged 65 years or less entails drinking more than 14 drinks per week or more than 4 drinks per occasion. Problem drinking entails use of alcohol accompanied by alcohol-related consequences but not meeting *International Statistical Classification of Diseases and Related Health Problems* (10th revision) or *Diagnostic and Statistical Manual of Mental Disorders* (4th edition, text revision; DSM-IV-TR) criteria (American Psychiatric Association [APA], 2000). Alcohol abuse (harmful use) according to DSM-IV-TR is significant impairment within 12 months with regard to failure to fulfill major role obligations, use in hazardous situations, alcohol-related legal problems, or social or interpersonal problems caused or exacerbated by alcohol (APA, 2000). **Alcoholism (alcohol dependence)** according to DSM-IV-TR is clinically significant impairment or distress in the presence of three or more of the following: (1) tolerance; (2) withdrawal; (3) a great deal of time spent obtaining alcohol, using alcohol, or recovering from its effects; (4) reducing or giving up important activities because of alcohol; (5) drinking more or longer than intended; (6) a persistent desire or unsuccessful efforts to cut down or control use of alcohol; and (7) continued use despite having a physical or psychological problem caused or exacerbated by alcohol (APA, 2000). The estimated annual costs attributable to alcohol use are approximately $185 billion (Harwood, 2000).

> *The estimated annual costs attributable to alcohol use are approximately $185 billion.*
>
> –Harwood (2000)

Fermentation is the basic process by which alcohol is made. Fermentation is the process where some yeasts act on sugar in cereal grains, fruits, and so on and recombines the carbon, hydrogen, and oxygen molecules of the sugar into ethyl alcohol and carbon dioxide. To increase the concentration of alcohol above 15%, distillation is done. Distillation is a process in which alcohol-containing solution is heated and the vapors collected and condensed into liquid form (Hart, Ksir, & Ray, 2009). The alcoholic content of the distilled beverages is expressed by the term *proof*. The proof number indicates how much percentage of alcohol by volume the drink contains and is twice the percentage of alcohol by volume. For example, 80-proof vodka is 40% alcohol.

Common alcoholic beverages are beer, wine, and distilled spirits. There are two types of wines in United States. The first are *generics*, named for their European origins, such as Chablis, Burgundy, and Rhine. The second are *varietals*, named after the variety of grape, such as Chardonnay, Merlot, and Zinfandel. Examples of distilled spirits are brandy, whiskey, gin, vodka, bourbon, and liqueurs.

Effects of Alcohol

When alcohol is consumed it is absorbed partly in the stomach and mainly in the small intestine. Alcohol is absorbed faster on an empty stomach than when it is consumed with food. Carbonated alcohol is also absorbed faster. After absorption the alcohol reaches the blood. The measure of concentration of alcohol in blood expressed in grams per deciliter is referred to as blood alcohol concentration (BAC) or blood alcohol level. Women consuming the same amount of alcohol tend to have higher BACs than men because women have a higher proportion of body fat. Likewise, a same-weight person with higher fat content will have higher BACs than a same-weight lean person. The enzyme alcohol dehydrogenase metabolizes alcohol. This enzyme is slower in women, and therefore women tend to have a higher BAC (Frezza et al., 1990).

The metabolism of alcohol takes place primarily in the liver, though some amount of alcohol is excreted unchanged in the breath and through skin and urine. First, alcohol is metabolized by alcohol dehydrogenase, which converts it into acetaldehyde. Then, the enzyme acetaldehyde dehydrogenase breaks down acetaldehyde into acetic acid. Several myths exist regarding alcohol metabolism that exercise or drinking coffee will hasten it, but this is not true. Alcohol interferes with the metabolism of several other drugs.

Alcohol's main effect is depressing the central nervous system (CNS). Alcohol acts primarily by enhancing the inhibitory effects of gamma-aminobutyric acid on gamma-aminobutyric acid receptors in the CNS. It also alters the effects of neurotransmitters: glutamate, dopamine, serotonin, and acetylcholine. In the past it was used as a general anesthetic agent, but it is no longer used for that purpose because better agents are available, its action was slow and uncontrolled, it makes blood slower to clot, and the dose required for anesthesia is very close to the lethal dose.

A *lcohol's main effect is depressing the central nervous system.*

The behavioral effects of alcohol depend on the BAC levels. At 0.05 g/dl BAC the person has lowered alertness, has some euphoria and feeling of relaxation, the cortical control releases inhibitions, and judgment is somewhat impaired. At 0.10 g/dl BAC reaction times are slowed, there is impaired motor function and ability to drive, and the person becomes reckless. At 0.15 g/dl BAC the reaction times get even slower, and the person may experience clumsiness and exaggerated emotions. At 0.20 g/dl the person is intoxicated. There is marked depression in sensory and motor functions. There may be unsteady gait and the person may demonstrate hostile or aggressive behavior. At 0.25 g/dl there is severe motor disturbance, and the person may have slurred speech and alterations in sensory perceptions. At 0.30 g/dl the person is in a stupor but is conscious. The person is confused, incapacitated, and has loss of feeling. At 0.35 g/dl the person is in a state of surgical anesthesia and is unconscious. At 0.40 g/dl 50% of the people would die from lung and heart failure. These effects are summarized in **Table 7.1**.

Toxicity of Alcohol

Alcohol is toxic and harmful both in the short and long term. Short-term effects are due to drinking and driving. Every year thousands of people die and are injured in traffic accidents involving alcohol. In 2009 there were 10,839 fatalities in alcohol-impaired driving crashes involving drivers with BACs over 0.08 g/dl (National Highway Traffic Safety Administration, 2010). These alcohol-related fatalities accounted for 32% of the total motor vehicle–related fatalities—a large proportion. Furthermore, among the 10,839 alcohol-related fatalities 7,281 (67%) involved drivers with a BAC of 0.08 g/dl or higher, 2,891 (27%) were motor vehicle occupants, and 667 (6%) were other people. Among alcohol-impaired drivers roughly 35% were between 21 and 24 years of age, 32% between 25 and 34 years, and 26% between 35 and 44 years (National Highway Traffic Safety Administration, 2010).

TABLE 7.1 Behavioral Effects of Alcohol Based on BAC Levels	
BAC (g/dl)	**Behavioral Effects**
0.05	• Lowered alertness
	• Some euphoria
	• Feeling of relaxation
	• Cortical control releases inhibitions
	• Judgment is somewhat impaired
0.10	• Reaction times get slower
	• Impaired motor function
	• Impaired ability to drive
	• Person becomes reckless
0.15	• Reaction times get even slower
	• May experience clumsiness
	• Exaggerated emotions
0.20	• Intoxicated
	• Marked depression in sensory and motor functions
	• Unsteady gait
	• Demonstrates hostile or aggressive behavior
0.25	• Severe motor disturbance
	• Slurred speech
	• Alterations in sensory perceptions
0.30	• Stuporous but conscious
	• Confused
	• Incapacitated
	• Loss of feeling
0.35	• State of surgical anesthesia
	• Unconscious
0.40	• Die from lung and heart failure

The number of deaths is only the tip of the iceberg. In 2008 more than 1.4 million arrests were made for driving under the influence of alcohol or narcotics (U.S. Department of Justice, Federal Bureau of Investigation, 2009). These arrests are a very small proportion of the number of people who drink and drive. Quinlan and colleagues (2005) found that 159 million Americans self-reported drinking and driving.

In addition to motor vehicle accidents, a person under the influence of alcohol is also prone to falling, drowning, and getting involved in accidents with cycling, boating, driving all-terrain vehicles, and operating machineries. These accidents can cause injuries and even deaths. In the short term alcohol can also cause toxicity due to overdose. Many people in the United States die from accidental alcohol poisoning. In developing countries people also die due to illicit liquor that is not properly made.

The long-term or chronic effects of alcohol are also profound. Alcohol use affects almost all organs of the body either directly or indirectly. Alcohol and its metabolite acetaldehyde are irritants to most tissues in the body. In addition, alcohol provides empty calories and therefore is often responsible for chronic malnutrition.

The brain is damaged by alcohol. There is an overall loss of brain tissue in heavy drinkers. It has been found that ventricles or internal spaces are enlarged and fissures (sulci) are widened in the cerebral cortex (Hart et al., 2009). Wernicke's encephalopathy is a classic organic brain damage syndrome due to chronic alcohol use and deficiency of thiamine (vitamin B_1) and is characterized by confusion, ataxia (lack of coordination of muscle movements, especially while walking), nystagmus (involuntary eye movements), ophthalmoplegia (paralysis or weakness of one or more of the muscles that control eye movement), and peripheral neuropathy (pain in nerves, loss of sensation, and an inability to control muscles) (Messing & Greenberg, 1995). Most patients with Wernicke's encephalopathy also have Korsakoff's psychosis, which is characterized by anterograde and retrograde amnesia or inability to remember recent events or to learn new information (Eisendrath & Lichtmacher, 2000). Because these two disorders often occur together they are called as Wernicke-Korsakoff syndrome.

The liver is also damaged by alcohol use (Reuben, 2008). Fatty acids and alcohol compete as the fuel for liver, and alcohol gets a higher priority. As a result fatty acids accumulate in the liver causing a condition called alcohol-related fatty liver, which is a reversible condition. Chronic inflammation of the liver tissue often leads to alcoholic hepatitis, a severe liver disease with a high mortality rate, even though it is also reversible. The clinical features of alcoholic hepatitis may range from an enlarged liver while asymptomatic to a severely ill person who dies quickly. Liver failure, gastrointestinal bleeding, and infection are the three main causes of death in patients with alcoholic hepatitis (Yu, Xu, Ye, Li, & Li, 2010). Alcoholic hepatitis leads to a condition of the liver called *cirrhosis*. The frequency of cirrhosis is around 8% to 15% among people who consume over 50 g of alcohol (4 oz of 100 proof whiskey, 15 oz of wine, or four 12 oz cans of beer) daily for over 10 years (Friedman, 2000). In cirrhosis liver cells are replaced with collagen, a fibrous tissue, that reduces blood flow, decreases functional cells, and leads to decreased ability of the liver to function. Cirrhosis is an irreversible disease with an age-adjusted death rate of 9.2 per 100,000 per year (Friedman, 2000). Cirrhosis may remain asymptomatic for years. Common initial symptoms are weakness, fatigability, disturbed sleep, muscle cramps, and weight loss. Later, anorexia develops with abdominal pain with ascites or fluid in the abdomen. In most cases the liver is enlarged. Complications from cirrhosis include bleeding from the upper gastrointestinal tract, liver failure, and greater chances of liver cancer.

Heavy alcohol use is related to increased mortality due to heart disease. This is often due to cardiomyopathy, or damage to the heart muscle, but heavy alcohol use also increases the chance of coronary heart disease. With regard to coronary heart disease, some observational studies found that individuals who consume alcohol within recommended limits may have a lower risk of coronary heart disease than do abstainers (Mukamal, 2010). Some prospective studies and international studies advocate that wine may be more protective against coronary heart disease than liquor or beer (Klatsky, 2010). However, there is conclusive evidence that heavy alcohol use is associated with definitive increase in incidence of coronary heart disease. If we define "heavy" drinking as three or more standard drinks per day, the alcohol–mortality relationship assumes a J-curve with risk being highest for heavy drinkers, lowest for light drinkers, and intermediate for abstainers (Klatsky, 2010). Increased risks from heavy drinking on coronary heart disease are due to its effect on (1) development of alcoholic cardiomyopathy, (2) development of systemic hypertension (high blood pressure), (3) contribution to heart rhythm disturbances, and (4) hemorrhagic stroke.

Chronic use of alcohol is also associated with increased risk for cancers of the mouth, tongue, pharynx, larynx, esophagus, breast, stomach, liver, lung, pancreas, prostate, colon, and rectum (Corrao, Bagnardi, Zambon, & La Vecchia, 2005; Gong et al., 2009; Raoul, 2008; Schuckit, 2009; Yi, Sull, Linton, Nam, & Ohrr, 2010). The possible mechanisms that cause cancers could be direct tissue damage caused by alcohol, nutritional deficiencies, or suppression of the immune system.

Alcohol use during pregnancy is especially harmful, producing a condition in the fetus called fetal alcohol syndrome. The manifestations of fetal alcohol syndrome include growth restriction, facial abnormalities, and serious CNS dysfunction (Crombleholme, 2000). Facial abnormalities include small head circumference, small eyes, retarded formation of the mid-facial area, flattened bridge and short length of the nose, and flattening of the vertical groove between the nose and the mouth, called the philtrum. CNS dysfunction includes abnormal neonatal behavior, mental retardation, attention deficit hyperactivity disorder, and other abnormal neurobehavioral developments. Toxicity is due to direct damage by alcohol and its metabolite acetaldehyde. The prevalence of fetal alcohol syndrome in the general population ranges from 0.2 per 1,000 births to 1.5 per 1,000 births (Floyd & Sidhu, 2004). Floyd and Sidhu (2004) also estimated that approximately one in eight pregnant women (approximately 500,000 per year) report alcohol use, of which approximately 80,000 reported binge drinking.

> *A*lcohol use during pregnancy is especially harmful. It produces a condition in the fetus called fetal alcohol syndrome.

Alcoholism

In simple terms alcoholism is the condition of physical dependence on alcohol to the extent that stopping alcohol use will bring on withdrawal symptoms. The following is the definition of alcohol dependence according to the DSM-IV-TR (APA, 2000, p. 213):

> A maladaptive pattern of alcohol use, leading to clinically significant impairment or distress, as manifested by three (or more) of the following seven criteria, occurring at any time in the same 12-month period:
>
> 1. Tolerance, as defined by either of the following:
>   a) A need for markedly increased amounts of alcohol to achieve intoxication or desired effect.
>   b) Markedly diminished effect with continued use of the same amount of alcohol.
> 2. Withdrawal, as defined by either of the following:
>   a) The characteristic withdrawal syndrome for alcohol (refer to DSM-IV for further details).
>   b) Alcohol is taken to relieve or avoid withdrawal symptoms.
> 3. Alcohol is often taken in larger amounts or over a longer period than was intended.
> 4. There is a persistent desire or there are unsuccessful efforts to cut down or control alcohol use.

5. A great deal of time is spent in activities necessary to obtain alcohol, use alcohol or recover from its effects.
6. Important social, occupational, or recreational activities are given up or reduced because of alcohol use.
7. Alcohol use is continued despite knowledge of having a persistent or recurrent physical or psychological problem that is likely to have been caused or exacerbated by the alcohol (e.g., continued drinking despite recognition that an ulcer was made worse by alcohol consumption).

Several screening instruments are available to help identify alcoholism. One such instrument is the CAGE questionnaire (Ewing, 1984). Another screening questionnaire is the Alcohol Use Disorder Identification Test (AUDIT) (Piccinelli et al., 1997). This is a slightly longer instrument with 10 items. A cut-off score of 5 on this instrument is associated with a sensitivity of 0.84, a specificity of 0.90, and a positive predictive value of 0.60.

The withdrawal syndrome associated with alcohol is quite severe, even leading to death if left untreated. It usually progresses in four stages. Stage 1 is characterized by tremors, rapid heart beat (tachycardia), hypertension, profuse sweating, anorexia or loss of appetite, and insomnia or difficulty in sleeping. Stage 2 is characterized by development of hallucinations or perceptions in the absence of a stimulus. These may be auditory, visual, or tactile hallucinations or a combination of these and are usually hallucinations of snakes, bugs, and so on. Stage 3 is characterized by delusions or false beliefs, disorientation, delirium, and amnesia or loss of memory. Stage 4 is characterized by seizures. Stage 3 and 4 are often referred to as **delirium tremens**.

Alcoholism has medical, economic, and psychosocial negative effects. Some of the medical complications include chronic brain syndromes, cerebellar degeneration, cardiomyopathy, and peripheral neuropathies.

Treatment of alcoholism encompasses the psychological, social, medical, and behavioral. Psychologically, the patient and his or her family must overcome denial and come to the stage of acceptance. Socially, involvement with groups such as Alcoholics Anonymous and other forms of social support are helpful. Medically, sometimes hospitalization may be necessary. Disulfiram is used as an aversive drug to discourage alcohol use. Naltrexone has also been used with good results. For withdrawal symptoms benzodiazepines are usually helpful. Finally, behaviorally, conditioning approaches are quite helpful.

Epidemiology of Alcohol Use

About 2 billion people all over the world consume alcoholic beverages, and 76.3 million have diagnosable alcohol-related disorders (World Health Organization [WHO], 2004). The global per capita consumption of alcohol in 2001 was 5.1 liters, of which beer accounts for 1.9 liters; wine, 1.3 liters; and spirits, 1.7 liters (WHO, 2004). Worldwide, alcohol was responsible for 1.8 million deaths (or 3.2% of total deaths) and 58.3 million (4% of total) disability-adjusted life years (WHO, 2008). Neuropsychiatric conditions account for close to 40% of the disability-adjusted life years. Unintentional injuries account for 32.0% of the total number of alcohol-attributable deaths; intentional injuries account for 13.7% (WHO, 2007a). Thus, injuries account for roughly half of all alcohol-related deaths. Between 10% and 18% of all emergency department visits are related to alcohol

(WHO, 2007a). On a global level, alcohol consumption has increased in recent decades, with a large majority of that increase occurring in developing countries. In terms of global gender distribution, men are more likely than women to drink, to consume a greater amount of alcohol, and to cause more problems associated with alcohol (Wilsnack, Wilsnack, & Obot, 2005).

Prevention and Control of Alcohol Abuse

Primary prevention strategies for combating alcohol abuse are based on policy and educational measures. The primary policy measure is reduction of the availability of alcohol (WHO, 2007b). This entails a wide range of governmental controls on the production, distribution, and sales of alcoholic beverages by either government monopolization of these activities or by issuing licenses that restrict the number of outlets for alcohol and their hours of operation. A related policy measure is restricting sales of alcohol. Moslem countries have a total ban on alcohol. Other countries ban sales to minors and have a minimum drinking age. The United States, for example, has a minimum drinking age of 21 years. Such measures are helpful in restricting the number of alcohol users. Another policy measure is increasing taxes on alcohol, thereby deterring its use by a large number of people. A further policy measure pertains to restricting alcohol advertisements, especially those that influence young people. This includes decreasing television and movie imagery supporting alcohol use and eliminating the promotion of sports and cultural events by alcohol companies.

Primary prevention strategies for combating alcohol abuse are based on policy and educational measures.

Another policy measure is the use of BAC laws regarding drinking and driving. Many countries, such as Hungary, Romania, and the Czech Republic, have instituted a zero-tolerance policy for drinking and driving (0.0 mg/ml BAC). The most liberal policy is found in some states in the United States that allow up to 1.0 mg/ml BAC as the permissible limit (International Center for Alcohol Policies, 2002). In Finland the BAC limit is 0.5 mg/ml, whereas in the United States it varies from 0.8 to 1.0 mg/ml (International Center for Alcohol Policies, 2002). Borkenstein (1976) found that alcohol was involved in 50% of highway deaths in the United States, whereas the comparable figure in Finland was only 27%. Similar comparisons can be made with other countries, and it is generally found that the more rigorous the BAC limits, the less deadly the consequences. Furthermore, it is well documented in scientific literature that even a minimal trace of blood alcohol can influence driving ability (Heifer, 1991).

Educational measures for primary prevention of alcohol start with school-based educational programs. Such programs should be delivered in middle and high school. Along with school-based educational programs, involvement of the mass media and educational community-based interventions are essential. All educational programs should be based on behavioral theories such as health belief model, social cognitive theory, theory of reasoned action, theory of planned behavior, or transtheoretical model. Another educational intervention is that of posting health warning signs on alcohol products. However, the WHO expert committee on problems related to alcohol consumption found that posting warning signs on alcohol products was not as effective as in the case of tobacco (WHO, 2007b).

Secondary prevention of alcohol abuse is done through early diagnosis and treatment. Along with the CAGE and AUDIT instruments mentioned above is the Michigan Alcoholism Screening Test (MAST), a 25-item questionnaire that takes approximately 25 minutes to complete (Storgaard, Nielsen, & Gluud, 1994). Two shortened versions of MAST are available: Short MAST (SMAST), with 13 items and a cut-off score of 3, and Brief MAST (b-MAST), with 10 items and a cut-off score of 6 (National Institute on Alcohol Abuse and Alcoholism, 1990). A geriatric version of MAST (MAST-G) is also available. All health care providers must regularly screen for alcohol use and possible hazardous alcohol drinking. Such screening should also be done at worksites. In addition to self-reports, laboratory markers such as gamma glutamyl transferase, mean corpuscular volume, aspartate aminotransferase, and carbohydrate-deficient transferring can be used; however, these lack desirable sensitivity and specificity. Research is ongoing for developing sensitive and specific laboratory-based markers, but none of these is yet available commercially (Dufour, 2010).

Pregnant women should be screened for alcohol use and warned of potential harms to the fetus. Interventions for alcohol-related problems should be available both in primary care settings and in specialized settings where more intensive treatment can be offered. Finally, tertiary prevention in the form of rehabilitation services for those recovering from severe alcohol dependence should be available. **Table 7.2** summarizes the measures for the prevention and control of alcohol abuse.

Examples of Public Health Interventions for Prevention and Control of Alcohol

The Australian Football League Central Australia's Responsible Alcohol Strategy, implemented in 2004, aimed at decreasing alcohol consumption at football matches and promoting healthy lifestyle messages to the youth of Central Australia participating in football (Mentha & Wakerman, 2009). An evaluation using a pretest–posttest design carried out from 2005 to 2007 found that volume of alcohol sold at matches decreased. It also found that alcohol-related violence decreased. The unintended consequences were decreased numbers of spectators attending matches, decreased sales in the canteen, and decreased sponsorship, which raised issues about sustenance of the intervention.

In the Netherlands, a community intervention for prevention and control of alcohol was carried out to try to reduce excessive drinking in young men on holiday in seaside camping resorts (van de Luitgaarden, Knibbe, & Wiers, 2010). The intervention was based on self-regulation. Data for evaluation were collected by self-reported questionnaires, interviews, observations by trained peers, and nuisance questionnaires completed by city residents.

The Pragmatics Project was implemented by undergraduate students at a large midwestern university (Buettner, Andrews, & Glassman, 2009). The approach was based on the student engagement model and was aimed at developing and implementing alcohol-prevention strategies such as reducing harm associated with high-risk drinking and off-campus parties. The intervention has replication potential to other courses in university settings.

The *Project Integrate* (Mello et al., 2009) used screening followed by brief intervention for prevention and control of alcohol abuse in the emergency department. Physicians

TABLE 7.2   Measures for Prevention and Control of Alcohol Abuse

Level of Prevention	Approach	Measure
Primary	Policy	Reduction of availability of alcohol
		• Governmental control
		• Licensing
		Restricting sales of alcohol
		• Total ban
		• Restricting sales to minors
		Increasing taxes on alcohol
		Restricting alcohol advertisements
		• Decreasing television and movie imagery supporting alcohol use
		• Eliminating promotion of sports and cultural events by alcohol companies
		Zero tolerance and maximum BAC laws
	Educational	School-based educational programs
		Mass media
		Community-based educational programs
		Posting health warning signs on alcohol products
Secondary	Early diagnosis and treatment	Screening
		Primary care interventions
		Intensive interventions in specialized settings
Tertiary	Rehabilitation	Rehabilitation centers

were involved in the screening, and a research assistant implemented the brief intervention. The challenge to acceptance of this model is the busy environment of the emergency department, but the model can be successful if other staff members such as research assistants are employed.

A comprehensive campus–community partnership intervention was introduced to reduce alcohol-related problems in a college population in Washington (Saltz, Welker, Paschall, Feeney, & Fabiano, 2009). The project's aim was to decrease disruptive off-campus parties by integrating students in the neighborhoods in which they lived, thereby increasing their accountability to these neighborhoods. The intervention also included increasing "party emphasis patrols" and collaborating with the city to develop a regulatory mechanism to reduce repeat problematic party calls to the same address. A website was also created to increase the knowledge and skills of students about living safely and legally in the community. Service learning projects were also implemented in the community. The evaluation entailed comparing it with another university that did not have such an intervention. The results showed that the prevalence of heavy episodic drinking was significantly lower at the experimental university. The intervention has potential for replication.

The Communities Mobilizing for Change on Alcohol (CMCA) is a community organizing program aimed at reducing teen (13–20 years) access to alcohol by changing community policies and practices (Wagenaar et al., 2000; Wagenaar, Murray, & Toomey, 2000). The goals of the CMCA were to limit access of youth to alcohol and to deliver the message to the community that underage drinking is inappropriate and unacceptable. The program had an important component of involving community members in seeking and achieving changes in local public policies and practices that affect underage youth's access to alcohol. The evaluation entailed a randomized 15-community trial. Data were collected at baseline and after 2.5 years of intervention. Data included surveys of youth, surveys of merchants, and direct testing of the tendency of alcohol outlets to sell to youth. Results demonstrated that the CMCA intervention favorably and significantly affected the behavior of 18- to 20-year-olds. It also favorably and significantly affected the practices of on-sale alcohol outlets. Alcohol merchants also increased age-identification checking and reduced tendency to sell to minors. But the intervention had little effect on younger adolescents. The Substance Abuse and Mental Health Services Administration identified this program in their National Registry of Evidence-Based Programs (http://nrepp.samhsa.gov).

FOCUS FEATURE 7.1 ALCOHOLICS ANONYMOUS

Alcoholics Anonymous (AA) is a worldwide organization and social support group for people with a desire to quit alcohol. The primary purpose of the organization is to help its members stay sober and to help other alcoholics achieve sobriety (Alcoholics Anonymous, 2010). It is not affiliated with or allied with any religion, sect, denomination, political viewpoint, organization, or institution. It does not support or oppose any cause. It does not have any membership dues or charge any money for its services. It is supported primarily by voluntary contributions of its members.

The origins of AA can be traced back the Oxford Group, a religious movement emphasizing self-improvement from the early 20th century in the United States and Europe. In the early 1930s in Vermont Rowland H. and Edwin T. joined the Oxford Group and were able to achieve sobriety by adhering to its principles. They were joined by Bill W. in the same experience. Bill went to Akron, Ohio and helped Dr. Bob quit alcohol. The date of Dr. Bob's last drink, June 10, 1935, is celebrated as the founding date of AA. They along with others formed the Alcoholic Foundation in 1938. Gradually, they came up with Twelve Steps and Twelve Traditions, which are the hallmarks of AA (Butler, 2010).

Twelve Steps

1. We admitted we were powerless over alcohol—that our lives had become unmanageable.
2. Came to believe that a Power greater than ourselves could restore us to sanity.
3. Made a decision to turn our will and our lives over to the care of God *as we understood* Him.
4. Made a searching and moral inventory of ourselves.
5. Admitted to God, to ourselves, and to another human being the exact nature of wrongs.
6. Were entirely ready to have God remove all these defects of character.
7. Humbly asked Him to remove our shortcomings.
8. Made a list of all persons we had harmed, and became willing to make amends to them all.
9. Made direct amends to such people wherever possible, except when to do so would injure them or others.
10. Continued to take personal inventory and when we were wrong promptly admitted it.
11. Sought through prayer and meditation to improve our conscious contact with God *as we understood Him*, prayer only for the power to carry that out.
12. Having had a spiritual awakening as a result of these steps, we tried to carry this message to alcoholics, and to practice these principles in all our affairs.

(continued)

Twelve Traditions

1. Our common welfare should come first; personal recovery depends on AA unity.
2. For our group purpose there is but one ultimate authority—a loving God as He may express Himself in our group conscience. Our leaders are but trusted servants; they do not govern.
3. The only requirement for AA membership is a desire to stop drinking.
4. Each group should be autonomous except in matters affecting other groups or AA as a whole.
5. Each group has but one primary purpose—to carry its message to the alcoholic who still suffers.
6. An AA group ought never endorse, finance or lend the AA name to any related facility or outside enterprise, lest problems of money, property and prestige divert us from our primary purpose.
7. Every AA group ought to be fully self-supporting, declining outside contributions.
8. Alcoholics Anonymous should remain forever non-professional, but our service centers may employ social workers.
9. AA, as such ought never be organized; but we may create service boards or committees directly responsible to those they serve.
10. Alcoholics Anonymous has no opinion on outside issues; hence the AA name ought never be drawn into public controversy.
11. Our public relations policy is based on attraction rather than promotion; we need always maintain personal anonymity at the level of press, radio and films.
12. Anonymity is the spiritual foundation of all our traditions, ever reminding us to place principle before personalities.

Several studies have been done to test the effectiveness of AA. Kaskutas (2009) performed a systematic review of these evaluations and noted that with regard to causal evidence of effectiveness of AA, five of six criteria are met. With regard to magnitude of effect, rates of abstinence in those who attend AA are about twice as high compared with those who do not. With regard to dose–response relationship, higher levels of attendance are related to higher rates of abstinence. With regard to the criterion of consistency, there is evidence for different samples and follow-up periods. Likewise, the criteria of temporality and plausibility are also substantiated. The only criterion that has mixed evidence is specificity. So, on the whole, AA can be considered an effective approach.

The Twelve Steps and Twelve Traditions are reprinted with permission of Alcoholics Anonymous World Services, Inc. ("AAWS") Permission to reprint the Twelve Steps and Twelve Traditions does not mean that AAWS has reviewed or approved the contents of this publication, or that AA necessarily agrees with the views expressed herein. AA is a program of recovery from alcoholism *only*—use of the Twelve Steps and Twelve Traditions in connection with programs and activities which are patterned after AA, but which address other problems, or in any other non-AA context, does not imply otherwise.

TOBACCO USE

Tobacco use entails smoking cigarettes, cigars, pipes, bidis or kreteks (clove cigarettes), or hookahs or using smokeless tobacco (snuff and chewing tobacco). Use of tobacco is associated with several chronic diseases. It has been implicated as a causative factor in coronary heart disease, peripheral vascular disease, cerebrovascular disease, lung cancer, oral cancer, laryngeal cancer, esophageal cancer, bladder cancer, renal cancer, pancreatic cancer, stomach cancer, cervical cancer, endometrial cancer, acute myeloid leukemia, chronic obstructive pulmonary disease, gastroesophageal reflux disease, and periodontitis (Doll, Peto, Boreham, & Sutherland, 2004; Giovino, 2007; Husten & Thorne, 2008). In addition, smoking by pregnant women has deleterious effects on the fetus. Smoking leads to low birth weight in infants. Infants born to women who smoke during pregnancy are on average 200 to 250 g lighter than infants born to nonsmokers (U.S. Department of Health and Human Services, 2001). Maternal smoking is also associated with preterm delivery and higher fetal, neonatal, and infant mortality.

Passive smoking, or exposure to secondhand smoke or environmental tobacco smoke, occurs when a person is in close proximity to a smoker and is associated with some of the same hazards associated with smoking. Passive smokers inhale mainstream smoke exhaled by smokers as well as sidestream smoke from the burning end of cigarettes (Kalucka, 2007). The smoke is very similar to the smoke inhaled by smokers and contains 4,000 chemicals, including 50 carcinogens. It is responsible for coronary heart disease (Law, Morris, & Wald, 1997) and lung cancer (Hackshaw, Law, & Wald, 1997).

Epidemiology of Tobacco Use

Tobacco companies manufacture about 5.5 trillion cigarettes a year, or about 1,000 cigarettes per person per year (Mackay & Eriksen, 2002). China consumes the most cigarettes (1,542 billion), followed by the United States (431 billion), Japan (328 billion), Russia (258 billion), and Indonesia (215 billion). Over 15 billion cigarettes are smoked every day worldwide.

Approximately 1 billion men and 250 million women in the world smoke (Mackay & Eriksen, 2002). Approximately 35% of men and 22% of women in developed countries and 50% of men and 9% of women in developing countries are smokers. The largest number of smokers is in China, where 300 million men smoke. With regard to smoking in men, trends in both developed and developing countries show that rates have peaked and there is a slow decline; however, smoking is nowhere near elimination. With regard to smoking in women, declining trends are seen in some developed countries, such as Australia, Canada, the United Kingdom, and the United States, but in several European countries these rates are increasing; in developing countries these rates have been stable (Mackay & Eriksen, 2002). The tobacco industry has especially marketed cigarettes to women in recent years as well as youth. Most smokers who begin smoking do so in their youth. If a person does not begin smoking by the end of his or her teens, the likelihood of that person starting smoking is very low. The highest rate of smoking in youth is found in central and eastern Europe, sections of India, and some of the western Pacific islands (Mackay & Eriksen, 2002). In addition to marketing by the tobacco industry, some factors influencing tobacco use among youth are accessibility to tobacco products at low price, peer pressure, lower self-image, the perception that tobacco use is "cool," and parental smoking. Because of the growing number of new smokers, the absolute number of smokers is likely to increase over the next couple decades even if the number of current smokers declines.

> *Approximately 1 billion men and 250 million women in the world smoke. It is estimated that 0.1 billion people died from tobacco use in the 20th century, and it is estimated that 1 billion people will die in the 21st century.*
>
> —Mackay & Eriksen (2002)

An estimated 0.1 billion people died from tobacco use in the 20th century, and it is estimated that 1 billion people will die in the 21st century (Mackay & Eriksen, 2002). There are more deaths attributed to tobacco than to HIV/AIDS, drugs, road accidents, murder, and suicide combined.

Prevention and Control of Tobacco Use

School-based education is an essential component of primary prevention, or preventing smoking initiation. Such programs should build refusal skills in youth and must be theory based. These programs should be targeted to grades 6 through 8, the time at which children are experimenting with smoking behavior. School-based educational programs should be combined with other strategies, such as legislation that bans advertisements that promote tobacco smoking. Comprehensive bans on all forms of tobacco promotion are an effective means to reduce tobacco use. This includes decreasing television and movie imagery supporting tobacco use, prohibiting the distribution of free tobacco products, and eliminating the promotion of sports and cultural events by tobacco companies (Novotny & Giovino, 1998). Cigarette packaging is also a tool for marketing, and many countries are advocating packaging cigarettes in plain packets (Mackay & Eriksen, 2002). Likewise, the marketing of cigarettes as "light" or "mild" is objectionable because it conveys a false impression that the cigarettes so labeled are less harmful.

A measure implemented by most countries around the world is to print health warnings on cigarette packs. Many countries still do not carry such health warnings, however, and in many countries the warnings are inconspicuous or not in the local language. Canada has some quite vivid warnings, which can be emulated by other countries. Legislation that restricts the sale of tobacco products to minors is also helpful in preventing the initiation of tobacco use. Countries such as the United States have implemented such laws. Increasing the price of tobacco products is also helpful in reducing tobacco use by youth (National Cancer Institute, 1993).

An example of a measure to reduce environmental tobacco smoke is legislation to ban smoking in public places. Banning smoking in workplaces is an effective means to reduce exposure to passive smoking as well as to reduce smoking by smokers, who consume fewer cigarettes per day. All major airlines are smoke free, and there are laws in most countries to make public buildings, hospitals, and other institutions smoke free.

Smokers should be detected early by routine questioning at the health care provider's office and should be directed to smoking cessation programs. Smoking cessation approaches include nicotine replacement therapy, bupropion therapy, social support, relaxation training, and problem-solving skills training. **Table 7.3** summarizes various prevention and control approaches to tobacco use.

DRUG MISUSE, ABUSE, AND DEPENDENCE

One definition for "drug" given in *Merriam Webster's Online Dictionary* is "a substance other than food intended to affect the structure or function of the body," and this is a generally acceptable definition in medicine and public health. Drugs are prescribed for diagnostic, therapeutic, preventive purposes, and those uses are all legal and legitimate. Sometimes drugs are misused or abused, or illegal drugs are used. It is these applications of drugs that we address in this chapter. The term **drug misuse** refers to using a drug for a purpose other than the one prescribed by a licensed health care provider or using amounts of a drug in greater quantity than normally used. For example, a person may

TABLE 7.3   Prevention and Control Measures for Tobacco Use

Type	Examples
Prevention	School-based education
	Legislations that ban advertisements that promote tobacco smoking
	• Decreasing television and movie imagery
	• Prohibiting free distribution of tobacco products
	• Eliminating promotion of sports and cultural events by tobacco companies
	• Plain packaging
	Cigarette packs to carry vivid health warnings
	Legislations that restrict sales of tobacco products to minors
	Increasing the price of tobacco products
	Ban smoking in public places
Smoking cessation	Nicotine replacement therapy
	Bupropion therapy
	Social support
	Relaxation training
	Problem-solving skills training

read in the newspaper that aspirin prevents heart attacks and begin taking two pills in the morning, two in the afternoon, and two in the evening; this is drug misuse. **Drug abuse** or **substance abuse** is the use of a substance in a way, quantity, or circumstances to cause problems or increase the propensity of occurrence of problems. These problems can be medical (such as dependence), social (such as broken family), legal (such as getting involved in crimes), occupational (such as missing work), psychological (such as craving), and physical (such as withdrawal symptoms). The DSM-IV-TR uses the following criteria for substance abuse (APA, 2000):

A. A maladaptive pattern of substance use leading to clinically significant impairment or distress, as manifested by one (or more) of the following occurring within a 12-month period:

1. Recurrent substance use resulting in failure to fulfill major role obligations at work, school, or home.
2. Recurrent substance use in situations in which it is physically hazardous.
3. Recurrent substance related legal problems.
4. Continued substance use despite having persistent or recurrent social or interpersonal problems caused or exacerbated by the effects of the substance.

B. The symptoms have never met the criteria for substance dependence for this class of substance.

Drug dependence or **substance dependence** is getting habituated to use of a drug to the extent that it is required in higher and higher doses and stopping it causes physical and psychological symptoms that require it to be used again and again. The DSM-IV-TR uses the following criteria for substance dependence (APA, 2000, p. 213):

A maladaptive pattern of substance use, leading to clinically significant impairment or distress, as manifested by three (or more) of the following, occurring at any time in the same 12-month period:

1. Tolerance as defined by either of the following:
   a. A need for markedly increased amounts of the substance to achieve intoxication or desired effect
   b. Markedly diminished effect with continued use of the same amount of the substance
2. Withdrawal, as manifested by either of the following:
   a. The characteristic withdrawal syndrome for the substance
   b. The same (or a closely related) substance is taken to relieve or avoid withdrawal symptoms
3. The substance is often taken in larger amounts or over a longer period than was intended.
4. There is persistent desire or unsuccessful efforts to cut down or control substance use.
5. A great deal of time is spent in activities necessary to obtain the substance.
6. Important social, occupational, or recreational activities are given up or reduced because of substance use.
7. The substance use is continued despite knowledge of having a persistent or recurrent physical or psychological problem that is likely to have been caused or exacerbated by the substance.
   • With physiological dependence: evidence of tolerance or withdrawal (i.e., either item 1 or 2 is present)
   • Without physiological dependence: no evidence of tolerance or withdrawal (i.e., neither item 1 nor 2 is present)

Commonly Abused Psychoactive Drugs

Stimulants are commonly abused psychoactive drugs that accelerate the CNS. Examples of stimulants include cocaine and amphetamines. **Cocaine** is a drug derived from the leaves of coca shrubs that stimulates the CNS by producing a feeling of euphoria. It has a long history of use in South American countries. In its earlier days the popular drink coca cola also contained cocaine, and cocaine was also used as a local anesthetic. In the United States cocaine abuse began in 1970s, and today it is the second most abused drug. There are about 1.7 million users or 0.7% of the population abuses cocaine (Office of National Drug Control Policy, 2003).

It is ingested (chewing of leaves), smoked (coca leaves + organic solvent), inhaled (free basing – heating with ether), snorted, and even taken intravenously. It blocks the reuptake of dopamine and serotonin, thereby prolonging their actions. It has a half-life of approximately 1 hour, but its metabolites have half-lives of up to 8 hours. The acute effects of cocaine are stimulation of the CNS, respiratory or cardiac arrest, and ventricular fibrillation. The chronic effects of cocaine include nasal inflammation, irritability, restlessness, paranoia, and auditory hallucinations.

Cocaine produces powerful psychological dependence. Quitting cocaine after regular use can produce abstinence syndrome in which initially the person is depressed. This phase lasts for days. The second phase is characterized by anxiety, boredom, amotivation (not taking any initiative), and anhedonia (the inability to gain pleasure from normally pleasurable experiences) and lasts for weeks. The third phase can be indefinite and entails craving with cues. Overdose can be lethal. The treatment of toxicity is done symptomatically in which propranolol is given for treatment of fibrillation and high blood pressure, haloperidol is given for psychotic symptoms, and diazepam is given for treatment of seizures. Antidepressants are used for abstinence syndrome. There is a role for post detox urine screening, exercise, contingency contracting, group therapy, and support groups.

> *C*ocaine is the second most abused drug in America, with about 1.7 million users, or 0.7% of the population, abusing cocaine.
>
> —Office of National Drug Control Policy (2003)

Amphetamines are synthetically prepared stimulants of the CNS. Common street names are "speed," "crank," "crystal," "meth," and "ice." Examples of these drugs are dextroamphetamine (Dexedrine), *d*-1-amphetamine (Benzedrine), and methamphetamine (Methedrine). The first amphetamine was patented in 1932 and used for narcolepsy treatment. Amphetamines are usually ingested or smoked. They stimulate production of norepinephrine, which makes the person alert and overcomes fatigue, and also produce euphoria. These drugs have beneficial effects in treatment of attention deficit hyperactivity disorder. Prolonged use of amphetamines is related to negative behaviors such as violence and paranoia. It also causes emotional distress and depression.

The second category of abused psychoactive drugs is **depressants**. Depressants are drugs that decelerate the CNS. Examples include barbiturates and benzodiazepines. There are three types of depressants: (1) sedatives, which reduce anxiety; (2) tranquilizers, which calm the system; and (3) hypnotics, which induce sleep. The earliest depressants were called nonbarbiturates and examples include chloral hydrate, paraldehyde, and bromide. These have several serious side effects and are not used any more. Barbiturates are commonly used today, and these are used for daytime sedation or to induce sleep and thus have high abuse potential. Development of tolerance, physical and psychological dependence, and fatal overdose are key drawbacks with barbiturates. **Table 7.4** summarizes some common barbiturates by their onset of action and duration of action.

TABLE 7.4 Common Barbiturates

Barbiturate Type	Onset of Action	Duration of Action
Short acting e.g., pentobarbital (Nembutal) secobarbital (Seconal)	15 min	2–3 hr
Intermediate acting e.g., aprobarbital (Alurate) amobarbital (Amytal) butabarbital (Butisol)	30 min	5–6 hr
Long acting e.g., mephobarbital (Mebaral) phenobarbital (Luminal)	1 hr	6–10 hr

Benzodiazepines are often prescribed and abused depressants. These cause less drowsiness and have a greater safety margin. They are used for treating insomnia and anxiety and also have anticonvulsant properties. Another type of depressants are inhalants, such as gaseous anesthetics (e.g., nitrous oxide, chloroform, ether, etc.), nitrites (e.g., isoamyl nitrite, isopropyl nitrite, butyl nitrite etc.), volatile solvents (e.g., petroleum), and aerosols (e.g., butane, propane etc.).

Psychotherapeutic drugs, or drugs used to treat mental disorders, are a third category of abused psychoactive drugs (discussed in greater detail in Chapter 8). These include major tranquilizers or antipsychotic drugs used to treat schizophrenia and other forms of psychosis. Some of these antipsychotic drugs are summarized in **Table 7.5**.

Antidepressants are used to treat depression. The first antidepressants were monoamine oxidase inhibitors, such as phenelzine (Nardil) and tranylcypromine (Parnate), and tricyclic antidepressants, such as amitriptyline (Elavil) and imipramine (Tofranil), but these drugs are not commonly used today because they have a number of side effects. Selective serotonin reuptake inhibitors such as fluxetine (Prozac), sertraline (Zoloft), paroxetine (Paxil), and venlafaxine (Effexor) are commonly used today.

Lithium is another type of psychotherapeutic drug that is used to prevent manic attacks. If taken in larger amounts it can lead to muscle weakness, confusion, dysarthria (difficulty in speech), vertigo, and rigidity.

Opium and its derivatives, or **opioids** (such as morphine, codeine, heroin, etc.), are the fourth category of abused psychoactive. These are derived from the plant *Papaver somniferum*. Opium and its derivates can be used subcutaneously, intramuscularly, intravenously, orally, and intranasally. They release endorphins and encephalins, which produce euphoria. They are used for their analgesic properties but have high psychological and physical dependence.

The fifth category of abused psychoactive drugs is the **hallucinogens**, or drugs that produce hallucinations or alter perception. Examples include LSD (lysergic acid diethylamide), "magic mushrooms" or psilocybin, morning glory seeds, dimethyltryptamine, mescaline or peyote cactus (*Lopophora williamsii*) derivative, 2,5-dimethoxy-4-methylamphetamine (DOM) or STP (serenity, tranquility, and peace), ecstasy, PCP (phencyclidine), and anticholinergic hallucinogens.

The sixth category of psychoactive drugs that is abused is **marijuana**. Marijuana is derived from the plant *Cannabis sativa, C. indica,* or *C. ruderalis*. The active ingredient is

TABLE 7.5 Examples of Antipsychotic Drugs	
Category of Antipsychotic Drug	**Examples**
Phenothiazines	Chlorpromazine (Thorazine), fluphenazine (Permitil)
Thioxanthenes	Chlorprothixene (Taractan)
Butyrophenones	Haloperidol (Haldol)
Dihydroindolone	Molindone (Moban)
Dibenzoxipene	Loxapine (Loxitane)
Atypical	Ziprasidone (Geodon)

THC (tetrahydrocannabinol). Various products are available, such as charas (pure resin extracted from surface of leaves and stem), hashish (less pure: 5–15% THC), ganja or sinsemilla (dried pistillate of female flowers before pollination: 5–10% THC), bhang (powder from the entire plant: 1% THC), and hash oil (boiled in alcohol: 50% THC). Marijuana is the most commonly used drug, with about 12.1 million users, or 5.4% of the population abusing this drug (Office of National Drug Control Policy, 2003). The most common routes of administration are ingestion and inhalation by smoking. Its half-life is 19 hours, and it takes 2 to 3 weeks for all its metabolites to get out of the system. Some of the physiological effects of marijuana are increased heart rate (tachycardia), reddening of eyes, dry mouth, and bronchodilation. Subjectively, it gives feelings of high and euphoria. It also causes rapid mood swings and produces physical and psychological dependence. It can impair driving behavior and with chronic use causes brain damage.

> *Marijuana is the most commonly used drug, with about 12.1 million users, or 5.4% of the population, abusing this drug.*
>
> –Office of National Drug Control Policy (2003)

The final category of abused psychoactive drugs is performance-enhancing drugs, such as anabolic steroids, female hormones, growth hormones, hormone receptor blockers, beta-2 agonists (Clenbuterol), and creatine. These drugs are mostly abused by athletes to enhance their performance in sports.

Prevention and Control of Substance Abuse

Primary prevention strategies for combating abuse of drugs problem are based on policy and educational measures. The primary policy measure is to reduce the availability and accessibility to drugs that have a potential for abuse. Most nations around the world have policies and legislations that ban use of harmful drugs. **Table 7.6** summarizes federal trafficking penalties for selected drugs in the United States.

Enforcement of these laws is needed universally. Some countries have less severe punishments, where others have even stricter punishments for those who break the laws. There is a need to tighten the laws in countries where punishments are lax.

Another category of primary prevention strategies are those programs aimed at young people who have not yet tried the substances in question or who may have tried alcohol or tobacco, the gateway drugs, a few times. These programs are often school based or sometimes after-school community based. The Drug Abuse Resistance Education (D.A.R.E.) program is delivered by police officers to elementary school students. This program began in the United States but is now available in many other countries as well. The effectiveness of this intervention is questionable. A recent meta-analysis showed "the effects of the D.A.R.E. program on drug use did not vary across the studies with a less than small overall effect while the effects on psychosocial behavior varied with still a less than small overall effect" (Pan & Bai, 2009, p. 270).

Secondary prevention programs are interventions designed for people who have experienced drugs but are not necessarily in need of treatment. Examples of these interventions are college-based programs, such as the multiple-behavior intervention developed by Werch and colleagues (2008). In this intervention marijuana-use behaviors were significantly improved. Secondary prevention also entails screening interventions and

TABLE 7.6 Federal Trafficking Penalties for Selected Drugs in United States.				
Drug (Schedule)	**Quantity**	**Penalties**	**Quantity**	**Penalties**
Cocaine (Schedule II)	500–4,999 g mixture	*First offense:* Not less than 5 yr and not more than 40 yr. If death or serious injury, not less than 20 or more than life. Fine of not more than $2 million if an individual, $5 million if not an individual	5 kg or more mixture	*First offense:* Not less than 10 yr and not more than life. If death or serious injury, not less than 20 or more than life. Fine of not more than $4 million if an individual, $10 million if not an individual.
Cocaine base (Schedule II)	5–49 g mixture		50 g or more mixture	
Fentanyl (Schedule II)	40–399 g mixture		400 g or more mixture	
Fentanyl analogue (Schedule I)	10–99 g mixture		100 g or more mixture	
Heroin (Schedule I)	100–999 g mixture		1 kg or more mixture	
LSD (Schedule I)	1–9 g mixture	*Second offense:* Not less than 10 yr and not more than life. If death or serious injury, life imprisonment. Fine of not more than $4 million if an individual, $10 million if not an individual.	10 g or more mixture	*Second offense:* Not less than 20 yr and not more than life. If death or serious injury, life imprisonment. Fine of not more than $8 million if an individual, $20 million if not an individual.
Methamphetamine (Schedule II)	5–49 g pure or 50–499 g mixture		50 g or more pure or 500 g or more mixture	
PCP (Schedule II)	10–99 g pure or 100–999 g mixture		100 g or more pure or 1 kg or more mixture	*Two or more prior offenses:* Life imprisonment

Source: United States Drug Enforcement Administration (n.d.). Federal trafficking penalties. Available at: http://www.justice .gov/dea/agency/penalties.htm. Accessed August 4, 2011.

interventions aimed at early diagnosis and treatment. Substance abuse has grown in prevalence during pregnancy. Approximately 225,000 infants per year are exposed prenatally to illicit substances (Keegan, Parva, Finnegan, Gerson, & Belden, 2010). Interventions for screening, education, and treatment are extremely important for this subgroup.

Tertiary prevention programs are interventions directed toward prevention of relapse after treatment, such as mindfulness-based relapse prevention (Witkiewitz & Bowen, 2010). Mindfulness-based practices teach alternative responses to emotional distress and decrease the learned response of craving and help overcome depressive symptoms. The types of prevention interventions for substance abuse are summarized in **Table 7.7**.

Examples of Public Health Interventions for Prevention and Control of Drugs

The Family Check-Up intervention is a primary prevention intervention delivered in schools that serve at-risk children and families (Stormshak & Dishion, 2009). The intervention is grounded in developmental theory and addresses risk factors such as substance

TABLE 7.7   Types of Prevention Interventions for Substance Abuse

Type of Prevention	Focus	Examples
Primary	Reduction of the availability and accessibility to drugs	Federal trafficking penalties
	School-based or sometimes after-school community-based programs	Drug Abuse Resistance Education (D.A.R.E.) program
Secondary	College-based programs	Multiple-behavior intervention
	Screening interventions and interventions aimed at early diagnosis and treatment	Screening, education, and treatment of pregnant women
Tertiary	Prevention of relapse	Mindfulness-based relapse prevention intervention

use, deviant peer affiliations, family management deficits, and problematic behaviors at school. This intervention has been in existence for over 20 years.

Across Ages is a school- and community-based program for children ages 9 to 13 (LoSciuto, Rajala, Townsend, & Taylor, 1996). This intervention pairs an older mentor (usually over 55 years) with children, especially those who are transitioning into middle school. The components of the intervention include (1) at least 2 hours per week of mentoring by older adults; (2) approximately 1 to 2 hours per week of community service by children such as visits to nursing homes; (3) monthly social and recreational activities for children, their families, and mentors; and (4) classroom instruction of twenty-six 45-minute social competence training lessons. Using an experimental design the intervention has been found to be effective.

Families and Schools Together is a multifamily group intervention designed to reduce substance abuse and build relationships between families, schools, and communities around elementary school children (Kratochwill, McDonald, Levin, Bear-Tibbetts, & Demaray, 2004). There are three components of the intervention: (1) outreach to parents, (2) eight weekly multifamily group sessions, and (3) ongoing monthly group reunions for up to 24 months to assist parents as the primary prevention agents for their children. The intervention has been tested using experimental design and found to be effective.

Guiding Good Choices is a drug use prevention program (Kosterman, Hawkins, Spoth, Haggerty, & Zhu, 1997; Mason, Kosterman, Hawkins, Haggerty, & Spoth, 2003) based on the research that consistent and positive parental involvement is essential for prevention of drug abuse. The intervention entails five-sessions: (1) preventing substance abuse in the family, (2) setting clear family expectations regarding drugs and alcohol, (3) avoiding trouble, (4) managing family conflict, and (5) strengthening family bonds. Using experimental designs the intervention has been found to be effective in preventing drug use.

FOCUS FEATURE 7.2 SHOULD MARIJUANA BE LEGALIZED?

There are two sides to this question. Some people believe medical marijuana should be legalized, whereas others are against this legalization. Those who favor legalization have the following reasons for

(continued)

their viewpoint. Marijuana is effective in controlling nausea, vomiting, and inability to eat for patients on chemotherapy. Persons suffering from cancer are put on chemotherapy, and one of the side effects is very severe nausea, which can be reduced by use of marijuana. These people also believe prohibition of alcohol has failed and so the prohibition of marijuana is bound to fail. They also argue that people can get prescriptions for more harmful and addicting drugs such as oxycodone (Oxycontin) and hydrocodone (Lortab). These people argue that according to some estimates taxpayers pay between $7.5 and $10 billion annually toward arrest and prosecution of marijuana cases, most of which involve mere possession (Bradshaw, 2006). In some states such as Alaska, Arizona, California, Colorado, Hawaii, Maine, Montana, Nevada, Oregon, Washington, and Vermont marijuana use is allowed for medical purposes (Gostin, 2005). The law is designed to ensure that "seriously ill" patients have access to marijuana for medical purposes to relieve suffering. The act exempts physicians, patients, and primary caregivers from criminal prosecution for possessing or cultivating marijuana for medicinal purposes with a physician's approval.

People who are against its legalization are concerned because it produces apathy, depression, and other harmful side effects. There has been a link between use of marijuana and psychosis (Drewe, Drewe, & Riecher-Rössler, 2004). They are also concerned because it is a gateway drug that can lead to use of other even more harmful drugs. They believe the negative aspects of this drug far outweigh any positives it might have. The U.S. Supreme Court has ruled that federal law enforcement authorities can criminally prosecute patients for possessing marijuana (Gostin, 2005). Further, because marijuana is inhaled and ingested its dose cannot be regulated. Before legalization of marijuana there is a need to ascertain the dose of THC and its standardized delivery mechanisms (Das, 2005). The drug dronabinol (Marinol) has THC as its active ingredient and is available in capsule form. It has been approved by the U.S. Food and Drug Administration to be taken with cancer chemotherapy and for stimulating the appetite in AIDS patients.

SKILL-BUILDING ACTIVITY

Imagine you have been asked to work with a group of pregnant women who are smokers to help them quit smoking. How would you go about designing a program for these women? What behavioral theory or model would you apply? What would be the key topics you will include in your program? What would be the duration of your program? You can take the help of an existing program from the literature to help you in your task.

SUMMARY

Alcohol use commonly involves the drinking of beer, wine, or spirits. CNS depressant is the main effect of alcohol. Alcohol is toxic and harmful both in the short and long term. The short-term harms include effects due to drinking and driving, falling, drowning, and getting involved in accidents. The long-term effects of alcohol include Wernicke's encephalopathy, Korsakoff's psychosis, fatty liver, hepatitis, cirrhosis, cardiomyopathies, fetal alcohol syndrome, and increased risk for cancers of the mouth, tongue, pharynx, larynx, esophagus, breast, stomach, liver, lung, pancreas, prostate, colon, and rectum. Alcoholism (alcohol dependence) according to DSM-IV-TR is clinically significant impairment or distress in the presence of three or more of the following: (1) tolerance; (2) withdrawal; (3) a great deal of time spent obtaining alcohol, using alcohol, or recovering from its effects; (4) reducing or giving up important activities because of alcohol; (5) drinking more or longer than intended; (6) a persistent desire or unsuccessful efforts to cut down or control use of alcohol; and (7) continued use despite having a physical or psychological problem caused or exacerbated by alcohol. Primary prevention strategies for combating alcohol abuse are based on policy and educational measures. Secondary prevention of alcohol abuse is done through early diagnosis and treatment. Tertiary prevention involves rehabilitation services for those recovering from severe alcohol dependence.

Tobacco use is causally linked to coronary heart disease, peripheral vascular disease, cerebrovascular disease, lung cancer, oral cancer, laryngeal cancer, esophageal cancer, bladder cancer, renal cancer, pancreatic cancer, stomach cancer, cervical cancer, endometrial cancer, acute myeloid leukemia, chronic obstructive pulmonary disease, gastro esophageal reflux disease, and periodontitis. Strategies for prevention and control of tobacco include school-based education, legislations that ban advertisements to promote tobacco use, legislations that restrict sales of tobacco products to minors, cigarette packs to carry vivid health warnings, increasing the price of tobacco products, banning smoking in public places, and facilitating smoking cessation.

Drug misuse refers to using a drug for a purpose other than the one prescribed by a licensed health care provider or using amounts of a drug in greater quantity than normally used. Drug abuse or substance abuse is the use of a substance in a way, quantity, or circumstances to cause problems or increase the propensity of occurrence of problems. Drug dependence or substance dependence is getting habituated to use of a drug to the extent that it is required in higher and higher doses and stopping it causes physical and psychological symptoms that require it to be used again and again. Commonly abused psychoactive drugs are stimulants, depressants, psychotherapeutic drugs, opioids, hallucinogens, marijuana, and performance-enhancing drugs. Primary prevention strategies for combating the drugs problem are based on policy and educational measures. Secondary prevention entails interventions designed for people who have experienced drugs but are not necessarily in need of treatment, screening programs, and early diagnosis and treatment programs. Tertiary prevention programs are interventions directed toward prevention of relapse after treatment.

REVIEW QUESTIONS

1. Summarize the effects of alcohol on the human body.
2. Discuss how alcohol is toxic to humans.
3. Define alcoholism. Name any two measures for screening alcoholism.
4. Discuss strategies for prevention and control of alcohol abuse.
5. Describe strategies for prevention and control of tobacco use.
6. Differentiate between drug misuse, drug abuse, and drug dependence.
7. Describe some commonly abused psychoactive drugs.
8. Discuss strategies for prevention and control of substance abuse.

WEBSITES TO EXPLORE

Alcoholics Anonymous (AA)

http://www.aa.org/

This is the official website of Alcoholics Anonymous (AA). Alcoholics Anonymous is "a fellowship of men and women who share their experience, strength and hope with each other that they may solve their common problem and help others to recover from alcoholism." The website has links such as information about AA, for the media, is AA for you?, for groups and members, archives and history, and how to find AA meetings. *Review the information. Using the "how to find AA meetings" find an AA meeting close to your home. Visit one of their meetings and write your impressions.*

Drug Abuse Resistance Education (D.A.R.E.)

http://www.dare.com/home/default.asp

This is the official website of the Drug Abuse Resistance Education (D.A.R.E.) program that provides children with the skills to avoid involvement in drugs, gangs, and violence. It was started in 1983 and is currently being implemented by 75% of the school districts in United States and in 43 other countries. *Review the various links this website has such as about D.A.R.E., D.A.R.E. dance, drug information, D.A.R.E. USA, international and news and bulletins. Prepare a summary of D.A.R.E.'s international activities.*

International Society for the Prevention of Tobacco Induced Diseases (ISPTID)

http://isptid.globalink.org/index.html

This is the website of the not-for-profit, academic, scientific and humanitarian organization of health professionals and scientists called International Society for the Prevention of Tobacco Induced Diseases (ISPTID). The website has information about this organization, news items related to tobacco, and information on meetings and publications. *Visit the links to "Facts" and "News." What new information did you learn?*

Narcotics Anonymous (NA)

http://www.na.org/

Narcotics Anonymous is an international, community-based organization comprised of recovering drug addicts. It holds approximately 43,900 weekly meetings in over 127 countries worldwide. The website has several links such as information about NA, service to members, find a meeting, and others. *Go to the periodicals and publications link and review the various publications of the organization. Which ones did you like?*

National Registry of Evidence-Based Programs

http://nrepp.samhsa.gov

This is the website maintained by Substance Abuse and Mental Health Services Administration (SAMHSA) and includes descriptions of public health interventions in the area of alcohol, tobacco, and other drugs found to be effective. This website is a searchable online registry. The interventions listed on this website have been rated by independent reviewers. *Using this website locate alcohol prevention interventions in the ages 6–12 and 13–17. Review these interventions and make a list of successful interventions.*

World Health Organization: Alcohol

http://www.who.int/topics/alcohol_drinking/en/

This is the website of World Health Organization that presents information on alcohol. It has links to facts and figures, question and answers, draft global strategy to reduce harmful use of alcohol, alcohol epidemiology and monitoring, and other links. *Review the information on the website and pay special attention to the draft global strategy to reduce the harmful use of alcohol link. Write a paper on how alcohol policy is made at world level.*

REFERENCES AND FURTHER READINGS

Alcoholics Anonymous. (2010). Information on Alcoholic Anonymous. Retrieved from http://www.aa.org/lang/en/subpage.cfm?page=1.

American Psychiatric Association (APA). (2000). *Diagnostic and Statistical Manual of Mental Disorders* (4th ed., text revision). Washington, DC: Author.

Borkenstein, R. F. (1976). Efficacy of law enforcement procedures concerning alcohol, drugs, and driving. *Modern Problems in Pharmacopsychiatry, 11,* 1–10.

Bradshaw, P. (2006). Should medical marijuana be legalized nationwide? *RN, 69*(10), 21–22.

Buettner, C. K., Andrews, D. W., & Glassman, M. (2009). Development of a student engagement approach to alcohol prevention: The Pragmatics Project. *Journal of American College Health, 58*(1), 33–37.

Butler, S. (2010). *Benign anarchy. Alcoholics Anonymous in Ireland.* Dublin: Irish Academic Press.

Corrao, G., Bagnardi, V., Zambon, A., & La Vecchia, C. (2005). A meta-analysis of alcohol consumption and the risk of 15 diseases. *Preventive Medicine, 38*(5), 613–619.

Crombleholme, W. R. (2000). Obstetrics. In L. M. Tierney, Jr., S. J. McPhee, & M .A. Papadakis (Eds.). *Current medical diagnosis and treatment 2000* (39th ed., pp. 758–782). New York: Lange Medical Books/McGraw-Hill.

Das, R. (2005). Regulation of medical marijuana [letter to the editor]. *Journal of the American Medical Association, 294*(24), 3091.

Doll, R., Peto, R., Boreham, J., & Sutherland, I. (2004). Mortality in relation to smoking: 50 years' observations on male British doctors. *British Medical Journal, 328*(7455), 1519.

Drewe, M., Drewe, J., & Riecher-Rössler, A. (2004). Cannabis and risk of psychosis. *Swiss Medical Weekly, 134*(45–46), 659–663.

Dufour, M. C. (2010). Alcohol use. In P. L. Remington, R. C. Brownson, & M. V. Wegner (Eds.), *Chronic disease epidemiology and control* (pp. 229–268). Washington, DC: American Public Health Association.

Eisendrath, S. J., & Lichtmacher, J. E. (2000). Psychiatric disorders. In L. M. Tierney, Jr., S. J. McPhee, & M. A. Papadakis (Eds.). *Current medical diagnosis and treatment 2000* (39th ed., pp. 1019–1078). New York: Lange Medical Books/McGraw-Hill.

Ewing, J. A. (1984). Detecting alcoholism: The CAGE questionnaire. *Journal of the American Medical Association, 252,* 1905–1907.

Floyd, R. L., & Sidhu, J. S. (2004). Monitoring prenatal alcohol exposure. *American Journal of Medical Genetics Part C Seminars in Medical Genetics, 127C*(1), 3–9.

Frezza, M., di Padova, C., Pozzato, G., Terpin, M., Baraona, E., & Lieber, C. S. (1990). High blood alcohol levels in women. The role of decreased gastric alcohol dehydrogenase activity and first-pass metabolism. *New England Journal of Medicine, 322*(2), 95–99.

Friedman, L. S. (2000). Liver, biliary tract, and pancreas. In L. M. Tierney, Jr., S. J. McPhee, & M. A. Papadakis (Eds.), *Current medical diagnosis and treatment 2000* (39th ed., pp. 656–697). New York: Lange Medical Books/McGraw-Hill.

Giovino, G. A. (2007). The tobacco epidemic in the United States. *American Journal of Preventive Medicine, 33*(6 Suppl.), S318–S326.

Gong, Z., Kristal, A. R., Schenk, J. M., Tangen, C. M., Goodman, P. J., & Thompson, I. M. (2009). Alcohol consumption, finasteride, and prostate cancer risk: Results from the Prostate Cancer Prevention Trial. *Cancer, 115*(16), 3661–3669.

Gostin, L. O. (2005). Medical marijuana, American federalism, and the Supreme Court. *Journal of the American Medical Association, 294*(7), 842–844.

Hackshaw, A. K., Law, M. R., & Wald, N. J. (1997). The accumulated evidence on lung cancer and environmental tobacco smoke. *British Medical Journal, 315*, 980–988.

Hart, C. L., Ksir, C., & Ray, O. (2009). *Drugs, society, and human behavior* (13th ed.). Boston: McGraw-Hill.

Harwood, H. J. (2000). *Updating estimates of the economic costs of alcohol abuse in the United States: Estimates, update methods, and data.* Bethesda, MD: National Institute on Alcohol Abuse and Alcoholism.

Heifer, U. (1991). Blood alcohol concentration and effect, traffic medicine characteristics and legal traffic relevance of alcohol limit values in road traffic [In German]. *Butalkohol, 28*, 121–145.

Husten, C. G., & Thorne, S. L. (2008). Tobacco: Health effects and control. In R. B. Wallace, N. Kohatsu, & J. M. Last (Eds.), *Wallace/Maxcy-Rosenau-Last public health and preventive medicine* (15th ed., pp. 953–998). New York: McGraw-Hill Medical.

International Center for Alcohol Policies. (2002). *Blood alcohol concentration limits worldwide* (ICAP Report No. 11). Washington, DC: Author.

Kalucka, S. (2007). Consequences of passive smoking in home environment. *Przeglad Lekarski, 64*(10), 632–641.

Kaskutas, L. A. (2009). Alcoholics Anonymous effectiveness: Faith meets science. *Journal of Addictive Diseases, 28*(2), 145–157.

Keegan, J., Parva, M., Finnegan, M., Gerson, A., & Belden, M. (2010). Addiction in pregnancy. *Journal of Addictive Diseases, 29*(2), 175–191.

Klatsky, A. L. (2010). Alcohol and cardiovascular health. *Physiology and Behavior, 100*(1), 76–81.

Kosterman, R., Hawkins, J. D., Spoth, R., Haggerty, K. P., & Zhu, K. (1997). Effects of a preventive parent-training intervention on observed family interactions: Proximal outcomes from Preparing for the Drug Free Years. *Journal of Community Psychology, 25*(4), 337–352.

Kratochwill, T. R., McDonald, L., Levin, J. R., Bear-Tibbetts, H. Y., & Demaray, M. K. (2004). Families and Schools Together: An experimental analysis of a parent-mediated multi-family group program for American Indian children. *Journal of School Psychology, 42*, 359–383.

Law, M. R., Morris, J. K., & Wald, N. J. (1997). Environmental tobacco smoke exposure and ischaemic heart disease: An evaluation of the evidence. *British Medical Journal, 314*, 973–980.

LoSciuto, L., Rajala, A. K., Townsend, T. N., & Taylor, A. S. (1996). An outcome evaluation of Across Ages: An intergenerational mentoring approach to drug prevention. *Journal of Adolescent Research, 11*(1), 116–129.

Mackay, J., & Eriksen, M. (2002). *The tobacco atlas.* Geneva: World Health Organization.

Mason, W. A., Kosterman, R., Hawkins, J. D., Haggerty, K. P., & Spoth, R. L. (2003). Reducing adolescents' growth in substance use and delinquency: Randomized trial effects of a preventive parent training intervention. *Prevention Science, 4*(3), 203–212.

Mayfield, D., McLeod, G., & Hall, P. (1974). The CAGE questionnaire: Validation of a new alcoholism screening instrument. *American Journal of Psychiatry, 131*(10), 1121–1123.

Mello, M. J., Baird, J., Nirenberg, T. D., Smith, J. C., Woolard, R. H., & Dinwoodie, R. G. (2009). Project integrate: Translating screening and brief interventions for alcohol problems to a community hospital emergency department. *Substance Abuse, 30*(3), 223–229.

Mentha, R., & Wakerman, J. (2009). An evaluation of the Australian Football League Central Australian Responsible Alcohol Strategy 2005–07. *Health Promotion Journal of Australia, 20*(3), 208–213.

Messing, R. O., & Greenberg, D. A. (1995). Alcohol and the nervous system. In M. J. Aminoff (Ed.), *Neurology and general medicine* (2nd ed.). New York: Churchill Livingstone.

Mukamal, K. J. (2010). A 42-year-old man considering whether to drink alcohol for his health. *Journal of the American Medical Association, 303*(20), 2065–2073.

National Cancer Institute. (1993). *The impact of cigarette excise taxes on smoking among children and adults: Summary report of a National Cancer Institute expert panel.* Washington, DC: Author.

National Institute on Alcohol Abuse and Alcoholism. (1990). NIAAA issues report on screening for alcoholism. *American Family Physician, 42*(6), 1664, 1666.

National Highway Traffic Safety Administration. (2010). Traffic safety facts 2009: Alcohol-impaired driving. Retrieved from http://www-nrd.nhtsa.dot.gov/Pubs/811385.PDF.

Novotny, T. E., & Giovino, G. A. (1998). Tobacco use. In R. C. Brownson, P. L. Remington, & J. R. Davis (Eds.), *Chronic disease epidemiology and control* (2nd ed., pp. 117–148). Washington, DC: American Public Health Association.

Office of National Drug Control Policy. (2003). Drug data summary. March 2003. Retrieved from http://www.whitehousedrugpolicy.gov/publications/factsht/drugdata/index.html.

Pan, W., & Bai, H. (2009). A multivariate approach to a meta-analytic review of the effectiveness of the D.A.R.E. program. *International Journal of Environmental Research and Public Health, 6*(1), 267–277.

Piccinelli, M., Tessari, E., Bortolomasi, M., Piasere, O., Semenzin, M., Garzotto, N., & Tansella M. (1997). Efficacy of the alcohol use disorders identification test as a screening tool for hazardous alcohol intake and related disorders in primary care: A validity study. *British Medical Journal, 314*(7078), 420–424.

Quinlan, K. P., Brewer, R. D., Siegel, P., Sleet, D. A., Mokdad, A. H., Shults, R. A., & Flowers, N. (2005). Alcohol-impaired driving among U.S. adults, 1993–2002. *American Journal of Preventive Medicine, 28*(4), 346–350.

Raoul, J. L. (2008). Natural history of hepatocellular carcinoma and current treatment options. *Seminars in Nuclear Medicine, 38*(2), S13–S18.

Reuben, A. (2008). Alcohol and the liver. *Current Opinion in Gastroenterology, 24*(3), 328–338.

Saitz, R. (2005). Unhealthy alcohol use. *New England Journal of Medicine, 352*, 596–607.

Saltz, R. F., Welker, L. R., Paschall, M. J., Feeney, M. A., & Fabiano, P. M. (2009). Evaluating a comprehensive campus-community prevention intervention to reduce alcohol-related problems in a college population. *Journal of Studies on Alcohol and Drugs, 16*(Suppl.), 21–27.

Schuckit, M. A. (2009). Alcohol-use disorders. *Lancet, 373*(9662), 492–501.

Storgaard, H., Nielsen, S. D., & Gluud, C. (1994). The validity of the Michigan Alcoholism Screening Test (MAST). *Alcohol and Alcoholism, 29*(5), 493–502.

Stormshak, E. A., & Dishion, T. J. (2009). A school-based, family-centered intervention to prevent substance use: The family check-up. *American Journal of Drug and Alcohol Abuse, 35*(4), 227–232.

U.S. Department of Health and Human Services. (2001). *Women and smoking: A report of the surgeon general.* Rockville, MD: U.S. Public Health Service, Office of the Surgeon General.

U.S. Department of Justice, Federal Bureau of Investigation (2009). 2008 Crime in the United States: Uniform Crime Reports. Table 29. Retrieved from http://www.fbi.gov/ucr/cius2008/data/table_29.html.

U.S. Drug Enforcement Administration (n.d.) Federal trafficking penalties. Retrieved from http://www.justice.gov/dea/agency/penalties.htm.

van de Luitgaarden, J., Knibbe, R. A., & Wiers, R. W. (2010). Adolescents binge drinking when on holiday: An evaluation of a community intervention based on self-regulation. *Substance Use and Misuse, 45*(1–2), 190–203.

Wagenaar, A. C., Murray, D. M., Gehan, J. P., Wolfson, M., Forster, J. L., Toomey, T. L., . . . , Jones-Webb, R. (2000). Communities Mobilizing for Change on Alcohol: Outcomes from a randomized community trial. *Journal of Studies on Alcohol, 61*(1), 85–94.

Wagenaar, A. C., Murray, D. M., & Toomey, T. L. (2000). Communities Mobilizing for Change on Alcohol (CMCA): Effects of a randomized trial on arrests and traffic crashes. *Addiction, 95,* 209–217.

Werch, C. E., Moore, M. J., Bian, H., DiClemente, C. C., Ames, S. C., Weiler, R. M., . . . , Huang, I. C. (2008). Efficacy of a brief image-based multiple-behavior intervention for college students. *Annals of Behavioral Medicine, 36*(2), 149–157.

Wilsnack, R. W., Wilsnack, S. C., & Obot, I. S. (2005). Why study gender, alcohol and culture? In I. S. Obot & R. Room (Eds.), Alcohol, gender and drinking problems: Perspectives from low and middle income countries (pp. 1–24). Retrieved from http://www.who.int/substance_abuse/publications/alcohol_gender_drinking_problems.pdf.

Witkiewitz, K., & Bowen, S. (2010). Depression, craving, and substance use following a randomized trial of mindfulness-based relapse prevention. *Journal of Consulting and Clinical Psychology, 78*(3), 362–374.

World Health Organization (WHO). (2004). Global status report on alcohol 2004. Retrieved from http://www.who.int/substance_abuse/publications/global_status_report_2004_overview.pdf.

World Health Organization (WHO). (2007a). Alcohol and injury in emergency departments: Summary of the report from the WHO Collaborative Study on Alcohol and Injuries. Retrieved from http://www.who.int/substance_abuse/publications/alcohol_injury_summary.pdf.

World Health Organization (WHO). (2007b). WHO Expert Committee on Problems Related to Alcohol Consumption: Second report (WHO Technical Report Series 944). Retrieved from http://www.who.int/substance_abuse/expert_committee_alcohol_trs944.pdf.

World Health Organization (WHO). (2008). Alcohol drinking. Retrieved from http://www.who.int/topics/alcohol_drinking/en/.

Yi, S. W., Sull, J. W., Linton, J. A., Nam, C. M., & Ohrr, H. (2010). Alcohol consumption and digestive cancer mortality in Koreans: The Kangwha Cohort Study. *Journal of Epidemiology, 20*(3), 204–211.

Yu, C. H., Xu, C. F., Ye, H., Li, L., & Li, Y. M. (2010). Early mortality of alcoholic hepatitis: A review of data from placebo-controlled clinical trials. *World Journal of Gastroenterology, 16*(19), 2435–2439.

CHAPTER 8

Essentials of Psychopharmacology and Treatment of Mental Health Disorders

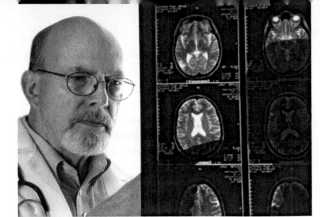

KEY CONCEPTS

- analysand
- analyst
- anterograde amnesia
- antianxiety agent
- antidepressant agent
- antipsychotic
- anxiolytic
- automatic thought
- behaviorism
- catastrophizing
- client-centered therapy
- cognitive behavioral therapy
- cognitive distortions
- cognitive triad
- couple and family therapy
- depot injection
- dialectical behavior therapy
- electroconvulsive therapy
- electroconvulsive treatment
- extinction
- eye movement desensitization and reprocessing
- family systems therapy
- family therapy
- Freudian psychology
- generic drug

- group psychotherapy
- hyperprolactinemia
- interpersonal deficits
- interpersonal psychotherapy
- interpersonal role disputes
- involuntary commitment
- magnification
- mind reading
- mindfulness
- minimization
- mood stabilizer
- neuroleptic
- operant conditioning
- overgeneralization
- partial hospitalization
- personalization
- phase I studies
- phase II studies
- phase III studies
- phase IV studies
- psychoanalysis
- psychoanalytic psychotherapy
- psychopharmacology
- punishment
- reinforcement
- retrograde amnesia

- Rogerian psychotherapy
- role transition
- split treatment
- systematic desensitization
- telepsychiatry

- therapeutic milieu
- transactional analysis
- transcranial magnetic stimulation
- transference

CHAPTER OBJECTIVES

After reading this chapter you should be able to
- Describe the different settings in which mental health services are delivered
- Discuss the basic classes of drugs available to treat mental illnesses
- Discuss the different phases of drug development
- Discuss the salient features of the different schools of psychotherapy

TREATMENT SETTINGS

Mental health services can be delivered via multiple different settings. These settings may range from very restrictive (inpatient) to least restrictive (care delivered in individual's home). Sometimes a combination approach may be required with home care combined with visits to a partial hospitalization program and so on.

Inpatient Treatment

A small fraction of individuals with psychiatric illnesses are treated in hospital settings because of the high cost of inpatient treatment. An individual is admitted when structure and safety of the individual or others around him or her cannot be ensured in the home or in community. Therefore, the most important goal of inpatient admission is to stabilize that individual's acute symptoms and bring him or her back to a level of functioning where treatment can be continued as an outpatient (Barry, 2002). For rapid resolution of symptoms psychotropic medications, psychotherapies, and group therapies may all be used.

Inpatient hospitalization of an individual with a psychiatric condition may be voluntary or involuntary. It becomes necessary when

- A rapid deterioration in mental status renders an individual a threat to him- or herself or to others
- The social environment/community of that individual cannot effectively support the emotional, physical, or psychological needs of that person

The average number of days of inpatient hospitalization has decreased continuously over the past several years due in part to legislation supporting community care of individuals with mental health needs and partly due to strict reimbursement mechanisms.

Therapeutic Milieu

The term *milieu* is derived from the French words *ma*, meaning "my," and *lieu*, meaning "place." A **therapeutic milieu** is a structured group setting in which the existence of the group is a key force in the outcome of treatment (Barry, 2002). Using the combined elements of positive peer pressure, trust, safety, and repetition the therapeutic milieu provides an idealized setting for group members to work through their psychological issues (Thomas, Shattell, & Martin, 2002). This term is typically used to refer to inpatient settings in which individuals learn healthy patterns of living through constant exposure to role models and strict expectations, but a therapeutic milieu can be developed with an outpatient group as well.

Community-Based Treatment Settings

Community-based treatments can be generally divided into outpatient treatment, partial hospitalizations, and home-based care. However, it is important to realize that the original Community Mental Health Act of 1963 defined a community mental health center as one that was accessible to the community and provided five basic services:

1. Inpatient treatment
2. Outpatient treatment
3. Partial hospitalizations
4. Emergency services
5. Consultation and education services to community agencies, groups, and individuals

Outpatient Treatment

A vast majority of individuals with mental health needs obtain treatment in public or privately funded clinic settings.

Partial Hospitalization

Partial hospitalization, also known as PHP (for partial hospitalization program), is a type of mental health program used to treat mental illness and substance abuse. In the setting of partial hospitalization the patient continues to reside at his or her home but commutes to a treatment center up to 7 days a week (Barry, 2002). PHPs are not used for individuals who are an acute threat to themselves or to others (such as acute suicidal depressed patients) because they are designed to focus on the overall treatment goals of the patient rather than on safety issues.

Two kinds of patients can best be managed in a PHP type setting:

1. Patients recently discharged from a psychiatric hospital but who require close supervision and ongoing support from a clinical team
2. Mentally ill individuals residing at home or the homeless who need such a setting to avoid inpatient hospitalization

Telepsychiatry

The use of electronic media has revolutionized ways in which individuals relate to each other and has had implications for all walks of human life. Its impact on health care has been profound. The phenomenon of remote communications with patients is a relatively recent development.

Telepsychiatry (a branch of telemedicine) is a specifically defined form of video conferencing that can provide psychiatric services to patients living in remote locations or otherwise underserved areas via the electronic transmission of images (American Psychiatric Association, 2010; Taintor, 2007). The first use of telepsychiatry dates back to 1957. Decreasing equipment and transmission costs and improvements in image quality have resulted in a wider adoption of telepsychiatry for particular populations.

Indications

Currently, telepsychiatry provides an assortment of services, such as diagnosis and assessment, medication management, and individual and group therapy. Consultative services between psychiatrists, primary care physicians, and other health care providers have also been facilitated by telepsychiatry. It has also been used in areas with shortage of mental health practitioners for providing second opinions (American Psychiatric Association, 2010).

Telepsychiatry holds promise as a means of getting patients into treatment who would not otherwise seek it. With a more widespread adoption of webcams, some patients have actually found telepsychiatry more convenient and less costly than traveling to a therapist's office (Taintor, 2007).

Future

Telepsychiatry has been shown to improve collaboration between health professionals. Research reveals that health care professionals believe telepsychiatry has given them a prospect to work more effectively as a team (Zaylor, Nelson, & Cook, 2001). Patient surveys indicate a higher level of satisfaction with regards to patient–physician communication and a belief that this is a reliable form of practice (Leonard, 2004). Overall, this new modality of care has helped to increase access to services and has helped to enhance the provision of services to families with homebound patients (Stamm, 1998).

However, there is an urgent need both for further research into the field and for randomized clinical trials of telemedicine applications. Until well-designed, randomized, controlled trials can evaluate the effectiveness of telepsychiatry, policy makers should be cautious about recommending increased use and investment in it.

There are a few barriers to providing telepsychiatry services. Reimbursement is still difficult to receive, especially through third-party payers, and licensure for practicing telepsychiatry may be difficult to obtain.

Involuntary Commitment

Involuntary commitment is the practice of admitting a person to a psychiatric hospital or ward against his or her will, in compliance with mental health laws of the country. Commitment is normally time-limited and requires reevaluation at fixed intervals.

In the United States involuntary commitment and the consequent deprivation of an individual's civil liberties is a serious matter indeed. Psychiatrists are in a unique position in that they have an ethical and legal responsibility to hospitalize patients against their will if they meet specific criteria. Even though individual states differ in their involuntary commitment procedures, the most important and virtually universal criteria include

- Dangerousness to self
- Dangerousness to others
- Serious impairment leading to an inability to care for oneself as a result of mental illness

A patient with severe mental illness cannot be committed to a psychiatric hospital if they are not at imminent risk of harm to themselves or to others. Family members, friends, police, or physicians can petition for the patient to be evaluated by a psychiatrist, at which point the psychiatrist determines the dangerousness of the patient's behavior.

If evaluated to be dangerous, the patient may then be hospitalized for a few days to a week, depending on the state's mental health laws. Within the designated time period the patient must present before a mental health court to determine whether he or she may be released or committed for longer treatment duration.

> *It is important to emphasize that mental illness is necessary but not sufficient for involuntary psychiatric hospitalization. Hearing voices (part of the diagnostic criteria for schizophrenia), for example, does not justify forced hospitalization.*

MEDICAL MEASURES INCLUDING DRUGS

Psychopharmacology

Psychopharmacology refers to the use of medications for the treatment of mental disorders. Plant extracts and naturally occurring substances have been used for centuries to influence mood and anxiety, to adjust sleep and arousal, to create euphoria, and to alter consciousness. Coffee, tea, and alcohol remain important examples.

The field of psychopharmacology underwent a rapid evolution during the second half of the 20th century, ushered in by discoveries of several medication classes. This led to the transformation of psychiatric treatment from a predominantly psychoanalytic to a biological orientation (Sussman, 2007a).

In the text below we discuss some of the major classes of psychiatric drugs, namely antipsychotic, antidepressant, antianxiety, and mood stabilizers. For further details on psychotropic medications, please refer to a textbook on psychopharmacology.

> *The first breakthrough in psychopharmacology occurred in the early 1950s with the discovery that chlorpromazine could cause dramatic control of psychotic symptoms. Chlorpromazine was released for clinical use in 1954 and was administered to more than 2 million patients within a short span of 8 months.*

Antipsychotic Drugs

An **antipsychotic** (or **neuroleptic**) is a psychotropic agent primarily used to treat psychosis. Some antipsychotic drugs have been around since the 1950s. These are called first-generation, conventional, or typical antipsychotics. The second-generation or atypical antipsychotics were developed much later, in the 1990s, with the sole exception of clozapine (discovered in the 1950s and introduced in 1970s). **Table 8.1** lists some of the common first- and second-generation antipsychotic medications (National Institute of Mental Health, 2010). The development of newer antipsychotic agents with fewer adverse

TABLE 8.1 Antipsychotic Medications	
	Drug
First-generation (conventional/typical) drugs	Chlorpromazine
	Haloperidol
	Perphenazine
	Fluphenazine
Second-generation (atypical) drugs	Risperidone
	Olanzapine
	Quetiapine
	Ziprasidone
	Aripiprazole
	Paliperidone

effects and greater relative effectiveness compared with existing agents is an area of active research (National Institute of Mental Health, 2010).

Usage   Antipsychotics are commonly used for schizophrenia, bipolar disorder, schizoaffective disorder, delusional disorder, substance-induced psychotic disorder, and psychotic disorders secondary to a medical condition. These medications can also be used for psychosis associated with a wide range of other diagnoses, such as psychotic depression. However, not all symptoms require heavy medication, and hallucinations and delusions should only be treated if they distress the patient or produce dangerous behaviors (Kammen, Hurford, & Marder, 2007; Marder, Hurford, & Kammen, 2007).

Antipsychotic medications are also used to treat nonpsychotic disorders. For instance, they are sometimes used off-label to manage some aspects of autism spectrum disorders. As an augmentation agent (an agent added to another to improve the effect of the latter) they have multiple off-label uses. Antipsychotic medications have been successfully used for the treatment of "treatment-resistant" depression (Kennedy & Lam, 2003) and obsessive-compulsive disorder (Fineberg, Gale, & Sivakumaran, 2006). This off-label use has expanded to increasing use as antidepressants, antianxiety drugs, mood stabilizers, cognitive enhancers, and antiaggressive, anti-impulsive, antisuicidal, and hypnotic (sleep) medications (Stafford, 2008).

Antipsychotics are occasionally used as a component of compulsory treatment via inpatient (hospital) commitment or outpatient commitment. This may involve various methods to persuade a person to take the medication, or actual force. Administration may rely on an injectable form of the drug rather than tablets. The injection may be of a long-lasting type known as a **depot injection**, usually applied at the top of the buttocks.

The prescription of neuroleptics involves six basic steps (Powers, 2008):

1. Initial assessment
2. Determination of potential medication side effects
3. Choice of an appropriate medication

4. Titration to the most favorable dose
5. Continuous monitoring of clinical efficacy and side effects
6. Assessment for dose reduction

Because of the chronic nature of the treated disorders and the fact that antipsychotic medications only control the symptoms and cannot cure the disease, once initiated these medications are seldom discontinued. The aim of the treatment is often to gradually reduce dosage to a minimum safe maintenance dose that is adequate to control the symptoms.

Side Effects   Antipsychotics are associated with a wide range of side effects. Many individuals discontinue their medications partly because of the adverse effects (Bellack, 2006). Extrapyramidal reactions include movement disorders, impotence, lethargy, seizures, intense dreams or nightmares, and **hyperprolactinemia** (abnormally high levels of prolactin, a hormone primarily associated with lactation, in the blood). Side effects from antipsychotics can be managed with a number of different drugs. For example, a class of medications called anticholinergics is often used to alleviate the motor side effects of antipsychotics (Healy, 2005). Some side effects only appear after the drug has been used for a long time.

Lowered life expectancy remains the most serious adverse effect associated with long-term antipsychotic use. This has sparked a controversy in regards to the usage of antipsychotics in dementia in older people, worsened by alleged use to control and sedate rather than the need to treat (Kammen et al., 2007; Marder et al., 2007). A 2009 systematic review of studies of schizophrenia also found decreased life expectancy associated with use of antipsychotics and argued that more studies were urgently needed (Weinmann, Read, & Aderhold, 2009). In "healthy" individuals without psychosis, doses of antipsychotics can produce the so-called negative symptoms (e.g., emotional and motivational difficulties) associated with schizophrenia (Healy, 2005).

Antipsychotics can alter the individual's perceptions of pleasurable sensations and lead to a severe reduction in the feelings of desire and motivation. This does not coincide with the apathy and lack of motivation experienced by the negative symptoms of schizophrenia. Detrimental effects on short-term memory have also been reported on high enough dosages. Because of these factors, these medications are believed to adversely affect creativity (Healy, 2005).

No discussion on antipsychotic medications can be complete without mentioning the two classes of medications that comprise the antipsychotic armamentarium. The debate centers on the benefits of using second-generation or atypical antipsychotics over first-generation drugs. **Table 8.2** explains some of the major differences between the two groups of medications (Kammen et al., 2007; Marder et al., 2007).

TABLE 8.2 Typical vs. Atypical Antipsychotics		
	Typical (Conventional or First Generation)	**Atypical (Second Generation)**
Efficacy	Comparable with that of second-generation compounds	Comparable with that of first-generation compounds
Side effects	Higher likelihood of side effects	Lower likelihood
Costs	Very low compared with second-generation compounds	Comparatively higher

Antidepressants

An **antidepressant** is a psychotropic agent used to treat mood disorders such as major depression and dysthymia. Antidepressants may also be used to treat anxiety disorders. The most important classes of antidepressants include the monoamine oxidase inhibitors, tricyclic antidepressants, tetracyclic antidepressants, selective serotonin reuptake inhibitors (SSRIs), and serotonin-norepinephrine reuptake inhibitors (SNRIs). The latter two categories, SSRIs and SNRIs, are currently the most favored of medications. These medications are among those most commonly prescribed by psychiatrists and other physicians, and their effectiveness and adverse effects are the subject of many studies and competing claims.

Most typical antidepressants have a delayed onset of action (2–6 weeks) and are usually administered from months to years. Depending on the chemical agent a slow titration both while initiating treatment, to avoid the development of side effects, and during discontinuation, to prevent the development of withdrawal symptoms, may be required.

Other classes of medications not classified as antidepressants, including antipsychotics in low doses (Wheeler-Vega, Mortimer, & Tyson, 2003) and benzodiazepines (Petty, Trivedi, Fulton, & Rush, 1995), may also be used to manage depression. The term *antidepressant* is sometimes loosely applied to any therapy (e.g., psychotherapy, electroconvulsive therapy, acupuncture) or process (e.g., sleep disruption, increased light levels, regular exercise) that can positively impact clinically depressed mood.

Prozac (fluoxetine) was the first SSRI to be approved for the treatment of depression in the United States in 1988.

Presently, the SSRIs are the most widely prescribed psychopharmacological agents for depression and anxiety. All the SSRIs (fluoxetine, sertraline, paroxetine, fluvoxamine, citalopram, and escitalopram) are equally effective. There may be significant differences in drug metabolism and factors such as time to action and so on (Sussman, 2007b).

One important social aspect of the introduction of SSRIs may have been some amelioration of the long entrenched stigma against depression and its treatment. Another important difference between SSRIs and older compounds was the markedly improved tolerability of these compounds. Side effects such as dry mouth, constipation, sedation, orthostatic hypotension, and tachycardia, all of which were commonly seen with the earlier antidepressant drugs (the tricyclics and monoamine oxidase inhibitors), were not seen with this group (Sussman, 2007b).

The extensive use of SSRIs is also due to approval by the U.S. Food and Drug Administration (FDA) for the following indications: major depression, obsessive-compulsive disorder, posttraumatic stress disorder, premenstrual dysphoric disorder, panic disorder, and social phobia (social anxiety disorder).

The SNRIs are a class of medications that block the neuronal uptake of both serotonin and norepinephrine, two chemicals used in neural transmission. The therapeutic effect of this class of drugs is attributable to this dual blockade. Hence, the SNRIs are also referred to as dual reuptake inhibitors (Thase, 2007).

Currently, three SNRIs are approved for use in the United States: venlafaxine (Effexor and Effexor XR), desvenlafaxine succinate (Pristiq), and duloxetine (Cymbalta). Venlafaxine is approved by the FDA for treatment of four therapeutic disorders: major depressive disorder, generalized anxiety disorder, social anxiety disorder, and panic disorder. Major depressive disorder is currently the only FDA-approved indication for desvenlafaxine (Thase, 2007).

Antianxiety Drugs

An **anxiolytic (antianxiety agent)** is a drug used for the treatment of anxiety and its attendant psychological and physical symptoms. Three classes of medications have gained prominence as anxiolytics: beta-receptor blockers, benzodiazepines, and certain antidepressants (both SSRIs and SNRIs discussed above).

Beta-receptor blockers, although not true anxiolytics, can help reduce the somatic symptoms of anxiety. These symptoms may include palpitations, shortness of breath, dizziness, and constriction of vision. Drugs such as propranolol have gained importance to counter some of the aspects of stage fright.

Benzodiazepines are a group of medications prescribed for short-term relief of severe and disabling anxiety. Benzodiazepines may also be indicated to cover the latent periods associated with the medications prescribed to treat an underlying anxiety disorder. They are used to treat a wide variety of conditions and symptoms and are usually a first choice when short-term central nervous system sedation is needed. Longer term uses include treatment for severe anxiety. There is a risk of a benzodiazepine withdrawal and rebound syndrome after continuous usage for longer than 2 weeks, and tolerance and dependence may occur in patients undergoing long-term treatment (Gelder, Mayou, & Geddes, 2005). Important benzodiazepines include alprazolam, clonazepam, diazepam, and lorazepam.

SSRIs and SNRIs are used more commonly as antidepressants, but their use has been extended to anxiety disorders. This class of drugs is classified mainly as antidepressants, and to be effective against anxiety disorders usually higher dosages are needed. Also, even though most SSRIs have anxiolytic properties, they are anxiogenic (anxiety provoking) when first introduced. For some individuals they may continue to be anxiety provoking. Hence, a low dose of a benzodiazepine is often used for several weeks when initiating SSRI/SNRI therapy to counteract the initial anxiety caused by the drugs until the therapeutic delay of the SSRI/SNRI is finished and the drug becomes effective.

Mood Stabilizers

A **mood stabilizer** is a psychotropic agent used to treat mood disorders characterized by sustained and extreme shifts in mood states, usually seen in bipolar disorders. Mood stabilizers prevent the swings between mania and depression. These drugs are also used in the treatment of borderline personality disorder and schizoaffective disorder (National Institute of Mental Health, 2010).

It is important to bear in mind that the term *mood stabilizer* refers to the final action of these drugs and encompasses some very different compounds with little or no structural similarity to each other. Common mood stabilizers are valproic acid, lamotrigine, carbamezipine, and lithium. Valproic acid, lamotrigine, and carbamezipine are sometimes referred to as "anticonvulsant mood stabilizers" mainly because these compounds also find utility in the treatment of seizure disorders. **Table 8.3** lists the mood stabilizers and their

TABLE 8.3 Mood Stabilizers	
Drug	**Common Side Effects**
Valproic acid	Drowsiness, diarrhea, constipation, unusual bruising or bleeding
Lamotrigine	Headaches, body aches, muscle pain, dizziness; rarely, a potentially fatal skin condition called Stevens-Johnson syndrome may develop
Carbamazepine	Drowsiness, headache, motor incoordination, stomach upset
Lithium	Restlessness, tremors, loss of appetite, stomach pain, hair loss, acne

common side effects. Some atypical antipsychotics (risperidone, olanzapine, quetiapine, and ziprasidone) have been found to have mood-stabilizing effects (Bowden, 2005) and are hence commonly prescribed even when psychotic symptoms are absent.

Drug Development and Approval

This section discusses, in brief, the major steps in the development and approval of a new drug. The development of a new pharmacological treatment of a psychiatric (or any other) disorder usually starts with animal investigations and lab testing of a compound in vitro. These preliminary investigations may be carried out before approaching the FDA. The few agents that are promising go forward in development.

Phases of Drug Development

Drug development to support a viable marketing application advances in somewhat overlapping phases. Nonclinical (also called preclinical) studies begin before human studies but continue throughout the clinical development period. Before each phase of human testing, animal testing is done to ensure the level of planned human exposure is safe. The usual temporal sequence proceeds from an initial classification of the drug to testing for efficacy and finally the exploration of potential side effects in the intended population of use.

Phase I   **Phase I studies** represent the initial introduction of the new drug in humans. The studies are closely monitored, conducted usually in healthy volunteers, and identify the properties of the drug and overt toxicities. These studies also establish tolerable doses for further testing. Phase I studies are conducted to obtain sufficient information about the drug to help design scientifically robust phase II studies. The total number of subjects generally ranges from 20 to 80.

Phase II   **Phase II studies** include carefully chosen patients with the disease or condition being studied. Phase II studies are closely monitored and optimized for the collection of efficacy data. Optimal doses of the drug and safety data regarding common short-term side effects are also obtained during this phase.

Phase III   After preliminary evidence suggesting effectiveness of the drug has been established in phase II trials, additional information about effectiveness and safety is needed to evaluate the overall risk-to-benefit relationship of the drug and to provide an adequate basis for product labeling. **Phase III studies** expand the information on the effectiveness and safety of the drug to assess the overall risk-to-benefit ratio. The study subjects are selected from a broader pool in comparison with phase II studies to help select a population that is more representative of the patients who will be exposed to the drug during marketing. Phase III studies may include from several hundred to several thousand subjects, including individuals with a broad range of typical comorbid conditions and concomitant medications seen in the target population.

Phase IV   **Phase IV studies** refer to the postmarketing activities conducted subsequent to the FDA approval of a drug. Active surveillance for rare adverse events and studies designed to look into approval for additional indications are two examples of phase IV studies.

Electroconvulsive Therapy

Even before the modern therapeutic era, convulsive therapies had been used at different times for the treatment of major psychiatric illnesses. Camphor was reportedly used as early as the 16th century, with several accounts of camphor convulsive therapies available from the late 1700s to the mid-1800s. Lucio Bini and Ugo Cerletti were interested in the use of electricity to induce seizures, and, after a series of animal experiments and observation of the use of electricity commercially, they safely pioneered the application of electric current across the heads of animals for that purpose (Prudic, 2007).

The first **electroconvulsive treatment** or **electroconvulsive therapy** (ECT) course was administered to a delusional and incoherent patient in 1938. The individual improved with the first treatment and remitted after 11. By the early 1940s electrical induction of convulsive therapy was made more reliable and shorter acting and virtually replaced chemically induced convulsive therapies. In 1940 the first use of ECT occurred in the United States.

Throughout the 1940s ECT enjoyed popularity as a first-line therapy. Efforts to improve the acceptability and safety profile of electrically induced convulsions continued in the following years. However, with the widespread use of pharmacological agents as first-line treatments for major psychiatric disorders, ECT is currently more commonly used for patients with resistance to those treatments. The only exception to this is life-threatening illness due to inanition, severe suicidal symptoms, or catatonia where ECT may be used as a first-line treatment.

ECT remains the most effective treatment for major depression and a rapidly effective treatment for life-threatening psychiatric conditions. Therefore, despite a decrease in the utilization of ECT since the middle of the 20th century it remains an active treatment for mental illnesses. Its use has shifted from public to private institutions, and it is estimated that approximately 100,000 patients have received ECT annually over the last few decades in the United States (Prudic, 2007).

Table 8.4 lists the common indications for the use of ECT.

Written informed consent is standard practice for ECT and involves a discussion of the risks and benefits of the treatment with the patient and/or legally sanctioned surrogate. Procedures for consent are locally regulated, particularly at the state level, and familiarity

TABLE 8.4	Indications for the Use of ECT
Criteria	**Indications**
Diagnostic	Major depression, both unipolar and bipolar
	Psychotic depression in particular
	Mania, including mixed episodes
	Schizophrenia with acute exacerbation
	Schizoaffective disorder
Clinical	Rapid response required on medical or psychiatric grounds or due to deterioration in patient's condition
	Risks of alternative treatments outweigh benefits
	Past history of poor response to psychotropics
	Past history of good response to ECT
	Patient preference
	Failure to respond to medications in the current episode
	Intolerance of pharmacotherapy in the current episode

with these regulations is essential. Consent can include both the anesthetic procedures and the electrical stimulation, although institutions may provide separate consents for each of these aspects of treatment. Consent forms generally cover several different areas and resemble the type of document used for comparable medical or surgical procedures. Descriptions of the procedure and expected benefits are detailed. Risks of the treatment, including possible medical and cognitive adverse effects, including death, should be documented.

Administration

Typically, ECT is given two to three times a week on nonconsecutive days. The latter frequency is common in the United States. Twice-weekly treatment is equally effective compared with thrice-weekly treatment, takes longer to reach efficacy, and is associated with fewer acute cognitive side effects. Daily treatment is rarely used. However, at one point daily treatment was believed to speed efficacy dramatically and was used in the most urgent situations, such as severe mania. The number of treatment sessions in a course of ECT should be individualized because patients vary in this requirement from a few sessions to more than 15, especially when changes in treatment technique have been made (Prudic, 2007).

ECT is the only treatment for major psychiatric syndromes that is discontinued when remission occurs. A significant number of patients relapse within the first few weeks of termination of ECT and may need further ECT. Often, additional ECT is given along with medications that are used for continuation and maintenance of remission.

Risks and Side Effects

Although ECT is generally safe, there are known risks and side effects. Some of the common side effects are confusion, memory loss, and physical side effects such as headache.

The confusion that occurs after an ECT treatment is usually immediate and may last from a few minutes to several hours. It is generally more noticeable in the elderly population. Memory loss secondary to ECT can manifest in different ways. **Retrograde amnesia**, or trouble remembering events that occurred before treatment began, may occur. Some people may complain of problems with memories of events that occur even after ECT has stopped, a phenomenon called **anterograde amnesia**. These memory problems usually improve within a couple of months (Prudic, 2007).

Coinciding with the ECT treatment, physical side effects such as nausea, vomiting, headache, jaw pain, muscle ache, or muscle spasms may occur. These are common and can easily be treated with medications. During ECT, heart rate and blood pressure increase and, in rare cases, lead to serious heart problems. In those with heart problems, ECT may be more risky.

PSYCHOTHERAPEUTIC APPROACHES

Behaviorism

Behaviorism is a philosophy of psychology based on the proposition that all actions taken by organisms can and should be regarded as behaviors (Skinner, 1984). It has also been called the learning perspective.

B. F. Skinner (1904–1990) remains undoubtedly the most influential behaviorist of our century. Skinner's basic concept was **operant conditioning**, in which behaviors are viewed as a function of the organism's history of reinforcement (Costa & McCrae, 2007).

Behaviorists, such as Skinner, refined and systematized the idea that animals could be taught tricks through rewards and punishments, using well-designed experiments to tease apart the effects of the amount and schedule of reinforcements, the use of reinforcers and punishers, and the difficulty of the discriminations required. Behaviors could be shaped, maintained, or eliminated by the judicious use of these principles.

A behavioral approach involves thinking about clinical symptoms as learned behaviors and developing treatment programs that help patients to learn new ways of behaving (and sometimes thinking) to reduce symptoms and improve quality of life. To develop an appropriate behavioral treatment plan, it is important to use behavioral assessment strategies to formulate a case conceptualization, which then guides the selection of specific treatment techniques. Behavior therapy does not always involve a simple matching of disorders and treatment techniques, although choosing appropriate approaches also occurs in the context of the scientific literature, that is, selecting treatment approaches from those that have been demonstrated to be effective in randomized clinical trials. Another key component of a behavioral approach involves identifying outcome measures that can be assessed over time to evaluate treatment efficacy and extent of change (Stanley & Beiderl, 2007).

Behavioral approaches have been used with many variations in techniques. However, all variations still share certain core principles (Skinner, 1984; Stanley & Beiderl, 2007):

- Maladaptive behaviors are acquired through learning, according to the same principles that govern the learning of adaptive behaviors.
- It is not essential to identify an underlying cause or motive for maladaptive behaviors.

- Learning principles can be used to modify maladaptive behavior.
- The focus of treatment is on factors that maintain current behavior rather than on historical issues.
- Therapists should be knowledgeable about scientific literature relevant to the patients they treat.
- It is important to set specific, measurable treatment goals and measure outcomes.

Exposure therapies are based on the premise that fears are acquired through associative learning (classical or operative conditioning). Interventions to eliminate fear use the same conditioning principles, and elimination of maladaptive fears requires exposure (contact) with the feared object, event, or situation. Exposure is a generic term used to depict a varied and complex set of procedures, all of which are capable of reducing or eliminating fear. **Table 8.5** explains some of the basic terminology associated with operant conditioning.

Systematic desensitization consists of two components: relaxation therapy and the presentation of fear-producing stimuli arranged within a hierarchy. The hierarchy consists of a series of situations (real or imagined) that represent successive approximations to the feared object, situation, or event. Conceptually, a hierarchy may be considered to be a ladder in which each rung brings one closer to the fearful stimulus. For example, the hierarchy for someone with an insect phobia might begin with holding a picture of an insect, then standing 6 feet from a covered, isolated bug, then progressively decreasing the distance, and so on. When constructing a fear hierarchy, it is advisable to adhere to three guidelines:

1. Items selected should be very similar to real-life experiences.
2. Items should be complete enough so the patient does not have to fill in the details.
3. Items should sample broadly from the domain of the situation in which the fear response might operate.

Cognitive Behavioral Approach

Cognitive behavioral therapy is a form of psychotherapy that attempts to treat problems concerning dysfunctional emotions, behaviors, and cognitions through a goal-oriented, systematic approach. A central tenet of the cognitive theory of emotional disorders is its stress on the **cognitive triad**, the psychological significance of people's beliefs about themselves, their personal world (including significant others), and their future. When people

TABLE 8.5 Definitions Associated with Operant Conditioning	
Term	**Definition**
Operant conditioning	Use of a behavior's antecedent and/or its consequence to influence the occurrence and form of behavior
Reinforcement	A consequence that causes a behavior to occur with greater frequency
Punishment	A consequence that causes a behavior to occur with less frequency
Extinction	Lack of any consequence following a behavior that leads to a decline in the frequency of that behavior

experience maladaptive subjective emotional distress the cognitive behavioral approach links it to their problematic, stereotypic, biased interpretations pertinent to this cognitive triad of self, world, and future. These biased interpretations are often called "**cognitive distortions**." For example, clinically depressed patients may believe themselves to be incompetent and powerless, view others as being disapproving and hypercritical, and see the future as miserable and unrewarding.

Although flawed and dysfunctional, the patient's viewpoints are perpetuated by cognitive processes that maintain them. For instance, depressed individuals may selectively focus on information suggesting that people do not care for them and ignore any evidence to the contrary. Because of such selective and biased information processing, depressed individuals often give up prematurely in trying to achieve important goals. This perpetuates the cycle of deepening pessimism, worsening mood, and further withdrawal from life goals (Newman & Beck, 2007).

Cognitive therapists teach their patients the skills of systematically identifying, examining, and modifying their maladaptive thinking styles (cognitive distortions). The ultimate goal is for the patient to develop a more objective and balanced view of his or her life situations, problems and potential solutions. Cognitive therapy is composed of a broad set of cognitive and behavioral techniques used strategically in the context of a comprehensive case conceptualization, facilitated by an understanding, accepting, and empathic therapeutic relationship (Newman & Beck, 2007). Cognitive therapists use homework assignments to reinforce these skills, so the patients learn and remember how to help themselves and thus maintain their therapeutic gains over the long term. Maintenance of clinical improvement and a comparatively huge research evidence base are the twin features that separate the cognitive behavioral approach from other contemporary psychotherapies.

Cognitive behavioral therapy practitioners teach their patients to view their excessively negative emotions and to ask themselves "what is going through my mind right now?" The goal is for patients to learn how to self-monitor their key automatic thoughts, perhaps leading to ascertaining deeper beliefs and schemas. An **automatic thought** (which can include both verbal ideas and images) occurs spontaneously and rapidly, representing an immediate interpretation of a situation. Most people are unaware that their automatic thoughts are associated with unpleasant feelings and behavioral problems. With some training and practice, however, patients increase their awareness of these thoughts and are able to pinpoint them with a high degree of regularity. It is possible to perceive a thought, focus on it, and evaluate it just as it is possible to identify and reflect on a sensation such as pain. Patients generally take for granted that their automatic thoughts are accurate and factual rather than view them as subjective representations of reality. In cognitive therapy patients learn to evaluate their automatic thoughts in a critical manner, with a nonjudgmental spirit. By changing their thoughts, patients can cope more effectively and devise ways to deal with the situation productively.

Depressed and anxious patients predictably interpret many situations in systematically biased ways despite the availability of more plausible interpretations. When asked to reflect on alternative explanations patients may realize their initial interpretations were based on doubtful premises. As patients learn to view their thoughts with greater objectivity, they begin to clarify and modify the meanings they have assigned to upsetting events.

Through a collaborative process the therapist helps to make gradual shifts in the patient's thinking that result in an increase in morale, improvement in hopefulness, and increase in self-efficacy (Newman & Beck, 2007).

Indications

Cognitive behavioral therapy is useful in several ways:

- *Mood disorders.* Cognitive therapy has been used successfully for the treatment of mood disorders (and in reducing the risk of suicide), anxiety disorders (e.g., phobias, panic disorder, social anxiety disorder, generalized anxiety disorder), psychotic disorders, personality disorders, substance abuse, and eating disorders.
- *Medical conditions.* This approach has also been evaluated as an adjunctive treatment for medical conditions such as chronic pain, health anxiety in cancer patients, and social competence after brain injury, among others.
- *Medication compliance.* One of the strengths of this therapy is its focus on modifying patients' maladaptive beliefs about taking medication (e.g., "If I feel well, I do not need to take medications for a longer duration"). The outcome is an improved synergy between cognitive therapy and pharmacotherapy, which benefits patients in multiple ways and leads to the best possible outcomes.

Table 8.6 describes some of the most common cognitive distortions that cognitive behavioral therapists address during their therapy sessions (Beck, 1995).

Psychoanalysis

Psychoanalysis (or **Freudian psychology**) is a body of ideas developed by Austrian neurologist Sigmund Freud that continually evolved in the decades that followed (Karasu & Karasu, 2007). The major application of psychoanalysis is to the study of human

TABLE 8.6   List of Common Cognitive Distortions

Term	Definition
Magnification	Distorting aspects of a memory or situation through magnifying them such that they no longer correspond to objective reality
Minimization	Distorting aspects of a memory or situation through minimizing them such that they no longer correspond to objective reality
Catastrophizing	Focusing on the worst possible outcome, however unlikely, without factoring in other possible (and less tragic) outcomes
Mind reading	Assuming knowledge of the intentions or thoughts of others without explicit communication of the same
Overgeneralization	Taking isolated cases and using them to make far-reaching generalizations
Personalization	Attribution of personal responsibility (or causal role) for events over which the individual has no control

Source: Data from Beck, J. S. (1995). *Cognitive therapy: basics and beyond.* New York: The Guilford Press.

psychological functioning and mental illnesses. Psychoanalysis has three main components (Karasu & Karasu, 2007; Moore & Fine, 1967):

1. A method of investigation of the mind and the way one thinks
2. A systematized set of theories about human behavior
3. A method of treatment of psychological or emotional illness

Freudian psychoanalysis refers to a specific type of treatment in which the **"analysand"** (the patient being analyzed) verbalizes thoughts, including free associations, fantasies, and dreams, from which the **analyst** (the psychotherapist trained in psychoanalysis) induces the unconscious conflicts causing the patient's symptoms and character problems and interprets them for the patient to create insight for resolution of the problems.

The specifics of the analyst's interventions typically include confronting and clarifying the patient's pathological defenses, wishes, and guilt. Through the analysis of conflicts, including those contributing to resistance and those involving transference onto the analyst of distorted reactions, psychoanalytic treatment can clarify how patients unconsciously are their own worst enemies: how unconscious, symbolic reactions that have been stimulated by experience are causing symptoms.

The basic method of psychoanalysis is interpretation of the patient's unconscious conflicts that are interfering with current-day functioning—conflicts that cause painful symptoms such as phobias, anxiety, depression, and compulsions. In patients who make mistakes, forget, or show other peculiarities regarding time, fees, and talking, the analyst can usually find various unconscious "resistances" to the flow of thoughts (sometimes called free association).

Psychoanalytic psychotherapy (also called psychodynamic psychotherapy or expressive psychotherapy) is based fundamentally on the application of techniques that derive from psychoanalysis. Psychoanalytic psychotherapy in its narrowest sense is the use of insight-oriented methods only. The primary distinction between psychoanalysis and other forms of therapy is in the handling of the transference. **Transference** is a phenomenon in psychoanalysis characterized by unconscious redirection of feelings from one person to another (Karasu & Karasu, 2007).

Indications

Generally speaking, chronic and mild cases of psychosis and all forms of symptomatic anxiety are considered the most amenable to psychoanalysis. More recently, its application to patients with depression has also been successful.

Psychoanalysis is precluded when dangerous behavioral or physical symptoms require more immediate attention or for virtually the entire realm of the psychoses, in which severe ego deficits and tenuous reality are apparent. For instance, it would not be advisable to recommend analysis for a patient who is acutely psychotic and a threat to others around him or her.

Patient Requisites

For psychoanalysis to succeed certain patient prerequisites should be met. In light of the intensity and the length of treatment, the patient should have a high degree of motivation. The patient must be willing to face issues of time and money and to endure the pain and frustration associated with sacrificing rapid relief in favor of future cure and with forego-ing the secondary gains of illness. Second, the patient should demonstrate the ability to form a relationship. The capacity to form and maintain, as well as to detach from, a trust-ing relationship is essential. The individual should also exhibit psychological mindedness (curiosity about oneself and the capacity for self-scrutiny), and finally the patient should exhibit adequate ego strength (ego strength helps us maintain emotional stability and cope with internal and external stress).

Limitations

Critics of psychoanalysis often question the credibility of the body of theory on which it is based. The validity of major psychoanalytic constructs has never been demonstrated through conventional research methodologies. The reliability of the case study method, which is considered the most subjective form of research observation in establishing effec-tiveness of psychoanalysis, has also been questioned.

Critics have also questioned the validity of interpretations, on which rests the very integrity of psychoanalysis as a clinical method (Karasu & Karasu, 2007). Economic con-straints, relating to the high cost in time and money, both for patients and in the training of future practitioners, are also potential roadblocks in the successful practice of psycho-analysis. Finally, because the technique of psychoanalysis delimits the potential patient population to an elite group, at least in theory (psychologically minded, high verbal and cognitive abilities, stable life situation), psychoanalysis may be unduly restricted to a diag-nostically, socioeconomically, or intellectually advantaged patient population.

Dialectical Behavior Therapy

Dialectical behavior therapy (DBT) is a form of psychotherapy originally developed for the treatment of individuals diagnosed with borderline personality disorder. DBT was for-mulated by Marsha M. Linehan, a psychology researcher at the University of Washington (Janowsky, 1999; Linehan & Dimeff, 2001). The technique of DBT combines standard cognitive behavioral techniques for emotion regulation and reality testing with concepts of distress tolerance, acceptance, and mindfulness. Some of these tenets have been derived from Buddhist meditative practice. Treatment strategies in DBT are based on the fusion of principles from behavioral learning theories with those of acceptance found in Eastern mindfulness and Western contemplative spiritual practices (Rosenthal & Lynch, 2007).

DBT may be the first therapy experimentally demonstrated to be generally effec-tive in treating borderline personality disorder (Linehan, Armstrong, Suarez, Allmon, & Heard, 1991; Linehan, Heard, & Armstrong, 1993). DBT has also found research support as an effective treatment for patients with different kinds of mood disorders, including self-injury. DBT treatment is divided into four primary modes:

1. Group skill training
2. Individual therapy
3. Phone consultation
4. Consultation team

Other, additional treatments that may be needed and are usually not controlled include pharmacotherapy and acute inpatient psychiatric hospitalization.

Skill training refers to a skill class rather than a traditional psychotherapy group and is conducted in a group format. The primary focus of the skill-building group is the acquisition of new coping skills. The basic assumption is that these patients must learn specific behavioral, emotional, cognitive, and interpersonal skills not acquired early on in life (Rosenthal & Lynch, 2007).

Mindfulness, considered the core set of skills in DBT, derives from both Western Christian contemplative and Eastern meditative traditions. It refers to the practice of paying attention in a particular way, to the present moment and without any judgment. Patients learn their behavior is a function of current emotions (emotion mind) or logical analysis (reasonable mind). This subjective knowledge often leads to suspension of short-term maladaptive and possibly harmful behaviors and their replacement by long-term gains in self-esteem and feelings of mastery (Linehan et al., 1991, 1993).

Borderline patients often experience intense emotional distress. Many such individuals may develop maladaptive behaviors as a means of reducing chronic and extreme distress. For example, self-mutilating behavior may serve to temporarily reduce subjective distress. The distress tolerance module, the second core set of skills taught through DBT, attempts to teach patients how to tolerate aversive emotional experiences without indulging in maladaptive behaviors. Other distress tolerance skills include awareness, breathing, and half-smile exercises as well as radical acceptance of reality in the current moment.

The emotion regulation skills module is designed to help patients to better comprehend their emotions, reduce emotional vulnerability, and decrease emotional suffering. Specific skills taught include increasing awareness of emotions, identifying and challenging distorted ways of thinking about emotions, identifying the connectedness of emotions with problem behaviors, accurately classifying emotions, understanding the functions emotions serve, reducing emotional vulnerability, increasing pleasant emotions, and acting opposite to behavioral urges linked with emotions (Rosenthal & Lynch, 2007).

One of the characteristic features of borderline personality disorder is chaotic interpersonal relationships. Consequently, the development of interpersonal skills is a crucial component in the treatment of this disorder. This skill module teaches group members how to identify factors that interfere with effective interpersonal interactions, confront common cognitive distortions associated with interpersonal situations, and determine the appropriate level of intensity for making requests or saying no in a given situation. Group members are encouraged to practice these skills in a wide variety of new situations to help strengthen newly acquired skills.

Interpersonal Therapy

Interpersonal psychotherapy (IPT) is a time-limited psychotherapy that focuses on the interpersonal dynamics and on building interpersonal skills (Guynn, 2007; Weissman, 2006). The basic premise upon which IPT is based is the belief that interpersonal factors may contribute significantly

Harry Stack Sullivan (1892–1949) is considered to be the Father of Interpersonal Psychiatry.

to psychological problems. IPT aims to change an individual's interpersonal behavior by promoting adaptation to current interpersonal roles and situations.

From the 1920s through the 1940s Harry Stack Sullivan developed his ideas as an alternative formulation to classic psychoanalytical theory (Guynn, 2007). Sullivan hypothesized that social interaction was the basis of everything that we consider human. He suggested there were two basic drives: (physical) satisfaction (i.e., food, warmth, shelter, sex) and (interpersonal) security.

Differences from Other Psychotherapies

A major difference between the different school of psychotherapies lies in the manner in which they conceptualize an individual patient's problems and in the typical length and focus of treatment. Although they use similar techniques, IPT differs from cognitive and behavioral approaches in that maladaptive or dysfunctional thoughts and behaviors are addressed only as they apply to problematic interpersonal relationships. The eventual goal is to change the relationship pattern rather than underlying cognitions (Weissman, 2006).

Timeline of Treatment

The typical course of IPT lasts 12 to 20 sessions over a 4- to 5-month period. The initial phase is dedicated to identifying the problem area that will be the target for treatment. The intermediate phase is devoted to working on the targeted problem area(s). Finally, the termination phase focuses on solidifying gains made during treatment and prepares the patient to separate from the therapist and to work independently (Guynn, 2007).

Utility of IPT

IPT seeks to identify and transform the maladaptive interpersonal context in which the psychiatric problem developed and is being sustained. IPT helps individuals identify and address interpersonal problems within four major social domains: grief, interpersonal role disputes, role transitions, and interpersonal deficits.

Grief is identified as the problem area when the onset of the patient's symptoms is associated with the death of a loved one, either recent or past. It can also result from the loss of a significant relationship or the loss of an important aspect of one's identity. The goals for treating complicated bereavement include facilitating mourning and helping the patient to find new activities and relationships to substitute for the loss.

Role transition includes any difficulties resulting from a change in life status. Common role transitions include a career change (promotion, firing, retirement), a family change (marriage, divorce, birth of a child), the beginning or end of an important relationship, a move, graduation from school, or diagnosis of a medical illness. The goals of therapy include mourning and accepting the loss of the old role, recognizing the positive and negative aspects of both the old and new roles, and restoring the patient's self-esteem by developing a sense of mastery in the new role.

Interpersonal role disputes are conflicts with a significant other (e.g., a partner, other family member, coworker, or close friend) that emerge from differences in expectations about the relationship. Treatment goals include a clear identification of the nature of the dispute and exploration of options to help resolve the dispute. It is important to determine the stage of the dispute; once the stage of the dispute becomes clear, it may be important to modify the patient's expectations and remedy faulty communication to bring about adequate resolution.

Interpersonal deficits refer to patients who are socially isolated or who are in chronically unfulfilling relationships. The goal is to reduce the patient's social isolation by helping him or her to enhance the quality of existing relationships and encouraging the formation of new relationships. To help these patients it is necessary to determine why they have difficulty in forming or maintaining relationships. Conducting a review of past significant relationships is very helpful in making this assessment.

Limitations

IPT has not been shown to be effective in treating substance abuse (Guynn, 2007). IPT was not developed to treat psychotic depression or other forms of psychosis, such as schizophrenia.

IPT is a fairly simple and elegant approach that is highly acceptable to patients. If a full course of IPT fails, treatment nonresponders should be evaluated for the possible recommendation of an alternative, evidence-based treatment (Guynn, 2007).

Group Psychotherapy

Group psychotherapy is an approach that uses a professionally trained therapist who organizes and guides a group of members to work together toward the maximal attainment of the goals for each individual in that group and for the group itself. Certain properties that are integral to a group, such as mutual support, can be exploited to help provide relief from psychological suffering. The group may also serve to provide a form of peer support to help offset the feeling of isolation experienced by many individuals who seek psychiatric help (Spitz, 2007). In a broader sense, group therapy can be understood to include any helping process that takes place in a group, including but not limited to support groups (for instance, Alcoholics Anonymous), skills training groups (such as anger management and DBT groups discussed earlier), and psychoeducation groups (Montgomery, 2002).

Utility of Group Psychotherapy

Therapy groups contain special properties that can be used for introducing change in group members. Some of these properties are unique to the group setting, whereas others are simply amplifications of more generic elements common to all effective psychotherapies (MacKenzie, 1997). Researchers and practitioners have tried to identify those therapeutic or "curative factors" present in groups to determine how they can be used to maximum effect (Spitz, 2007). For instance, catharsis is an emotional response that produces a state of relief in the patient and is often manifested during the interactions in a group therapy session.

Small sized and homogenous groups may be ideal for the distribution of accurate information about a condition shared by the group members. Such conditions could be medical illness, substance abuse, and chronic and persistent severe psychiatric conditions, including schizophrenia and major affective disorders (Spitz, 2007).

Family and Couples Psychotherapy

Definition

Family therapy is a kind of psychotherapy that focuses on families and couples to foster change and development. Also referred to as **couple and family therapy** and **family systems therapy**, this branch of psychotherapy emphasizes family relationships as an important factor in psychological health. Family therapy focuses on the underlying dynamics within the families and visualizes change in terms of the interaction among different family members (or spouses in the case of couple's therapy). Such changes in interpersonal interaction can help an individual cope more effectively (Carson, 2000). Family therapy is an assortment of many techniques, all of which have the final goal of direct alteration of maladaptive family processes.

Differences from Other Psychotherapies

One of the major differences between traditional individual psychotherapies and family therapy is the relationship between the therapist and the patient. In the former, it is the interaction between the therapist and the patient that forms the basis for driving the change in the individual. The therapist's allegiance lies toward the patient and unless mandatory all information revealed during sessions is considered strictly confidential, even from family members. In family and couple therapy the opposite is the case. Because of complex histories predating the therapy, the initial job of the therapist is to stabilize the family system by decelerating the intensity of interactions. Also, adequate rapport has to be formed with all members seeking treatment. The family therapist has to find a point of entry into the current family configuration and gradually work from there (Spitz & Spitz, 2007).

Indications for Family and Couple Therapy

Both family and couple therapy have specific indications. **Table 8.7** enumerates some of these indications (Spitz & Spitz, 2007).

Contraindications for Family and Couple Therapy

Certain characteristics of the family unit preclude family therapy: presence of an emotionally unstable member; history of violence in the family; inflexible, rigid, and unwilling to change members; severity of mental illness (acutely suicidal family members); cases of physical or sexual abuse of a child (reportable offenses); family belief system runs counter to therapy; and essential members refuse to participate in the family therapy (Spitz & Spitz, 2007). Factors precluding couple therapy include unequal levels of motivation between the two partners, threat of domestic violence, severity of mental illness, and when one of the members has an ongoing, active relationship with someone other than the partner.

Client-Centered Therapy

Client-centered therapy (also called **Rogerian psychotherapy**) is a fairly widely used model of psychotherapy wherein the therapist creates a relaxed, nonjudgmental environment

TABLE 8.7   Indications for Family and Couple Therapy

Therapy	Indication
Family	• Problems across generational boundaries, for instance, conflicts between two generations, more than one generation living in the same space, etc.
	• Serious medical or mental illness in a family member
	• Familial stress secondary to cultural or religious differences or societal differences, e.g., interracial or same-sex partnerships
	• Sibling issues beyond parental control
	• A child/adolescent being treated for a psychiatric illness and having behavioral issues
Couple	• Specific psychosocial stressors for couples: possibility of a divorce or breakup, disclosure of an affair
	• Communication problems
	• Termination of partnerships: when relationships are ending and children are involved (to minimize harm to children)

Source: Data from Spitz, H. I., & Spitz, S. (2007). Family and couple therapy. In B. J. Sadock, V. A. Sadock, & P. Ruiz (Eds.), *Kaplan and Sadock's comprehensive textbook of psychiatry* (pp. 2846–2857). Philadelphia: Lippincott Williams & Wilkins.

by demonstrating genuineness, empathy, and unconditional positive regard toward their patients while using a nondirective approach. This facilitates the individual undergoing therapy in generating solutions to their problems. The model was created by Carl Rogers, a psychologist in 1940 (Prochaska & Norcross, 2007).

Rogerian psychotherapy is based on the idea that each person has the ability to solve psychological problems and that feeling understood and highly appreciated helps the forces within to solve those problems (Altshuler & Brenner, 2007). At the time when this method was published, ideas such as an instinct toward self-realization and limitless inner powers had huge appeal.

Indications

The general indications for client-centered therapy are when individuals perceive discrepancies in themselves or see that their behavior is out of control. The theory ensures that a trial of this form of therapy is unlikely to be harmful (Altshuler & Brenner, 2007).

Transactional Analysis

Transactional analysis (or transactional psychotherapy) was conceived by Eric Berne, a psychiatrist trained in the psychoanalytic tradition. Berne departed from conventional psychoanalytic teachings to focus on social interaction during therapy. He published two books, *Transactional Analysis in Psychotherapy* in 1961 and *Games People Play* in 1964. The underlying premise for transactional analysis is that humans seek intimacy, comfort, or recognition through social interactions. They get such intimacy and recognition through mutual exchanges Berne called "strokes." Harmonious and realistic transactions foster mental health, whereas transactions rooted in ulterior motives lead to discomfort and disharmony

(Altshuler & Brenner, 2007). Because it focuses on communication, transactional analysis has also been successfully applied in the analysis of organizations and systems.

FOCUS FEATURE 8.1 PSYCHOSURGERY

Psychosurgery refers to neurosurgical treatment of mental disorders. Introduced in the early 1930s, psychosurgery has been a controversial approach to treating the mentally ill. Portuguese neurologist Egas Moniz is usually credited with being the originator of psychosurgery, although there had been previous attempts to operate on the brains of mentally ill people. The practice of psychosurgery was popularized in the United States by Walter Freeman. Freeman modified the original surgeries to devise a procedure he called lobotomy. Further refinements called transorbital lobotomies involved anesthetizing a patient with electroconvulsive shock and hammering an ice pick–like instrument through the eye socket. The procedure was widely adopted and in certain instances abused. With the development of psychotropic agents, the procedure was largely shunned. Other forms of psychosurgery survived but on a smaller scale. Presently, psychosurgical procedures are banned in most countries and heavily regulated in others and reserved for a small number of patients with depression or obsessive-compulsive disorder who have failed other treatment options.

During a psychosurgical procedure a small piece of brain is destroyed or removed using a stereotactic needle. The lesions are made by heat, radiation, freezing, or cutting. Approximately one-third of patients show major symptomatic improvement. Although recent advances in surgical technique have led to a huge reduction in the incident of death and major side effects, the procedure may still have significant morbidity in the form of seizures, incontinence, decreased drive and initiative, weight gain, and cognitive and problems.

NEWER APPROACHES

Transcranial Magnetic Stimulation

Transcranial magnetic stimulation (TMS) is the application of a rapidly changing magnetic field to the superficial layers of the cerebral cortex thereby inducing locally changing small electric currents called "eddy" currents. TMS can be visualized as electrical stimulation without an electrode because it uses magnetic fields to indirectly induce electrical pulses (Rowny & Lisaby, 2007). TMS devices deliver strong magnetic pulses via a coil that is held on the scalp. TMS exemplifies noninvasive stimulation of focal regions of the brain and can be used for research or therapeutically without the need for anesthesia (Barker, Jalinous, & Freeston, 1985).

The use of TMS in the treatment of major depressive disorder has been the most-studied therapeutic application of this technique. Evidence from a growing number of randomized, controlled trials suggests a significant antidepressant effect with TMS applied to the dorsolateral prefrontal cortex. Not all studies have been positive, however, and the average effect size in depression is moderate—less than with ECT but comparable with that seen with traditional pharmacotherapy.

Use of TMS in the treatment of schizophrenia has yielded some promising results in experimental studies that used low-frequency TMS to inhibit temporal-parietal areas of the cortex linked to hyperactivity during hallucinations. TMS is also being actively studied and has shown some early positive results as a treatment modality in anxiety disorders, including applications for obsessive-compulsive disorder and panic and Tourette's disorders.

TMS is not currently approved by the FDA as a clinical treatment modality. However, it is being considered for use as an indication of depression. If it is approved as an effective and safe treatment, it might be preferable to more invasive modalities like ECT.

TMS and other forms of magnetic stimulation hold tremendous promise in psychiatric treatment due to their focality and noninvasiveness. However, much research is needed to replicate preliminary findings, improve optimal dosing, establish the patient characteristics that predict response, and examine the influence of concomitant medications on TMS effect (Barker et al., 1985; Rowny & Lisaby, 2007).

Two more recent additions to brain stimulation methods, deep brain stimulation (DBS) and vagus nerve stimulation (VNS), were introduced about a decade after the first trials of TMS. Both were first approved by the FDA in 1997 in the realm of treating sequelae of neurological syndromes. DBS was initially approved for the treatment of essential tremor and Parkinson's tremor, whereas VNS was approved for the treatment of epilepsy. Five years later, in 2002, indications for DBS were expanded to include treatment of all symptoms of Parkinson's disease, including tremor, slowness, and stiffness, as well as involuntary movements induced by medications (Rowny & Lisaby, 2007).

TMS, DBS, and VNS originated in the field of neurology. Psychiatrists quickly saw the potential for those tools in the treatment of psychiatric conditions, however, and as a result of clinical trials in depression, VNS subsequently received FDA approval for the adjunctive long-term treatment of chronic or recurrent depression in adults. In addition, human studies designed to validate the efficacy of DBS in the treatment of depression and obsessive-compulsive disorder are underway.

Eye Movement Desensitization and Reprocessing

Eye movement desensitization and reprocessing (EMDR) is a comprehensive, integrative psychotherapy approach (Shapiro, 2001). EMDR has been described as an eclectic approach that combines elements of many different psychotherapy styles in structured protocols that are designed to maximize treatment effects. These include psychodynamic, cognitive behavioral, interpersonal, experiential, and body-centered therapies (Shapiro, 2002). Even though it is a kind of psychotherapy, EMDR is a novel technique and hence discussed in this subsection.

EMDR psychotherapy attends to the past experiences that have set the groundwork for pathology; the current situations that trigger dysfunctional emotions, beliefs, and sensations; and the positive experience needed to enhance future adaptive behaviors and mental health (Shapiro, 2001, 2002).

During treatment various procedures and protocols are used to address the entire clinical picture. One of the procedural elements is "dual stimulation" using bilateral eye movements, tones, or taps. During the reprocessing phases the client attends momentarily to past memories, present triggers, or anticipated future experiences while simultaneously focusing on a set of external stimulus. During that time clients generally experience the emergence of insight, changes in memories, or new associations (Shapiro, 2001, 2002). The clinician assists the client to focus on appropriate material before initiation of each subsequent set.

Even though eye movements are the most distinctive element of EMDR, it is, in itself, a complex psychotherapy that blends multiple components thought to contribute to the treatment effects. Eye movements are used to engage the client's attention to an external stimulus while the client is simultaneously focusing on internal distressing material. Shapiro describes eye movements as "dual attention stimuli" to identify the process in which the client attends to both external and internal stimuli (Shapiro, 2001, 2002).

Utility

EMDR has been used for trauma such as that resulting from natural disaster, wars, or terrorism. EMDR has an impact on intrusive imagery (such as nightmares and flashbacks), numbing, and hyperarousal symptoms of posttraumatic stress disorder as well as on associated grief and depression (American Psychiatric Association, 2004).

COSTS ASSOCIATED WITH MENTAL HEALTH CARE

General Trends

The past few decades have seen rapid developments in the treatment of mental illnesses. Advances have been made in the field of both psychotherapies and psychotropic agents. Key innovations have occurred with psychotropic agents used to treat depression, schizophrenia, and bipolar disorder. Predictably, these developments led to huge increases in expenditures on psychotropic medications. From 1996 to 2001 spending on psychotropic drugs almost tripled from $5.9 million to $14.7 million (Zuvekas, 2005).

A study by the National Alliance on Mental Illness (2006) found that the cost for treating depression is three times higher for U.S. citizens with limited access to treatment. The annual out-of-pocket costs for medication, psychotherapy, and other treatment averaged $4,312 for those with restricted access versus $1,496 for those with good health insurance.

Costs Associated with Pharmaceuticals

The cost of a psychotropic medication depends on whether it is available as a generic formulation or not. Per the FDA (2010, para. 1), "A **generic drug** [bold added] is identical—or bioequivalent—to a brand name drug in dosage form, safety, strength, route of administration, quality, performance characteristics and intended use." Usually, when a drug company markets a psychotropic drug it owns the patent rights to the drug for a predetermined number of years. The cost of that drug is unusually high during those years and falls dramatically once the drug can be marketed in a generic form.

Tables 8.8 and 8.9 enumerate the costs of some of the common antidepressants and antipsychotic medications, respectively. **Table 8.8** provides the list of common antidepressants and the cost of a months' supply for the lowest strength of that medication. If a generic version of that antidepressant is available, the cost for the generic has been provided. The chemical compound of that antidepressant is mentioned within parenthesis.

Table 8.9 provides a list of common antipsychotic medications and the cost of a months' supply for the lowest strength of that medication. If a generic version of that drug is available, the cost for the generic has been provided. The chemical compound in that antipsychotic is mentioned within parenthesis. Interestingly, the first three agents are all first-generation antipsychotic compounds that have been around for decades, whereas the

TABLE 8.8 Cost of Antidepressant Medications

Antidepressant	Generic	Cost for 30-Day Supply
Prozac (fluoxetine), 10-mg capsules	Y	$14.99
Celexa (citalopram), 10-mg tablets	Y	$16.99
Remeron (mirtazapine), 7.5-mg tablets	Y	$49.99
Lexapro (escitalopram), 5-mg tablets	N	$99.99
Pristiq (desvenlafaxine), 50-mg tablets	N	$141.99
Cymbalta (duloxetine), 20-mg capsules	N	$145.99

last three are second-generation compounds and relatively recent entrants into the psychotropic market.

Therapy-Related Costs

Due to pressures from managed care companies, there has been a trend in favor of psychotropic medications and against psychotherapy despite the fact that the efficacy of most psychotherapies has been demonstrated time and time again. In a randomized, controlled trial on recurrent major depression, 75 outpatients were randomly assigned to three arms: acute and maintenance treatment with antidepressants, acute and maintenance cognitive therapy, and acute antidepressants followed by maintenance cognitive therapy. Cognitive therapy proved as effective as medication in both the acute and maintenance phases, with a trend favoring cognitive therapy's long-term efficacy (Blackburn & Moore, 1997). In another study researchers randomly assigned 40 patients who had been successfully treated with medication for recurrent major depression into two groups: clinical management or cognitive behavioral therapy. After 20 weeks antidepressant medications were tapered off and eventually discontinued in both groups. Two years later only 25% of the patients who received cognitive behavioral therapy had relapsed compared with 80% of the other group (Fava, Rafanelli, Grandi, Conti, & Belluardo, 1998). A cost-effectiveness analysis of cognitive behavioral therapy, Prozac, and combination therapy factored in issues such

TABLE 8.9 Cost of Antipsychotic Medications

Antipsychotic Agent	Generic	Cost for 30-Day Supply
Haldol (haloperidol), 0.5-mg tablets	Y	<$5
Prolixin (fluphenazine), 1-mg tablets	Y	<$5
Thorazine (chlorpromazine), 10-mg tablets	Y	<$10
Zyprexa (olanzapine), 2.5-mg tablets	N	$275.99
Abilify (Aripiprazole), 2-mg tablets	N	$531.98
Geodon (ziprasidone), 20-mg capsules	N	$250.00

TABLE 8.10 Cost of Psychotherapy			
No. of Sessions	Psychiatrist (MD) (US Dollars)	Psychologist (US Dollars)	Social Worker (US Dollars)
15	1,331	1,053	898
10	893	703	598
10	456	353	299

Source: Data from Dewan, M. (1999). Are psychiatrists cost-effective? An analysis of integrated versus split treatment. *American Journal of Psychiatry, 156,* 324–326.

as lost productivity, wages, taxes, and community service during treatment (Antonuccio, Thomas, & Danton, 1997). This analysis concluded that providing Prozac alone would cost an estimated 33% more than cognitive behavioral therapy over a 2-year period and that providing combination therapy would cost an estimated 23% more. **Table 8.10** provides some of the projected costs for outpatient psychotherapy visits (Dewan, 1999). As can be seen from these data, the cost of the sessions depends largely on whether it is being delivered by a psychiatrist, a psychologist, or a social worker.

Split Treatment

Split treatment refers to a model of care in which fragmented care is encouraged by two or more providers instead of a single mental health practitioner who can deliver comprehensive holistic mental health care (i.e., the psychiatrist) (Dewan, 1999). Under such a fragmented model the psychiatrist provides medications while a psychotherapist delivers the therapy. The integrated biopsychosocial model practiced by psychiatry is both theoretically and economically the preferred model when combined treatment is required.

SKILL-BUILDING ACTIVITY

Select any mental health condition. Then, research the evidence-based treatments (both psychopharmacology and psychotherapeutic) available for that condition. Compile your findings in a brochure, including a brief paragraph on the major presenting features of that diagnoses. Also compare the costs of providing psychopharmacological and psychotherapeutic treatments.

SUMMARY

Mental health services can be delivered via multiple different settings ranging from very restrictive (inpatient) to least restrictive (care delivered in individual's home). A therapeutic milieu is a structured group setting in which the existence of the group is a key force in the outcome of treatment. Using the combined elements of positive peer pressure, trust, safety, and repetition the therapeutic milieu provides an idealized setting for group members to work through their psychological issues.

The use of electronic media has revolutionized ways in which individuals relate to each other and has had implications for all walks of human life. Its impact on health care has been profound. The phenomenon of remote communications with patients is a relatively recent development. Telepsychiatry (a branch of telemedicine) is a specifically defined form of video conferencing that can provide psychiatric services to patients living in remote locations or otherwise underserved areas via the electronic transmission of images.

Involuntary commitment is the practice of placing a person in a psychiatric hospital or ward against his or her will, in compliance with mental health laws of the country. Commitment is normally time-limited and requires reevaluation at fixed intervals. In the United States involuntary commitment and the consequent deprivation of an individual's civil liberties are serious matters indeed. Psychiatrists are in a unique position in that they have an ethical and legal responsibility to hospitalize patients against their will if they meet specific criteria. Even though the individual states differ in their involuntary commitment procedures, the most important and virtually universal criteria include dangerousness to self, dangerousness to others, or serious impairment leading to an inability to care for oneself as a result of mental illness.

Psychopharmacology refers to the use of medications for the treatment of mental disorders. Plant extracts and naturally occurring substances have been used for centuries to influence mood and anxiety, to adjust sleep and arousal, to create euphoria, and to alter consciousness. Coffee, tea, and alcohol remain important examples. The text discusses antipsychotics (psychotropic agent primarily used to treat psychosis), antidepressants (psychotropic agents used to treat mood disorders such as major depression and dysthymia), antianxiety (drugs used for the treatment of anxiety and its attendant psychological and physical symptoms), and mood stabilizers (psychotropic agents used to treat mood disorders characterized by sustained and extreme shifts in mood states, usually seen in bipolar disorders).

Drug development to support a viable marketing application advances in somewhat overlapping phases. Nonclinical (also called preclinical) studies begin before human studies but continue throughout the clinical development period. Before each phase of human testing, animal testing is done to ensure that the level of planned human exposure is safe. The usual temporal sequence proceeds from an initial classification of the drug to testing for efficacy and finally the exploration of potential side effects in the intended population of use. It is divided into four overlapping phases, from phase I through phase IV.

The first electroconvulsive treatment or ECT course was administered to a delusional and incoherent patient in 1938. Throughout the 1940s ECT enjoyed popularity as a first-line therapy. Efforts to improve the acceptability and safety profile of electrically induced convulsions continued in the following years. However, with the widespread use of pharmacological agents as first-line treatments for major psychiatric disorders, ECT is currently more commonly used for patients with resistance to those treatments. The only exception to this is life-threatening illness due to inanition, severe suicidal symptoms, or catatonia where ECT may be used as a first-line treatment.

There are different schools of psychotherapy. Some of these are behaviorism, cognitive behavioral therapy, psychoanalysis (or Freudian psychology), DBT, IPT, group psychotherapy, family therapy, client-centered therapy (also called Rogerian psychotherapy), and transactional analysis (or transactional psychotherapy). TMS, DBS, and VNS are novel modalities of treatment available for the treatment of psychiatric conditions.

The past few decades have seen rapid developments in the treatment of mental illnesses. Advances have been made both in the field of psychotherapies and psychotropic agents. This has predictably led to huge increases in expenditures on psychotropic medications. Costs associated with mental health care can be divided into costs pertaining to medications and costs associated with provision of psychotherapy. Split treatment refers to a model of care where instead of a single mental health practitioner who can deliver comprehensive holistic mental health care (i.e., the psychiatrist), fragmented care is encouraged by two or more providers.

REVIEW QUESTIONS

1. Enumerate the different settings in which mental health services are delivered.
2. Describe the drug development process in the United States.
3. What do you understand by the term "involuntary commitment"?
4. Discuss the indications for electroconvulsive therapy.
5. Enumerate the indications for interpersonal therapy. How is it different from other therapies?

WEBSITES TO EXPLORE

U.S. Food and Drug Administration (FDA)

http://www.fda.gov/drugs/developmentapprovalprocess/default.htm

This is the website for the U.S. Food and Drug Administration, an agency of the U.S. Department of Health and Human Services. The FDA is responsible for protecting and promoting the public health by ensuring the safety, effectiveness, and security of human and veterinary drugs, vaccines and other biological products, medical devices, the nation's food supply, cosmetics, dietary supplements, and products that give off radiation. *Review the information. An energy drink called 4-Loco received considerable attention and eventually was banned by FDA. Compile a chronology of events that led the FDA to pull this product of the market.*

New York Psychoanalytic Society & Institute

http://www.psychoanalysis.org/

The New York Psychoanalytic Society is one the oldest psychoanalytic organization in the United States. While remaining faithful to the old psychoanalytic traditions, the Institute has modernized its curriculum and greatly increased the number of programs it offers. The institute offers formal training in psychoanalysis. *Review the website and compile a list of minimum requirements needed to complete psychoanalytic training from this institute.*

REFERENCES AND FURTHER READINGS

Altshuler, K. Z., & Brenner, A. M. (2007). Other methods of psychotherapy. In B. J. Sadock, V. A. Sadock, & P. Ruiz (Eds.), *Kaplan and Sadock's comprehensive textbook of psychiatry* (pp. 2911–2922). Philadelphia: Lippincott Williams & Wilkins.

American Psychiatric Association. (2004). *Practice guideline for the treatment of patients with acute stress disorder and posttraumatic stress disorder*. Arlington, VA: American Psychiatric Association.

American Psychiatric Association. (2010). Topic 4: Telepsychiatry. Retrieved from http://www .psych.org/Departments/HSF/UnderservedClearinghouse/Linkeddocuments/telepsychiatry.aspx.

Antonuccio, D. O., Thomas, M., & Danton, W. G. (1997). A cost-effectiveness analysis of cognitive behavior therapy and fluoxetine (prozac) in the treatment of depression. *Behavior Therapy, 28*(2), 187–210.

Barker, A. T., Jalinous, R., & Freeston, I. L. (1985). Non-invasive magnetic stimulation of human motor cortex. *Lancet, 1*(8437), 1106–1107.

Barry, P. D. (2002). *Mental health and mental illness*. Philadelphia: Lippincott Williams & Wilkins.

Beck, J. S. (1995). *Cognitive therapy: Basics and beyond*. New York: Guilford Press.

Bellack, A. S. (2006). Scientific and consumer models of recovery in schizophrenia: Concordance, contrasts, and implications. *Schizophrenia Bulletin, 32*(3), 432–442.

Blackburn, I. M., & Moore, R. G. (1997). Controlled acute and follow-up trial of cognitive therapy and pharmacotherapy in out-patients with recurrent depression. *British Journal of Psychiatry, 171*, 328–334.

Bowden, C. L. (2005). Atypical antipsychotic augmentation of mood stabilizer therapy in bipolar disorder. *Journal of Clinical Psychiatry, 66*(Suppl 3), 12–19.

Carson, V. B. (2000). *Mental health nursing: The nurse-patient journey*. Philadelphia: W. B. Saunders.

Costa, P. T., & McCrae, R. R. (2007). Approaches derived from philosophy and psychology. In B. J. Sadock, V. A. Sadock, & P. Ruiz (Eds.), *Kaplan and Sadock's comprehensive textbook of psychiatry* (pp. 870–873). Philadelphia: Lippincott Williams & Wilkins.

Dewan, M. (1999). Are psychiatrists cost-effective? An analysis of integrated versus split treatment. *American Journal of Psychiatry, 156*, 324–326.

Fava, G. A., Rafanelli, C., Grandi, S., Conti, S., & Belluardo, P. (1998). Prevention of recurrent depression with cognitive behavioral therapy: Preliminary findings. *Archives of General Psychiatry, 55*, 816–820.

Fineberg, N. A., Gale, T. M., & Sivakumaran, T. (2006). A Review of antipsychotics in the treatment of obsessive compulsive disorder. *Journal of Psychopharmacology, 20*(1), 97–103.

Gelder, M., Mayou, R., & Geddes, J. (2005). *Psychiatry* (3rd ed.). New York: Oxford.

Guynn, R. W. (2007). Dialectical behavior therapy. In B. J. Sadock, V. A. Sadock, & P. Ruiz (Eds.), *Kaplan and Sadock's comprehensive textbook of psychiatry* (pp. 2873–2883). Philadelphia: Lippincott Williams & Wilkins.

Healy, D. (2005). *Psychiatric drugs explained* (4th ed.). London: Elsevier.

Janowsky, D. S. (1999). *Psychotherapy indications and outcomes*. Washington, DC: American Psychiatric Press.

Kammen, D. P., Hurford, I., & Marder, S. R. (2007). First-generation antipsychotics. In B. J. Sadock, V. A. Sadock, & P. Ruiz (Eds.), *Kaplan and Sadock's comprehensive textbook of psychiatry* (pp. 3105–3127). Philadelphia: Lippincott Williams & Wilkins.

Karasu, T. B., & Karasu, S. R. (2007). Psychoanalysis and psychoanalytic psychotherapy. In B. J. Sadock, V. A. Sadock, & P. Ruiz (Eds.), *Kaplan and Sadock's comprehensive textbook of psychiatry* (pp. 2746–2774). Philadelphia: Lippincott Williams & Wilkins.

Kennedy, S. H., & Lam, R. W. (2003). Enhancing outcomes in the management of treatment resistant depression: a focus on atypical antipsychotics. *Bipolar disorders, 5*, 36–47.

Leonard, S. (2004). The development and evaluation of a telepsychiatry service for prisoners. *Journal of Psychiatric Mental Health Nursing, 11*(4), 461–468.

Linehan, M. M., Armstrong, H. E., Suarez, A., Allmon, D., & Heard, H. L. (1991). Cognitive-behavioral treatment of chronically parasuicidal borderline patients. *Archives of General Psychiatry, 48*, 1060–1064.

Linehan, M. M., & Dimeff, L. (2001). Dialectical behavior therapy in a nutshell. *California Psychologist, 34*, 10–13.

Linehan, M. M., Heard, H. L., & Armstrong, H. E. (1993). Naturalistic follow-up of a behavioral treatment of chronically parasuicidal borderline patients. *Archives of General Psychiatry, 50*(12), 971–974.

MacKenzie, K. R. (1997). *Time managed group psychotherapy*. Washington, DC: American Psychiatric Press.

Marder, S. R., Hurford, I., & Kammen, D. P. (2007). Second-generation antipsychotics. In B. J. Sadock, V. A. Sadock, & P. Ruiz (Eds.), *Kaplan and Sadock's comprehensive textbook of psychiatry* (pp. 3206–3241). Philadelphia: Lippincott Williams & Wilkins.

Montgomery, C. (2002). Role of dynamic group therapy in psychiatry. *Advances in Psychiatric Treatment, 8*(1), 34–41.

Moore, B. E., & Fine, B. D. (Eds.). (1967). *Glossary of psychoanalytic terms and concepts*. New York: American Psychoanalytic Association.

National Alliance on Mental Illness. (2006). National survey finds depression costs nearly tripled for individuals with limited access to care. Retrieved from http://www.nami.org /Template.cfm?Section=Press_July_2006&Template=/ContentManagement/ContentDisplay .cfm&ContentID=36184.

National Institute of Mental Health. (2010). Borderline personality disorder. Retrieved from http:// www.nimh.nih.gov/health/publications/borderline-personality-disorder-fact-sheet/index.shtml.

Newman, C. F., & Beck, A. T. (2007). Cognitive therapy. In B. J. Sadock, V. A. Sadock, & P. Ruiz (Eds.), *Kaplan and Sadock's comprehensive textbook of psychiatry* (pp. 2857–2874). Philadelphia: Lippincott Williams & Wilkins.

Petty, F., Trivedi, M. H., Fulton, M., & Rush, A. J. (1995). Benzodiazepines as antidepressants: Does GABA play a role in depression? *Biological Psychiatry, 38*(9), 578–591.

Powers, R. E. (2008). Choosing the right neuroleptic for a patient. *Bureau of Geriatric Psychiatry*. Retrieved from http://www.google.com/url?sa=t&source=web&cd=1&ved=0CBsQFjAA&url= http%3A%2F%2Fwww.alcouncil.com%2Fdocs%2F2008Conference%2Fhandouts%2Fpo wers%2FChoosing%2520the%2520right%2520neuroleptic%2520for%2520a%2520patient .pdf&ei=OY1ATpP6M--ksQLc8tzSBg&usg=AFQjCNGnc61ejHaJ-k5RcNvNRIxasWfmxw.

Prochaska, J. O., & Norcross, J. C. (2007). *Systems of psychotherapy: A transtheoretical analysis* (6th ed.). Belmont, CA: Thompson Brooks/Cole.

Prudic, J. (2007). Electroconvulsive therapy. In B. J. Sadock, V. A. Sadock, & P. Ruiz (Eds.), *Kaplan and Sadock's comprehensive textbook of psychiatry* (pp. 3285–3301). Philadelphia: Lippincott Williams & Wilkins.

Rosenthal, M. Z., & Lynch, T. R. (2007). Dialectical behavior therapy. In B. J. Sadock, V. A. Sadock, & P. Ruiz (Eds.), *Kaplan and Sadock's comprehensive textbook of psychiatry* (pp. 2884–2893). Philadelphia: Lippincott Williams & Wilkins.

Rowny, S. B., & Lisaby, S. H. (2007). Other brain stimulation methods. In B. J. Sadock, V. A. Sadock, & P. Ruiz (Eds.), *Kaplan and Sadock's comprehensive textbook of psychiatry* (pp. 3285–3301). Philadelphia: Lippincott Williams & Wilkins.

Shapiro, F. (2001). *Eye movement desensitization and reprocessing: Basic principles, protocols, and procedures.* New York: Guilford Press.

Shapiro, F. (2002). *EMDR as an integrative psychotherapy approach: Experts of diverse orientations explore the paradigm prism.* Washington, DC: American Psychological Association Books.

Skinner, B. F. (1984). The operational analysis of psychological terms [Reprint]. *Behavioral and Brain Sciences* 7(4), 547–553.

Spitz, H. I. (2007). Group psychotherapy. In B. J. Sadock, V. A. Sadock, & P. Ruiz (Eds.), *Kaplan and Sadock's comprehensive textbook of psychiatry* (pp. 2832–2844). Philadelphia: Lippincott Williams & Wilkins.

Spitz, H. I., & Spitz, S. (2007). Family and couple therapy. In B. J. Sadock, V. A. Sadock, & P. Ruiz (Eds.), *Kaplan and Sadock's comprehensive textbook of psychiatry* (pp. 2846–2857). Philadelphia: Lippincott Williams & Wilkins.

Stafford, R. S. (2008). Regulating off-label drug use–rethinking the role of the FDA. *New England Journal of Medicine, 358,* 1427–1429.

Stamm, B. H. (1998). Clinical applications of telehealth in mental health care. *Professional Psychology Research and Practice, 29,* 536–542.

Stanley, M. A., & Beiderl, D. C. (2007). Behavior therapy. In B. J. Sadock, V. A. Sadock, & P. Ruiz (Eds.), *Kaplan and Sadock's comprehensive textbook of psychiatry* (pp. 2781–2800). Philadelphia: Lippincott Williams & Wilkins.

Sussman, N. (2007a). Other methods of psychotherapy. In B. J. Sadock, V. A. Sadock, & P. Ruiz (Eds.), *Kaplan and Sadock's comprehensive textbook of psychiatry* (pp. 2965–2982). Philadelphia: Lippincott Williams & Wilkins.

Sussman, N. (2007b). Selective serotonin reuptake inhibitors. In B. J. Sadock, V. A. Sadock, & P. Ruiz (Eds.), *Kaplan and Sadock's comprehensive textbook of psychiatry* (pp. 3190–3205). Philadelphia: Lippincott Williams & Wilkins.

Taintor, Z. (2007). Electronic media in psychiatry. In B. J. Sadock, V. A. Sadock & P. Ruiz (Eds.), *Kaplan & Sadock's comprehensive textbook of psychiatry* (1059–1070). Philadelphia: Lippincott Williams & Wilkins.

Thase, M. E. (2007). Selective serotonin-norepinephrine reuptake inhibitors. In B. J. Sadock, V. A. Sadock, & P. Ruiz (Eds.), *Kaplan and Sadock's comprehensive textbook of psychiatry* (pp. 3185–3190). Philadelphia: Lippincott Williams & Wilkins.

Thomas, S. P., Shattell, M., & Martin, T. (2002). What's therapeutic about the therapeutic milieu? *Archives of Psychiatric Nursing, 16*(3), 99–107.

U.S. Food and Drug Administration (FDA). (2010). Information for consumers: Questions & answers. Retrieved from http://www.fda.gov/Drugs/ResourcesForYou/Consumers/QuestionsAnswers/ucm100100.htm.

Weinmann, S., Read, J., & Aderhold, V. (2009). Influence of antipsychotics on mortality in schizophrenia: Systematic review. *Schizophrenia Research, 113*(1), 1–11.

Weissman, M. M. (2006). A brief history of interpersonal psychotherapy. *Psychiatric Annals, 36*(8), 553–557.

Wheeler-Vega, J. A., Mortimer, A. M., & Tyson, P. J. (2003). Conventional antipsychotic prescription in unipolar depression. I. An audit and recommendations for practice. *Journal of Clinical Psychiatry, 64*(5), 568–574.

Zaylor C., Nelson, E. L. & Cook, D. J. (2001). Clinical outcomes in a prison telepsychiatry clinic. *Journal of Telemedicine and Telecare,* 7 (Suppl. 1), 47–49.

Zuvekas, S. H. (2005). Prescription drugs and the changing patterns of treatment for mental disorders. *Health Affairs, 24*(1), 195–205.

CHAPTER 9

Mental Health Promotion for Children and Adolescents

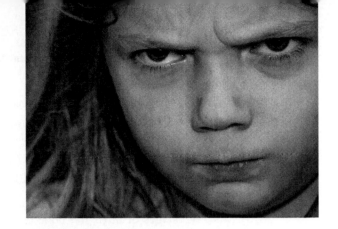

CHAPTER OBJECTIVES

After reading this chapter you should be able to
- Identify various milestones of mental health development through infancy, childhood, and adolescence
- Describe the difference between gender and sex
- Describe four basic parenting styles
- Discuss different types of play

- Identify various eating disorders
- Discuss various community and school-based interventions aimed to prevent mental health problems among children and adolescents

NATURE OF INFANTS, CHILDREN, AND ADOLESCENTS

Although there is no universal definition, a **child** generally refers to an individual between the stages of birth and puberty. In the United States we commonly refer to children as **"minors"** or people under the age of adulthood. The age an individual moves into adulthood (and thus is no longer a minor) is 18 years; however, there still can be exceptions and limits placed on younger adults. For example, to consume alcohol in the United States adults must be at least 21 years of age. According to the United Nations Convention on the Rights of the Child, a child is "a human being below the age of 18 years unless under the law applicable to the child" (United Nations General Assembly, 1989).

As individuals progress through childhood they go through three distinct stages, known as infancy, childhood, and adolescence. The Centers for Disease Control and Prevention (CDC) classifies infancy lasting from approximately ages 0 to 3 years, childhood lasting approximately from ages 4 to 11 years, and adolescence lasting from approximately ages 12 to 19 years (CDC, 2011). As individuals progress through these stages, it is expected they reach both physical milestones (e.g., appropriate height and weight) and developmental milestones (psychosocial and cognitive) (**Table 9.1**). However, it is important to note that children develop at different rates; therefore, these milestones can only act as guidelines. It can also be difficult to identify whether children have developmental problems as they age. Parents should closely monitor their children to ensure they are reaching important milestones for their ages. Recognizing a problem early allows for earlier intervention, which can ultimately favor children's mental health.

Important Milestones for Infants (Ages 0–3 Years)

Infants develop at their own pace, so it is difficult to predict when they will learn a given skill. By 3 months infants should be able to raise their head and chest when lying on their stomach, open and shut their hands, grasp and shake hand toys, follow moving objects with their eyes, recognize familiar objects and people from a distance, smile at the sound of a familiar voice, and imitate sounds through babble. By 7 months infants should enjoy social play, respond to other people's expressions of emotion, explore with hands and mouth, recognize emotions through tones, roll both ways (front to back, back to front), transfer objects from hand to hand, and start to respond to key words, such as their own name and phrases such as "no."

By 1 year infants become shy or anxious with strangers, display fear or unease in the absence of their parent or guardian, feed themselves finger foods, explore objects in different ways (i.e., shaking, banging, throwing, and dropping), start to say simple words such as "mama" or "dada," and respond to simple verbal requests. In year 2 infants become more self-aware, imitate behaviors of others, become more excited about the company of other children, demonstrate increasing independence, and begin to show defiant behavior. In the third year infants can imitate adults and playmates, can take turns in games, understand the

TABLE 9.1 Important Cognitive Milestones for Infants, Children, and Adolescents

Age	Milestones
Infants 0–3 yr	• Smile at the sound of a familiar voice • Enjoy social play • Respond to other people's expressions of emotion • Recognize emotions through tones • Cry in the absence of their parent or guardian • Imitate behaviors of others • Become more excited around other children • Express affection more openly
Children 4–11 yr	• Cooperate with other children • Participate in fantasy play • Become more like their friends • Show more independence • Have stronger sense of right and wrong • Give more attention to friendships and teamwork • Peer pressure becomes stronger
Adolescents 12–19 yr	• Greater focus on self • Increased moodiness • Become more interested and influenced by peer groups • Better able to express their feelings through talking • Increased independence from parents • Develop a deeper capacity for caring and sharing

Source: Centers for Disease Control and Prevention (CDC). (2010). Developmental milestones. Available at: http://www .cdc.gov/ncbddd/actearly/milestones/index.html; Middle childhood (6–8 years old): Developmental milestones. Available at: http://www.cdc.gov/ncbddd/childdevelopment/positiveparenting/middle.html; Middle childhood (9–11 years old): Developmental milestones. Available at: http://www.cdc.gov/ncbddd/childdevelopment/positiveparenting/middle2.html; Developmental milestones. Available at: http://www.cdc.gov/ncbddd/childdevelopment/positiveparenting/adolescence .html; Middle adolescence (15–17 years old): Developmental milestones. Available at: http://www.cdc.gov/ncbddd /childdevelopment/positiveparenting/adolescence2.html. Accessed August 10, 2011.

concept of possession (what is mine vs. what is yours), express affection more openly, and can separate from parents more easily (CDC, 2010a).

Important Milestones for Children (Ages 4–11 Years)

As infants age into childhood, more complex social, emotional, and cognitive milestones are reached. During the fourth year of life children become interested in new experiences, can cooperate with other children, participate in "fantasy play" where they assume the roles of others, can follow three-part commands, and try to solve problems from a single point of view. By age 5 children want to please friends, become more like their friends, are more likely to agree to rules, show more independence, are aware of gender, and can distinguish between fantasy and reality (CDC, 2010a). During the ages of 6 and 8 rapid mental development occurs, and important milestones include a stronger sense of right and wrong, having an awareness of the future, attending more to friendships and teamwork, and having a desire to be liked or accepted by friends (CDC, 2010b). By middle childhood (9–11 years old) children are growing more independent, and because friendships are very important, peer pressure can become strong during this time. During these years children start to form more complex friendships and peer relationships/networks, become more independent from their family, become aware of their body (especially as they approach puberty), and face more academic challenges at school (CDC, 2010c).

Important Milestones for Adolescents (Ages 12–19 Years)

Adolescence is a time in which many mental, emotional, and physical changes occur. In early adolescence (ages 12–14 years) body image becomes a greater concern, and **adolescents** at this age focus on self, go back and forth between high expectations and low confidence, display increasing moodiness, become more interested and influenced by peer groups, show less affection and attention toward family members, and are better able to express their feelings through talking (CDC, 2010d). During middle adolescence (ages 15–17 years) most girls become physically mature, whereas boys continue to mature. During this time adolescents show an increased interest in the opposite sex, have less conflict with parents, display increased independence from parents, develop a deeper capacity for caring and sharing with developing more intimate relationships, and start to have concerns about future educational and vocational plans. Finally, during the final years of adolescence they begin to realize the importance of their parents to a greater extent, peer groups become less important and are replaced with fewer, closer friendships, and unrealistic fantasies from early adolescence are replaced with more realistic plans (CDC, 2010e).

DETERMINANTS AND INFLUENCES ON MENTAL HEALTH OF INFANTS, CHILDREN, AND ADOLESCENTS

Several factors influence the mental health of infants, children, and adolescents as they develop. These factors are displayed in **Figure 9.1** and discussed below.

Gender and Sex

Although the terms "gender" and "sex" may appear to be synonymous, they are in fact distinct from one another. **Sex** refers to the biological factors of being a man or a woman. For example, humans typically have 46 pairs of chromosomes, with the 23rd pair determining sex: two X chromosomes produce a female and an X and Y chromosome produce a male. However, **gender** refers to the social dimensions of being a man or a woman and is often more flexible. There are two aspects of gender: gender identity and gender role.

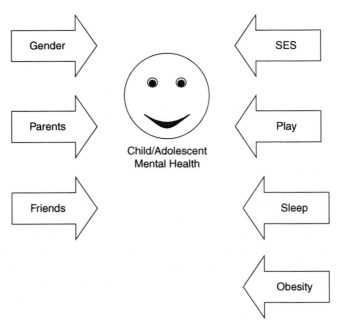

FIGURE 9.1   Determinants of child/adolescent mental health.

Gender identity refers to the sense of belongingness to one sex, and **gender role** refers to a set of expectations one believes a certain sex should fulfill. Differences in mental health among sexes can come from several factors, including both (1) may experience different environmental risk factors, (2) experience different levels of the same environmental risk factor, (3) have different biological processes, (4) require different thresholds of biological or genetic risk for mental health problems, and (5) experience environmental and biological interactions differently (Zahn-Waxler, Shirtcliff, & Marceau, 2008).

During infancy there do not appear to be many differences in problematic behaviors between girls and boys. Studies with infants and toddlers have shown no difference in aggression, activity levels, or difficult temperament between sexes. After infancy and into early childhood, however, differences are more likely to emerge. Boys are 3 to 10 times more likely to experience externalizing problems such as conduct disorders, language disorders, defiant disorder, physical aggression, and attention deficit hyperactivity disorder than girls, and girls are more likely to experience adolescent-onset, internalizing problems such as emotional disorders, depression, mood disorders, anxiety disorders, and eating disorders than boys (Crick & Zahn-Waxler, 2003). Adolescent boys continue to engage in greater physical aggression and violence (i.e., criminal behavior) more so than girls (Loeber & Stouthamer–Loeber, 1997).

> *Gender and sex are commonly used interchangeably; however, they can mean something different. Gender is more of a social variable, whereas sex is a biological variable.*

Parents

Parents and their parenting styles can affect the mental health of their children. As of 2010, 69% of children lived with two parents (including biological, step, or adoptive parents), 27% lived with only one parent, and 4% did not live with either parent (Federal Interagency Forum on Child and Family Statistics, 2010). Although parents can exhibit a variety of parenting styles, there are four basic styles based on two dimensions: *responsiveness* and *demandingness* (Baumrind, 1991) **(Table 9.2)**. The **authoritarian parenting style** is restrictive, places firm boundaries on the child, and does not allow children to have much say in decisions (highly demanding and direct but low responsiveness). Children living with parents who enforce this style have reported greater feelings of unhappiness, fearfulness, and anxiety. The **authoritative parenting style** encourages children to be independent thinkers and gives them choices among a defined set a boundaries (both highly demanding and responsive). Children living with parents who enforce this style have reported greater feelings of cheerfulness, self-control, and self-reliance and are overall more socially competent. The **neglectful parenting style** is one in which parents are uninvolved with their children (neither demanding nor responsive). Children living with parents who enforce this style are typically socially incompetent and lack a sense of self-control, and children growing up in this environment are generally least competent of all styles. Finally, the **permissive parenting style** is one in which parents are highly involved in their children's life but few demands are placed on them (highly responsive, but not demanding). Children living with parents who enforce this style are typically socially incompetent and lack self-control.

Using these four parenting styles there is a possibility of 16 different parent dyads for children and adolescents who live with both parents. A study on adolescents found those with both parents using the authoritative style had the best mental health outcomes. It also found that in households with one authoritative parent, in most cases, that parent buffered the child from the consequences of living in a household with neglectful and permissive parenting styles (Simons & Conger, 2007).

Friends

Several behavioral theories consider the extent to which friends and peer relationships contribute to mental health. In the transtheoretical model a key process of change is *helping relationships*, which refer to developing caring, open, and accepting relationships. In the

TABLE 9.2   Parenting Styles by Responsiveness and Demandingness

	Demandingness	
	High	**Low**
Responsiveness		
High	Authoritative	Permissive
Low	Authoritarian	Neglectful

Source: Data from Baumrind, D. (1991). The influence of parenting style on adolescent competence and substance use. *Journal of Early Adolescence, 11,* 56–95.

theory of planned behavior an important construct is *subjective norms*, which suggests that the thoughts and opinions of significant others in an individual's life will influence his or her behaviors (Sharma & Romas, 2008).

Friendships during childhood serve six major functions: companionship, stimulation, physical support, ego support, social comparison, and intimacy/affection. Companionship refers to having a familiar partner or peer with whom one spends time and engages in activities. Stimulation refers to activities shared with friends that are interesting, exciting, and amusing. Physical support refers to time, resources, and assistance friends often provide. Ego support refers to emotional support and encouragement, which in turns allows the individual to see him- or herself as competent, attractive, and interesting. Social comparison allows children to compare the ways they act toward others, to determine whether their behavior is considered normal. Finally, intimacy and affection refer to trusting relationships with friends in which self-disclosure takes place (Santrock, 2002).

The quality and quantity of friends are especially important in childhood. One study showed that shy and withdrawn children were as likely as nonaggressive and nonwithdrawn children (control) to have mutual stable best friendships; however, withdrawn children's friends were more withdrawn and victimized than other children's friends. Similarities in social withdrawal and peer victimization were also shown for withdrawn children and their friends. Withdrawn children also have reported lower friendship quality than nonwithdrawn children (Rubin, Wojslawowicz, Rose-Krasnor, Booth-LaForce, & Burgess, 2006). Another study found children who were more accepted in kindergarten were less likely to be chronically abused by peers from kindergarten to fourth grade, were less likely to be chronically excluded by peers, and those rated as more acceptable by their peers in kindergarten were likely to have higher standardized achievement scores. Chronically excluded children were also more likely to be disengaged in their school classrooms, which can lead to lower achievement outcomes (Buhs, Ladd, & Herald, 2006). One study evaluated whether friendship was a moderator between peer victimization and internalizing difficulties (such as being withdrawn, lack of humor, or self-esteem) and externalizing behavioral problems (lashing out, aggression, disruptiveness). Researchers found that having a friend decreased children's risk of being victimized over the school year, and children without friends typically had greater internalizing and external behavioral problems (Hodges, Boivin, Bukowski, & Vitaro, 1999).

The quality and quantity of friends are especially important in childhood.

Play

"Playing" in childhood is important in that it has been shown to contribute to the cognitive, physical, social, and emotional well-being of children. Play serves many purposes, including allowing children to socialize with peers, release tension, increase curiosity, and advance in their cognitive development. The United Nations Convention on the Rights of the Child, article 31, states children have the right to engage in rest, leisure, play, and recreation activities (United Nations General Assembly, 1989). Play can be described as a spontaneous activity in which children engage to amuse and to occupy themselves (Burdette & Whitaker, 2005). However, play is limited among some children because of neighborhood violence, poverty, and, in some countries, an increased reliance on child labor.

Children are also being raised in a "hurry up and go" environment, whereby busy parents and academic pressures make it difficult for children to find extra time to play. This is evident in our own public schools. With the No Child Left Behind legislation, schools and school districts are under increased pressure to focus efforts on academic areas that are tested through standardized examinations that excludes physical education classes and recess, which give children the opportunity to play.

Bergin (1998) describes five types of play among children. **Sensorimotor play** is often displayed in infants and is any behavior that derives pleasure from exercising existing sensorimotor schema. **Practice play** is similar; however, this starts in childhood and includes any repetition of behavior when learning new skills or when physical or mental mastery are needed for games or sports. **Pretense or symbolic play** is when children transform their surroundings into symbols. **Social play** involves any type of play performed with peers. **Constructive play** is a combination of sensorimotor play, practice play, and symbolic play. Finally, **games** are activities that can be played alone or with others and typically include a defined set of rules and competition with others.

Play is also used as a type of therapy for children, known as play therapy. This type of therapy is unique to children because many younger than age 11 do not have the ability for abstract thought, which is needed for identifying underlying causes to mental health issues (Bratton, Ray, & Rhine, 2005). Therefore, unlike adults, who can communicate through talk therapy, children can best express themselves through play and activity therapy. During play therapy, play is seen as a means for communication between the child and the therapist. It is assumed that children will use play in such a way that directly or symbolically shows their feelings, thoughts, and experiences. Play therapy has been shown to be effective across different age groups, genders, and target problem behaviors (Bratton et al., 2005).

While playing children have the opportunity to practice and demonstrate many skills and tasks that prepare them for more complex situations as they get older. For example, when children play in groups they sustain relationships, learn teamwork, engage in sharing, negotiate, and use conflict resolution skills. While playing they also encounter opportunities for decision making, which stimulate problem-solving skills, creative thinking, and imagination. Problem solving can also promote executive functioning—a higher level skill that integrates attention and other cognitive functions such as planning, organizing, sequencing, and decision making (Burdette & Whitaker, 2005). Physical activity and play are often interchangeable with children. One study found aerobic capacity, which is a measure of physical activity, was positively associated with reading achievement, math achievement, and total academic achievement, whereas body mass index (BMI) was inversely related to these areas of academic achievement (Castelli, Hillman, Buck, & Erwin, 2007).

Sleep and Sleep Patterns

Adequate sleep is essential for mental health. Current studies suggest that 25% to 40% of children and adolescents experience some type of sleep problem (Mindell & Meltzer, 2008). Sleep problems can range from physiological, such as obstructive sleep apnea, to behavioral, such as insomnia. Sleep recommendations in infancy, childhood, and adolescence greatly vary. According to the National Sleep Foundation (2009) newborns (0–2 months) require 12 to 18 hours, infants (3–11 months) require 14 to 15 hours, toddlers (1–3 years) require

12 to 14 hours, preschoolers (3–5 years) require 11 to 13 hours, school-age children (5–10 years) require 10 to 11 hours, and teens (10–17 years) require 8.5 to 9.25 hours.

In one study designed to measure the association between habitual sleep duration and cognitive functioning in healthy, non–sleep-deprived children, researchers found that longer habitual sleep duration in healthy children was associated with better performance on measures of perceptual reasoning, overall IQ, and reported measures of competence and academic performance (Gruber et al., 2010). A study done with infants and young children (ages 1.5–5 years) found that nighttime sleep duration and hyperactivity were significantly associated, in that children with shorter nighttime sleep duration had higher rates of hyperactivity (Touchette et al., 2009).

Also, certain conditions are greatly associated with sleep disturbances from infancy to adolescence, such as learning disability, cerebral palsy, visual impairment, psychiatric disorders such as attention deficit hyperactivity disorder (ADHD), abuse-related trauma and depressive symptoms, developmental disorders such as autism, and general psychological problems (Wiggs & France, 2000). A study conducted in Taiwan found adolescents with a childhood diagnosis of ADHD were more likely to have current and lifetime sleep problems and sleep disorders including insomnia, sleep terrors, nightmares, bruxism, and snoring (Gau & Chiang, 2009).

> *Approximately 25% to 40% of children and adolescents experience some type of sleep problem.*
>
> —Mindell & Meltzer (2008)

Socioeconomic Status

Socioeconomic status (SES) is a measure of an individual's economic and social position in society. SES is typically composed of three variables: income, educational attainment, and current employment status. However, some studies may only use one indicator of SES to describe an individual, such as poverty status. In 2008, 14.1 million of all children (19%) lived in poverty, which is the highest rate since 1998. African American children made up the largest percentage of those children (35%), whereas Hispanics were not far behind (31%) and Whites were much lower (11%) (Federal Interagency Forum on Child and Family Statistics, 2010). Low SES neighborhoods commonly have high unemployment rates and a large percentage of families on welfare. These neighborhoods are also more dangerous for children. Crime and violence rates are higher in lower SES communities, and the air and water quality are usually worse, due to outdated municipal services (Evans, 2004).

Academic disparities are also found among children from low and high SES families. On a national literacy assessment students from lower SES households scored much lower than students from higher SES households (Lee, Grigg, & Donahue, 2007). These disparities are attributable to factors that occur before and during the time children spend in school. Before school, children from lower SES households tend to have fewer literary opportunities, including fewer books in their homes, and they attend lesser quality preschools that tend to emphasize academic activities less. While attending school, children from lower SES households typically take classes from more inexperienced teachers, have low amounts of family involvement with their academics, and have less overall resources, such as computers. Children from lower SES household also are often exposed to more family conflicts and violence, are separated from their family members, and live in unstable homes. Parents of children in lower SES households are also often less support-ive and less responsive and tend to use the authoritarian parenting style (Evans, 2004).

FOCUS FEATURE 9.1 KIDSCREEN STUDY FROM 12 EUROPEAN COUNTRIES

As you have learned in this chapter, there is a great prevalence of child and adolescent mental health problems. These problems burden the individual by leading to lower academic achievement, and these problems can burden the family by increasing the stress and frustration of family members involved. Such mental health problems can persist into adulthood; therefore, there is great need to promote prevention efforts. Mental health issues can be difficult to define and measure in populations. The aim of the European KIDSCREEN Project is to examine the cross-national differences in the prevalence of children's and adolescents' mental health problems and identify associated problems of mental health issues. The project involved 12 European countries: Austria, Switzerland, Czech Republic, Germany, Spain, France, Greece, Hungary, the Netherlands, Poland, Sweden, and the United Kingdom. This study was comprehensive and used various methods of measurements as described in **Table 9.3**.

TABLE 9.3   Measurements and Scales Used in the KIDSCREEN Study

Name of Scale	Measures
The Strength and Difficulties Questionnaire (SDQ) (Goodman, 1997)	Evaluated mental health symptoms and positive attitudes
Family Affluence Scale (FAS) (Currie, Elton, Todd & Platt, 1997)	Evaluated SES
Oslo Three-Item Support Scale (Brevik & Dalgard, 1996)	Evaluated children's level of social support
Short Form 12 Health Survey (SF-12) (Ware, Kosinski, & Keller, 1996)	Evaluated parents' well-being and mental problems
KIDSCREEN-10 (Ravens-Sieberer et al., 2005)	Evaluated health-related quality of life (i.e., mood, emotions, autonomy, satisfaction with relationships)

The final sample of children enrolled in this study was 15,945, with countries' response rates varying from as high as 91.2% (Sweden) to as low as 24.2% (Spain). Mental health problems varied consider-ably across nations, with the highest prevalence found in the United Kingdom, Czech Republic, France, Hungary, and Greece. Factors found to be associated with higher mental health problems in childhood and adolescence included lower SES, poor social support, poor parental relations, and parental mental health problems. The largest and most stable risk factor for mental health issues was social support. Gender displayed only a small association with health problems; however, there were differences across gender in the types of mental health issues: girls reported higher emotional symptoms, whereas boys reported higher levels of conduct problems (Ravens-Sieberer et al., 2008).

Obesity and Overweight

Among youth, overweight and obesity are defined using growth charts published by the CDC. Children (ages 2–20) with a BMI for age and sex greater or equal to the 95th per-centile are classified as obese, and overweight is defined as a BMI for age and sex greater or equal to 85th percentile (CDC, 2010g). During the past three decades the prevalence of child and adolescent obesity has tripled, and disparities are commonly noted among minority groups. Currently, 16.9% of children (ages 2–19) are obese and 31.7% are overweight. (Ogden, Carroll, Curin, Lamb, & Flegal, 2010.)

As reported in the 2009 American Heart Association Childhood Obesity Research Summit Report, overweight children and adolescents consistently experience greater psychological distress such as high rates of depression, low reported self-esteem, social marginalization, and negative body image compared with their normal weight peers (Daniels, Jacobson, McCrindle, Eckel, & Sanner, 2009). Misconceptions are commonly placed on obese youth that may reinforce a negative body image that include personal traits such as laziness, selfishness, and lower intelligence (Wilkinson, 2008). Adolescence is also a time when individuals have heightened sensitivity about their perceived body image. In a study with adolescents measuring perceptions of body weight, 8.8% of the youth were measured as obese, but 12.7% self-reported themselves as "fat." Obesity rates were also higher among males; however, females were more likely to consider themselves "fat" (De Sousa, 2008).

In a study examining the relationship of depression and obesity among adolescents in grades 7 through 12, those with the highest BMIs were found to have the highest rate of depression (Goodman & Whitaker, 2002). After a 1-year follow-up, sustained elevated BMIs were again positively associated with higher depression rates. Another study found obese female adolescents (as compared with nonobese female adolescents) were less likely to associate with friends, more likely to report feelings of hopelessness, more likely to report serious emotional problems, and more likely to report a suicide attempt within the past week (Olds, 2009).

Overweight and obese adolescents also tend to engage in harmful health behaviors to either lose weight or cope with stress. The 2009 Youth Risk Behavior Survey reported that 4.0–10.6% of adolescents engage in unhealthy dietary practices (i.e., food restricting; purging; using laxatives/diuretics; consuming diet pills, powders, or liquids); however, these behaviors increase with age and are more common with overweight adolescents than normal weight adolescents (Eaton et al., 2010). Female adolescents may also be more vulnerable than males for such behaviors. In another study researchers reported 18% of overweight females engaged in unhealthy dietary behaviors such as taking diet pills and laxatives/diuretics and vomiting (Jasik & Lustig, 2008).

Bullying is another issue that faces obese and overweight adolescents, as the two are generally predictive of one another. Weight-based teasing has also been negatively associated with usage of unhealthy weight control methods, decreased body satisfaction and self-concept, and depressive symptoms. In turn, higher body dissatisfaction has also been noted to be associated with higher rates of depression and anxiety (Daniels, et al., 2009).

Autism

Autism is another important determinant of mental health among children and adolescents. The way in which the word *autism* is used in today's society can be misleading. Autism is formally known as **autism spectrum disorder** (ASD) and includes a group of developmental deficits across three domains: social interaction, communication, and repetitive or stereotypic behavior (Newschaffer et al., 2007). The term *spectrum disorder* signifies that ASD affects individuals in different ways, which can make them difficult to diagnose. The three main types of ASDs are autistic disorder, Asperger syndrome, and pervasive developmental disorder not otherwise specified. **Autistic disorder** (or classic autism) describes those who have significant language delays, social and communication challenges, unusual behaviors and interests, and often intellectual disabilities. **Asperger syndrome** is typically seen as a milder version of autistic disorder. Individuals with this diagnosis are likely to have social challenges and unusual behaviors or interests without the intellectual disabilities associated with autistic disorder. Finally, **pervasive developmental disorder not otherwise specified** (or atypical autism) describes individuals who only meet some of the criteria for autistic disorder and Asperger syndrome but typically have fewer and milder symptoms (CDC, 2010h).

Throughout the 1980s ASDs were considered rare; however, today they are the second most commonly diagnosed developmental disability among children, with mental retardation being the first (Newschaffer et al., 2007). ASDs are found equally among all racial, ethnic, and socioeconomic groups, but boys are four times more likely to be diagnosed than girls (CDC, 2010h). Diagnosing ASDs can be difficult because there is no biological or blood test that health professionals can use. Rather, health professionals rely on objective evaluations, such as the achievement of developmental milestones, and subjective evaluations, such as evaluating a variety of behavioral characteristics commonly associated with ASDs like social responsiveness, communication, and play (Landa, 2008). ASDs are also commonly diagnosed with other conditions that affect mental health such as mental retardation, behavioral difficulties (i.e., perseveration, obsessiveness, aggression), hyperactivity, and psychiatric symptoms such as anxiety and depression (CDC, 2010h).

MALADAPTIVE BEHAVIORS IN CHILDHOOD

Conduct Disorder and Oppositional Defiant Disorder

Conduct disorders are defined in the *Diagnostic and Statistical Manual of Mental Disorders*, 4th edition, text revision (DSM-IV-TR), as a "repetitive and persistent pattern of behavior in which the basic rights of others or major age-appropriate societal norms or rules are violated" (American Psychiatric Association [APA], 2000, p. 98). Diagnosis of conduct disorders includes the engagement in at least three behaviors that fall into four main categories (APA, 2000):

1. Aggressive conduct that causes or threatens physical harm to other people or animals (i.e., physical harm toward others or animals)
2. Nonaggressive conduct that causes property loss or damage (i.e., deliberately causing fire with the intent to harm others)
3. Deceitfulness or theft
4. Serious violations of rules (i.e., skipping school or staying out late despite parental prohibition)

These disturbances must also cause clinically significant impairments to social, academic, or occupational functioning (APA, 2000).

Along with conduct disorders, **oppositional defiant disorders** are the most common reasons for referral of children and adolescents to outpatient mental health clinics and residential treatment centers (Kimonis & Frick, 2010). Oppositional defiant disorders are similar to conduct disorders; however, they are commonly seen as a precipitating behavior and less serious. Oppositional defiant disorders are defined in the DSM-IV-TR as a "recurrent pattern of negativistic, defiant, disobedient, and hostile behavior toward authority figures that persists for at least 6 months" (APA, 2000, p. 100). Diagnosis of oppositional defiant disorders includes the engagement in at least four of the following behaviors (APA, 2000):

1. Losing temper
2. Arguing with adults
3. Actively defying or refusing to comply with the requests or rules of adults
4. Deliberately doing things that will annoy other people
5. Blaming others for his or her own mistakes or misbehavior
6. Being touchy or easily annoyed by others
7. Being angry and resentful
8. Being spiteful or vindictive

Using data from the National Comorbidity Survey Replication, researchers estimate the lifetime prevalence of conduct disorders to be 9.5%, affecting significantly more males (12.0%) than females (7.1%). Individual conduct disorder symptoms also greatly varied, from as high as 32.8% for those who reported repeatedly staying out at night without parental permission to as low as 0.3% who reported forcing sexual activity upon others (Nock, Kazdin, Hiripi, & Kessler, 2006). The estimated lifetime prevalence of oppositional defiant disorders was estimated to be 10.2%; however, rates were not significantly different between males (11.2%) and females (9.2%) (Nock, Kazdin, Hiripi, & Kessler, 2007). Data from the National Comorbidity Survey Replication also indicated that conduct disorders and oppositional defiant disorders are significantly associated with an increased risk of all other mental disorders including (but not limited to) alcohol abuse or dependence, drug abuse or dependence, and any mood or anxiety disorder. The only exception was conduct disorders were not significantly associated with an increase risk of agoraphobia (Nock et al., 2006, 2007).

Youth Violence and Bullying

Currently, violence is the second leading cause of death among youth (ages 10–24), with approximately 5,764 deaths associated annually (CDC, 2010i). **Youth violence** can include many forms of behavior that lead to serious injury, emotional harm, and even death. Behaviors can include violent acts, such as bullying, slapping, or punching; verbal altercations, such as harassment or yelling; and life-threatening acts, such as assault with a deadly weapon. Nationwide, 17.5% of high schools students reported carrying a weapon (i.e., gun, knife) at least once a month. Rates are higher among males (27.1%) compared with females (7.1%) and higher among Whites (18.6%) and Hispanics (17.2%) compared with African Americans (14.4%). Also, 31.5% of high school student reported being in at least one physical fight in the past month. Rates were higher among males (39.3%) compared with females (22.9%) and higher among African Americans (41.4%) and Hispanics (36.2%), compared with Whites (27.8%) (Eaton et al., 2010).

Violence affects all youth to some extent; however, some groups are more vulnerable to violence and victimization than others. Four distinct types of risk factors can increase the chances youth are involved with violence: interpersonal, family, peer/social, and community. Individual risk factors include a history of victimization; ADHD or other learning disorders; a history of aggressive behavior; involvement with drugs, alcohol, or tobacco; lower IQ; poor self-control; deficits in social cognitive or information-processing abilities; stress; preexisting emotional problems; and antisocial behaviors. Family risk factors include parents who use authoritarian parenting styles, disengaged or uninterested parent, parents living in poverty, parental engagement in substance abuse or criminal activities, and overall poor family functioning. Peer/social risk factors include having delinquent friends, gang involvement, social rejection by peers, low involvement in community activities, poor academic performance, and low commitment to school. Finally, community risk factors include living in low SES areas, low levels of community participation, and living in socially disorganized neighborhoods (Eaton, et al., 2010; Resnick, Ireland, & Borowsky, 2004; Stith-Prothrow, 1995).

Youth violence holds obvious physical consequences such as injury or death, but it also can lead to serious mental health–related consequences. For example, adolescents who are victimized are at greater risk of developing psychological and behavioral problems, such as depression, alcohol abuse, anxiety, and suicidal behaviors (Krug, Mercy, Dahlberg, & Zwi, 2002). Being a victim of bullying has been shown to be associated with (1) low psychological well-being, which includes feelings of general unhappiness, low-self esteem, anger, and sadness; (2) poor social adjustment, which refers to feelings of aversion toward your social environment, loneliness, or absenteeism; (3) psychological distress, which is more serious than the first area and includes higher levels of anxiety, depression, and suicidal thoughts; and (4) physical unwellness, which includes signs of physical disorders (Rigby, 2003).

Violence is the second leading cause of death among youth (ages 10–24).

Suicide

Suicide is the third leading cause of death among youth (ages 10–24), with approximately 4,400 deaths associated annually (CDC, 2009). The World Health Organization (2007) describes **suicide** as "the result of an act deliberately initiated and performed by a person in the full knowledge or expectation of its fatal outcome". Suicidal behaviors are often prevalent among adolescents and are often distinguished between suicidal ideation and attempted suicide. **Suicidal ideation** refers to thoughts of harming or killing oneself. **Attempted suicide** refers to a nonfatal, self-inflicted destructive act with explicit or implicit intent to die. Finally, **suicidality** refers to all suicide-related behaviors and thoughts including completing or attempting suicide, suicidal ideation, or communications (Bridge, Goldstein, & Brent, 2006; Goldsmith, Pellmar, Kleinman, & Bunney, 2002).

Suicide affects all youth, but some groups are at higher risk than others. Suicide rates are much greater in male compared with female adolescents. For example, the suicide mortality rates (per 100,000) for children and young adolescents is 1.0 for boys and 0.3 for girls, and rates among older adolescents and young adulthood (15–24) are 16.1 for boys compared with 3.5 for girls (WHO, 2002). Suicide attempts, however, are more common among female adolescents. Data from the National Comorbidity Survey found among young suicide attempters, 64% were female and 36% were male (Nock et al., 2006). The 2007 Youth

Risk Behavior Surveillance System found that among high school students (9th through 12th grades) 14.5% had suicide ideation, 11.3% had made a suicide plan, 6.9% had attempted suicide, and 2% had been treated by a physician or nurse from harmful effects of their suicide attempt (Eaton et al., 2008).

Suicide rates are also higher among homosexual adolescents. A study using data from the National Longitudinal Study of Adolescent Health found that 17.2% of lesbian, gay, and bisexual (LGB) adolescents reported suicidal ideation, whereas only 6.3% of non-LGB adolescents reported such thoughts. Furthermore, 4.9% of LGB adolescents reported suicide attempts, whereas only 1.6% of non-LGB adolescents reported suicide attempts (Silenzio, Pena, Duberstein, Cerel, & Knox, 2007).

The top methods used for suicide among adolescents are firearms (46%), suffocation (37%), and poisoning (8%). The most commonly reported method for suicide attempts is the ingestion of pills (Shain, 2007). Risk factors associated with suicide among children and adolescents include history of previous suicide attempts, family history of suicide, history of depression or other mental condition, alcohol or drug abuse, stressful life events, easy access to lethal methods, exposure to the suicidal behavior of others, incarceration, and physical or sexual abuse (CDC, 2009; Hawton & James, 2005; Nock et al., 2006).

Many consequences are associated with suicidal behaviors. One longitudinal study following Dutch children for 11 years found childhood suicide ideation highly predicted suicide ideation in adulthood, greater lifetime history of suicide attempt, and increased likelihood for mood and anxiety disorder in adulthood (Herba, Ferdinand, Ende, & Verhulst, 2007). Another study found that suicidality among a large cohort of Australian youth (ages 13–15; including suicidal thoughts, plans, and threats) was negatively associated with perceived academic performance, self-esteem, and locus of control (Martin, Richardson, Bergen, Roeger, & Allison, 2005).

Suicide is the third leading cause of death among youth (ages 10–24).

Attention Deficit Hyperactivity Disorder

Attention Deficit Hyperactivity Disorder (ADHD) has been associated with many developmental, cognitive, emotional, social, and academic impairments among children and adolescents (Wehmeier, Schacht, & Barkley, 2010). It has been estimated that 4.5 million children between the ages of 5 and 17 years have been diagnosed with ADHD, and rates have dramatically increased in the last few decades (Bloom & Cohen, 2007). For example, the average annual increase in the percentage of children diagnosed with ADHD was 3% from 1997 to 2006 (Pastor & Reuben, 2008). The CDC (2010f) describes ADHD as individuals "who have trouble paying attention, controlling impulsive behaviors (might act without thinking about what the result will be), and in some cases, are overly active." Sometimes ADHD is referred to as ADD (attention deficit disorder), but these terms are used interchangeably. ADHD is diagnosed using the DSM-IV-TR (APA, 2000). To diagnose ADHD children must display six or more behaviors from one of two groups of symptoms for attention deficit, hyperactivity, or impulsivity, and impairment must be present in at least two domains of life (APA, 2000).

ADHD affects all youth, but some groups are at higher risk than others. For example, ADHD rates are much greater in male compared with female adolescents. Using a nationally representative sample, it was found that overall 8.4% of children have been diagnosed with ADHD; however, 10.7% of boys had been diagnosed and 6.6% of girls had been diagnosed (Pastor & Reuben, 2008). ADHD rates also appear to increase with age: 7.1% of youth ages 6 to 11 have been diagnosed with ADHD, whereas 9.6% of youth ages 12–17 years have been diagnosed with ADHD (Pastor, et al., 2008). There are also reported disparities between race, with non-Hispanic Whites (9.8%) having the highest rates, followed by non-Hispanic Blacks (8.6%), and Hispanics (5.3%) reportedly have the lowest rates (Pastor, et al., 2008). The family environment also appears to be a risk factor: children living with only their mothers have been shown to have higher rates of diagnosis (11.2%), compared with children who live with both parents (7.1%) (Pastor, et al., 2008). ADHD greatly varies by region as well, with Colorado (~5%), California (~5.5%), and Utah (~5.5%) having the three lowest prevalences among states, and Alabama (~11%), Louisiana (~10.5%), and West Virginia (10.5%) having the three highest prevalence rates. Finally, ADHD appears to affect children living in families of lower SES more often (9.6%) than children living in families with a higher SES (7.4%) (Visser & Lesesn, 2005).

Children and adolescents diagnosed with ADHD also have a high probability of remaining ADHD as they enter adulthood. It has been reported that up to 65% of children diagnosed with ADHD remained so into adulthood (Wolraich, et al., 2005). There are also reported consequences associated with ADHD. More than 80% of children with ADHD are likely to have at least one other psychiatric disorder, and 50% are likely to have two or more disorders (Wehmeier, Schacht, & Barkley, 2010). Learning disorders are more common among children with ADHD, which can contribute to lower self-esteem and create problems with peer relationships (Wehmeier, et al., 2010). All problems associated with ADHD have been shown to affect the quality of life for both the children who are diagnosed and the families with whom they live (Wehmeier, et al., 2010).

In a report using a nationally representative sample of children, researchers found those with a history of ADHD were six times more likely to have academic difficulties than children without a history of ADHD, as well as higher emotional and conduct problems (Strine et al., 2006). Children with ADHD were also nine times more likely to have an overall emotional and behavioral problem compared with children without ADHD and have difficulties with home life, peer relationships, classroom learning, and leisure activities. Parents also see the effects ADHD has on their children. Parents have reported that children with ADHD have 3 times as many peer problems than those without ADHD and are almost 10 times more likely to have difficulties that interfere with their friendships (Strine et al., 2006).

Eating Disorders

Many adolescents suffer from disordered eating. Eating disorders include a variety of behaviors that lead to abnormal eating behaviors. The most common eating disorders are anorexia nervosa and bulimia nervosa. **Anorexia nervosa** (AN) is a psychiatric illness whereby the patient refuses to maintain a body weight within normal guidelines. Criteria for diagnosing AN using the DSM-IV-TR include maintaining a body weight greater than or equal to 85% of ideal body weight, intense fear of become fat or gaining weight, disturbances in the way an individual assesses his or her own body weight (i.e., views themselves as fat/overweight when they are not), and amenorrhea for postmenarchal women. **Bulimia nervosa** (BN) is an illness whereby the patient consumes a large amount of calories at one sitting and then engages in a compensatory behavior in an attempt to alleviate his or her body from these calories. Compensatory methods can include purging (i.e., vomiting, use of laxatives) or nonpurging (i.e., excessive exercise, periods of starvation). Criteria for diagnosing BN using the DSM-IV-TR include recurrent episodes of binge eating, a sense of lack of control during the episode, recurrent inappropriate compensatory behaviors (i.e., vomiting, misuse of laxatives, diuretics, enemas, fasting, or excessive exercise), and self-evaluation is heavily influenced by body shape and weight. Finally, eating disorders that have not been classified by the DSM-IV-TR fall into the category of **eating disorder not otherwise specified**. The most common eating disorder that falls into this category is **binge eating disorder**, which is similar to BN but the inappropriate compensatory behaviors are not typically present (APA, 2000).

Eating disorders affects all youth, but some groups are at higher risk than others. For example, 17.9% of girls have been diagnosed with some eating disorder in their lives, compared with only 6.5% of boys. Specifically, the lifetime prevalence of AN was 0.7% for girls and 0.2% for boys, of BN was 1.2% for girls and 0.4% for boys, of eating disorder not otherwise specified was 14.6% for girls and 5.0% for boys, and of binge eating disorder was 1.5% for girls and 0.9% for boys (Kjelsas, Bjornstrom, & Gotestam, 2004). Age at onset for AN and BN are also different. AN can develop earlier from about 8 years of age, whereas BN is rare below the age of 13. AN also reaches its peak around ages 15 to 18 years, whereas BN becomes more common than AN by young adulthood (Gowers, 2008). Another study found that boys and girls with ADHD were at higher risk for BN symptoms than children without ADHD (Mikami et al., 2010).

Eating disorders have many consequences. Body dissatisfaction has been identified as an important risk factor for eating disorders and contributes significantly to poor self-esteem and depression among adolescents. It has been reported that as many as 46% of girls and 26% of boys are dissatisfied with their body size and shape, whereas only 12% of girls and 17% of boys report they are satisfied with their body size and shape (Presnell, 2007). This dissatisfaction is related to overall distress and unhealthy weight control behaviors and can lead to extreme methods of altering ones appearance, such as cosmetic surgery and steroid use. One study found that children who first attempted to lose weight below the age of 12 years were more likely to be overweight in adulthood, and the odds of having a binge eating disorder in adulthood was three times greater among those earlier dieters (Rubinstein, McGinn, Wildman, & Wylie-Rosett, 2010). Children and adolescents who attempt weight loss also have increased odds of having unhealthy eating behaviors as an adult. It has also been reported that poor self-esteem, feelings of ineffectiveness, depression, anxiety, impaired concentration, and obsessional symptoms are frequently present in adolescents with eating disorders (Gowers, 2008). If adolescents lose weight while having an eating disorder, they may also become more socially withdrawn and isolated from peers (Gowers, 2008). Longer term medical complications can also be detrimental to adolescents who are still physically developing. For example, adolescents with AN often have disturbances in their linear growth, have a higher risk for osteoporosis, and are at risk for structural and functional brain changes. These complications are serious, as they may not be completely reversible and the impact later in life is unknown (Katzman, 2005).

MENTAL HEALTH INTERVENTIONS FOR CHILDREN AND ADOLESCENTS

Many interventions have been implemented in the community and in schools that target mental health issues among children and adolescents. A study on middle-school children in Italy implemented two interventions to evaluate which approach to improving mental health would yield better results: an intervention designed to promote overall psychological well-being (WBT group) and an intervention designed to remove distress from daily living activities (AM group). Both interventions were 6 weeks long and met once per week. Researcher reported that among the WBT group, significant improvements were made for autonomy and physiological anxiety, whereas among the AM group, anxiety and worrying significantly decreased. Researchers concluded that both interventions were essentially equally effective (Tomba et al., 2010).

Another study evaluated two interventions designed to reduce depressive symptoms among middle-school students. Researchers randomized students into one of three different school-based intervention conditions: The Penn Resiliency Program (PRP), the Penn Enhancement Program (PEP), and a control program (CON). The PRP was a group intervention that aimed to teach students cognitive behavioral and social problem solving skills by linking beliefs, feelings and behaviors; by cognitive restructuring; and by using cognitive styles. While in the program students also learned techniques for coping and problem solving, such as assertiveness, relaxation strategies, and negotiation skills and how to apply these strategies to their own lives. The PEP was a group intervention that aimed to teach students how to identify and deal with stressors in their lives, such as peer pressure, trust and betrayal, friendships, and family conflict. This intervention differed from the PRP in that it did not have aspects of cognitive behavioral therapy. The CON was a control group, and students in this group completed all the evaluations the other groups completed but received no intervention. Students in the PRP and PEP groups met once after school per week for 12 weeks. Overall, there was no reported intervention effect for reducing depressive symptoms in either the PRP or PEN intervention compared with the CON condition; however, there were inconsistent effects for the PRP group, as two of the three PRP groups significantly reduced depressive symptoms (Gillham et al., 2007).

Another example is the FRIENDS intervention, a school-based intervention aimed at the prevention and control of emotional disorders among school children. The intervention was based on evidence-based emotional health cognitive behavior therapy and implemented by school nurses. Evaluations were collected by self-reported questionnaires, interviews, and observations by trained peers. After 3 months of completing the intervention children reported significantly higher levels of self-esteem and lower levels of anxiety. Researchers also examined the effects of the intervention among the most severe children (i.e., highest anxiety scores) and found these children significantly benefited from the intervention (Stallard, Simpson, Anderson, Hibbert, & Osborn, 2007).

Another study evaluated an intervention that aimed to reduce eating disorders among middle-school children. The Healthy Schools-Healthy Kids intervention was a comprehensive, universal intervention implemented in four schools in Canada. The 8-month intervention was multicomponent and included parent education (i.e., workshops, and newsletters), an in-class curriculum implemented to all students, a Girl Talk peer support group implemented by nurses for female students only, a one-session focus group for male students covering topics such as bullying and positive coping skills, a play performed by high school students emphasizing media and peer pressures on body image, and posters and video presentations that were made throughout the school year. The intervention was successful for reducing weight-loss behaviors among students; however, this effect was not found at the 6-month follow-up. Researchers also reported that high-risk students appeared to benefit more from the intervention than low-risk students, with regards to having better body satisfaction, reducing disordered eating, and internalizing media ideas (McVey, Tweed, & Blackmore, 2007).

A study evaluated two interventions designed to reduce depressive symptoms among high-school students. Researchers randomized students into one of three different intervention conditions. The first intervention was based on cognitive behavior therapy, which aims to teach students to (1) monitor their daily moods; (2) identify events that cause stress; (3) discover, challenge, realistically evaluate, and revise negative beliefs; (4) recognize the connections among stressful events, beliefs, and consequences; and (5) learn problem-solving and coping techniques. The second intervention was an interpersonal psychotherapy–adolescent skills training program (IP-AST), which is an extension of interpersonal therapy, found to be effective in the treatment of depression in adolescents. This type of therapy aims to teach adolescents how to communicate appropriately and have adequate social skills to develop and maintain positive relationships, which in turn will prevent depression. The final group was a control group that attended a standard health class. At the end of the interventions adolescents in the cognitive behavior and IPT-AST groups did not differ with regards to improvements in depression scores; however, both groups reported significantly lower depression scores than the control group. Adolescents with the highest reported depression scores also did significantly better than those with lower baseline depression scores in both intervention groups. Improvements, however, were not retained after a 6-month follow-up period (Horowitz, Garber, Ciesla, Young, & Mufson, 2007).

Another example is the 5-2-1 Go! intervention, which was implemented to promote healthy eating behaviors and physical activity to reduce the prevalence of overweight and prevent disordered eating habits to middle-school students. The intervention was a school-wide program implemented over a 2-year period to 808 middle-school students from six different schools. Researchers found that after a 30-day follow-up period the odds of disordered weight control methods were reduced by two-thirds in the treatment condition, compared with the control condition, and significantly more girls (3.6%) reported disordered weight control behaviors in a control intervention, compared with students receiving the 5-2-1 Go! intervention (1.2%). There was no difference, however, for these behaviors in boys in both interventions (Austin et al., 2007).

Another study evaluated an intervention aimed to reduce depressive symptoms among middle-school children by reducing risk factors for depression. The LISA intervention was a primary prevention intervention implemented in Germany. The 10-week intervention was based on the social information processing model and cognitive behavioral therapy and included modules on (1) illustrating the relationship between cognition, emotion, and behavior; (2) exploring and changing dysfunctional cognitions; (3) assertiveness training; and (4) social competence training. Researchers compared students in the LISA intervention with children in a control intervention and found the LISA intervention to be more successful. Student in the LISA intervention sustained lower levels of depression symptoms, whereas students in the control intervention had higher levels of depression symptoms, and students in the LISA intervention reported larger social network sizes. Researchers also reported the intervention was more beneficial for students with baseline low self-efficacy compared with those with baseline high self-efficacy in terms of having fewer depressive symptoms at the 3-month follow-up (Possel, Baldus, Horn, Groen, & Hautizinger, 2005).

The RAP-Kiwi intervention was implemented in New Zealand to prevent depression among middle-school children. The intervention consisted of 11 sessions based on cognitive behavior therapy implemented to 392 middle-school students from two different schools. Researchers found that after the intervention depression was significantly lower in children receiving the intervention, compared with children who received a control intervention. Depression scores were also consistently lower in the RAP-Kiwi intervention group during follow-up measures taken at 6, 12, and 18 months (Merry, McDowell, Wild, Bir, & Cunliffe, 2004).

Another example of an intervention to promote mental health among youth was done with the Los Angeles Unified School District to reduced posttraumatic stress disorder among middle-school children who had experienced or been exposed to high levels of violence. Adolescents attending two middle schools were randomly assigned to a treatment or delayed treatment group and received a 10-week cognitive-based therapy intervention. After the intervention youth in the intervention group had significantly lower posttraumatic stress disorder symptoms (as measured by a Child PTSD Symptom Scale), depression (as measured by a Child Depression Inventory), and parent-reported psychosocial dysfunction (as measured by a Pediatric Symptom Checklist) than youth in the delayed treatment group (Stein et al., 2003).

Finally, the Problem Solving for Life intervention was implemented in Australia to prevent depression among adolescents. The intervention consisted of eight sessions targeting problem-solving skills, positive problem-solving orientation, and optimistic thinking styles implemented over the course of 8 weeks. Researchers compared children receiving the PSFL intervention with children in a control intervention not focused on problem-solving skills and found from before to after the intervention students with initially elevated depression scores (high risk) did significantly better in the PSFL intervention compared with students in the control intervention. Also, significantly less high-risk students in the PSFL intervention retained their high-risk status at the end of the intervention. Significant effects were also seen among students with lower initial depression scores (low risk). Low-risk students in the PSFL group showed a small and significant decrease in depression at the end of the intervention, whereas students in the control condition experienced an increase in depression by the end of the intervention (Spence, Sheffield, & Donovan, 2003).

SKILL-BUILDING ACTIVITY

Imagine you have been asked to work with a group of at-risk children. How would you go about assessing their risk for mental health problems? What factors would you look for? What would be the key topics for your program? What would be the duration of your program? You can take the help of an existing program from this chapter to help you in your task.

SUMMARY

There is no universal definition for term "child", but it generally refers to an individual between the stages of birth and puberty. The three distinct stages of childhood are known as infancy, childhood, and adolescence. There are no set definitions for these time periods, but the CDC classifies infancy as lasting from approximately ages 0 to 3 years, childhood lasting approximately from ages 4 to 11 years, and adolescence lasting from approximately ages 12 to 19 years. As individuals progress through these stages, it is expected they reach both physical and developmental milestones; however, children develop at different rates and therefore these milestones can only act as inexact guidelines.

There are many important determinants to mental health among children and adolescents, including gender, sex, parenting styles, the quality and quantity of friends, playing, sleeping, SES, and obesity. Although the terms "gender" and "sex" may appear to be synonymous, they are in fact distinct. Sex refers to the biological factors of being a man or woman, and gender refers to the social dimensions of being a man or woman. There are two aspects of gender: gender identity, which refers to the sense of belongingness to one sex, and gender role, which refers to a set of expectations one believes a certain sex should fulfill.

The four basic parenting styles are authoritarian, authoritative, neglectful, and permissive. These parenting styles are based on two dimensions: responsiveness and demandingness. Friendships serve six major functions: companionship, stimulation, physical support, ego support, social comparison, and intimacy/affection. Play also serves many purposes, including allowing children to socialize with peers, releasing tension, increasing curiosity, and advancing cognitive development. There are five types of play among children: sensorimotor play/practice play, pretense/symbolic play, social play, constructive play, and games.

Adequate sleep is also essential for mental health. Sleep can affect mental health and such problems can range from physiological, such as obstructive sleep apnea, to behavioral, such as insomnia. Sleep recommendations during infancy, childhood, and adolescents greatly vary.

SES is typically composed of three variables: income, educational attainment, and current employment status. Low SES neighborhoods commonly have high unemployment rates and a large percentage of families on welfare, which have been associated with child and adolescent mental health.

It has been consistently reported that overweight children and adolescents experience greater psychological distress such as high rates of depression, low reported self-esteem, social marginalization, and negative body image compared with their normal weight peers.

Maladaptive behaviors in childhood result from mental health issues, including violence, bullying, suicide, ADHD, and eating disorders. Youth violence is the second leading cause of death among youth (ages 10–24) and can include many forms of behavior that lead to serious injury, emotional harm, and even death. Suicide is the third leading cause of death among youth (ages 10–24). Suicidal behaviors include suicidal ideation, which refers to thoughts of harming or killing oneself, and attempted suicide, which refers to a nonfatal, self-inflicted destructive act with explicit or implicit intent to die.

ADHD has been associated with many developmental, cognitive, emotional, social, and academic impairments among children and adolescents (Wehmeier, Schacht, & Barkley, 2010). Some 4.5 million children between the ages of 5 and 17 years have been diagnosed with ADHD, and rates have dramatically increased in the last few decades.

Eating disorders include any behavior that leads to abnormal eating behaviors. The most common eating disorders are AN, which is a psychiatric illness, whereby the patient refuses to maintain a body weight within normal guidelines, and BN, which is an illness whereby the patient consumes a large amount of calories at one sitting and then engages in a compensatory behavior in an attempt to alleviate his or her body from these calories. Eating disorders that have not been classified are known as eating disorder not otherwise specified, the most common being binge eating disorder. Binge eating disorder is similar to BN but the inappropriate compensatory behaviors are not typically present.

Primary interventions that aim for the prevention of mental heath issues and promoting overall good health are typically implemented in the school and community setting. Many of these interventions are based on cognitive behavior therapy, interpersonal psychotherapy, and enhancing problem-solving skills. Interventions ranged from as short as 8 weeks to as long as 2 years and were implemented in a variety of ways, including after-school activities, curriculum integration in an existing health class, integration in the entire schools activities, and programs by school nurses. Overall, these interventions were found to be effective for preventing the onset of mental health issues and reducing current mental health issues.

REVIEW QUESTIONS

1. Summarize the important mental health milestones experienced by infants, children, and adolescents.
2. Explain how sex and gender are similar and different.
3. Define the four parenting styles. What are the two major factors used in determining these parenting styles?
4. Discuss the major functions friends serve in childhood.
5. Describe the consequences children and adolescents may face if they do not receive adequate sleep.
6. Describe various risk factors that lead to youth violence.
7. Differentiate between suicide, suicide ideation, suicide attempt, and suicidality.
8. Describe the three major types of eating disorders.

WEBSITES TO EXPLORE

International Bullying Prevention Association (IBPA)

http://www.stopbullyingworld.org/

The International Bullying Prevention Association is a nonprofit association with the mission to support and enhance research related to bullying and bullying prevention to create principles and practices that achieve a safe school, work, and community environment. On this website there are links to many types of resources, including articles, websites, books, bullying prevention materials, policy guidelines, and videos. *Click on the link for one or more of these resources. On a separate piece of paper, write your impressions.*

National Eating Disorders Association (NEDA)

http://www.nationaleatingdisorders.org/

This is the official website of the National Eating Disorders Association (NEDA), a non-profit organization dedicated to supporting individuals dealing with eating disorders and families dealing with loved ones with eating disorders. This organization advocates for improved access to care for those dealing with an eating disorder and to increase research in this area to understand effective prevention and treatment strategies. NEDA also started an annual *NEDAwareness* week, a national eating disorders awareness week, which kicks off with a walk-a-thon, hosted in several cities across the United States. *Review the various links to programs and events listed on this website. If an event is in your area, attend one and write a reflection of your experience. If no events are in your area, prepare a summary of the various programs and activities.*

Active Minds

http://www.activeminds.org/

Active Minds is a student-run organization on college campuses across the United States to increase mental health awareness, education, and advocacy for all students. This organization utilizes peer-to-peer outreach to promote its mission and works to give students a voice to change the conversation about mental health, to encourage students to seek help as soon as needed, and to serve as a liaison between students and the mental health community. *Explore this website. Does this organization have a presence at your university? If so, contact an officer of the program to learn more. Also, check out the resources for which this website provides links. What new information did you learn?*

Striving to Reduce Youth Violence Everywhere (STRYVE)

http://www.safeyouth.gov

Striving to Reduce Youth Violence Everywhere, or STRYVE, is a national program led by the Centers for Disease Control and Prevention, aimed at the prevention of youth violence. STRYVE takes a public health approach to preventing youth violence and to achieve its three goals, which are to increase the awareness of youth violence, promote the most effective youth violence prevention efforts, and help communities prevent youth violence. This website also provides online training in a three-part series to help individuals understand what youth violence is and how to prevent it. *Go to the website and watch the three modules. Write a reflection for what you learned. What were your impressions?*

National Federation of Families: For Children's Mental Health

http://www.ffcmh.org/

This is a website for the National Federation of Families for Children's Mental Health, a national, family-run organization that serves to provide advocacy at the national level for the rights of children and youth with mental health problems, provide leadership and assistance to a network of family run organizations, and to collaborate with families and other organizations to transform mental health care in the United States. This organization has local chapters in every state and also holds an annual meeting each year.

Using this website locate an organization near you. Try to attend a local meeting or the annual national meeting and write a reflection for what you learned.

Suicide Prevention Action Network USA (SPAN USA)

http://www.spanusa.org/

This is a website for the Suicide Prevention Action Network USA (SPAN USA), a network of affiliates and volunteer organizations working together to promote and advocate for suicide prevention. SPAN USA is a nonprofit organization with 32 community-based chapters and invests in educational campaigns, innovative demonstration projects, and policy work. *Locate the "Quick Facts" link on this website and read through the information. What surprised you the most? Also, locate the "Survivor Stories" link and read through two or three stories. Write your impressions about the story that touched you the most.*

REFERENCES AND FURTHER READINGS

American Psychiatric Association (APA). (2000). *Diagnostic and statistical manual of mental disorders* (4th ed.), text revision. Washington, DC: American Psychiatric Association.

Austin, S. B., Kim, J., Wiecha, J., Troped, P. J., Feldman, H. A., & Peterson, K. E. (2007). School-based overweight preventive intervention lowers incidence of disordered weight-control behaviors in early adolescent girls. *Archives of Pediatrics & Adolescent Medicine, 161*(9), 865–869.

Baumrind, D. (1991). The influence of parenting style on adolescent competence and substance use. *Journal of Early Adolescence, 11,* 56–95.

Bergin, D. (1998). *Readings from . . . Play as a medium for learning and development* (1st ed.). Olney, MD: Association for Childhood Education International.

Bloom, B., & Cohen, R. A. (2007). Summary Health Statistics for U.S. Children: National Health Interview Survey, 2006. National Center for Health Statistics. *Vital Health Statistics, 10*(234).

Bratton, S. C., Ray, D., & Rhine, T. (2005). The efficacy of play therapy with children: A meta-analytic review of treatment outcomes. *Professional Psychology: Research and Practice, 36*(4), 378–390.

Bridge, J. A., Goldstein, T. R., & Brent, D. A. (2006). Adolescent suicide and suicidal behavior. *Journal of Child Psychology and Psychiatry, 47,* 372–394.

Brevik, J. I., & Dalgard, O. S. (1996). *The Oslo Health Profile Inventory.* Oslo, Norway: University of Oslo.

Buhs, E. S., Ladd, G. W., & Herald, S. L. (2006). Peer exclusion and victimization: Processes that mediate the relation between peer group rejection and children's classroom engagement and achievement? *Journal of Educational Psychology, 98*(1), 1–13.

Burdette, H. L., & Whitaker, R. C. (2005). Resurrecting free play in young children: Looking beyond fitness and fatness to attention, affiliation and affect. *Archives of Pediatric and Adolescent Medicine, 159,* 46–50.

Castelli, D. M., Hillman, C. H., Buck, S. M., & Erwin, H. E. (2007). Physical fitness and academic achievement in third- and fifth-grade students. *Journal of Sport & Exercise Psychology, 159,* 46–50.

Centers for Disease Control and Prevention (CDC). (2009). Suicide prevention: Youth suicide. Retrieved from http://www.cdc.gov/violenceprevention/pub/youth_suicide.html.

Centers for Disease Control and Prevention (CDC). (2010a). Developmental milestones. Retrieved from http://www.cdc.gov/ncbddd/actearly/milestones/index.html.

Centers for Disease Control and Prevention (CDC). (2010b). Middle childhood (6–8 years old): Developmental milestones. Retrieved from http://www.cdc.gov/ncbddd/childdevelopment /positiveparenting/middle.html.

Centers for Disease Control and Prevention (CDC). (2010c). Middle childhood (9–11 years old): Developmental milestones. Retrieved from http://www.cdc.gov/ncbddd/childdevelopment /positiveparenting/middle2.html.

Centers for Disease Control and Prevention (CDC). (2010d). Early adolescence (12–14 years old): Developmental milestones. Retrieved from http://www.cdc.gov/ncbddd/childdevelopment /positiveparenting/adolescence.html.

Centers for Disease Control and Prevention (CDC). (2010e). Middle adolescence (15–17 years old): Developmental milestones. Retrieved from http://www.cdc.gov/ncbddd/childdevelopment /positiveparenting/adolescence2.html.

Centers for Disease Control and Prevention (CDC). (2010f). Attention-deficit/hyperactivity disorder (ADHD). Retrieved from http://www.cdc.gov/ncbddd/adhd/research.html.

Centers for Disease Control and Prevention (CDC). (2010g). Basics about childhood obesity. Retrieved from http://www.cdc.gov/obesity/childhood/basics.html.

Centers for Disease Control and Prevention (CDC). (2010h). Autism spectrum disorders (ASDs). Retrieved from http://www.cdc.gov/ncbddd/autism/index.html.

Centers for Disease Control and Prevention (CDC). (2010i). Injury prevention & control: Violence prevention. Retrieved from http://www.cdc.gov/violenceprevention/youthviolence/.

Centers for Disease Control and Prevention (CDC). (2011). Parent information. Retrieved http:// www.cdc.gov/parents/index.html.

Crick, N. R., & Zahn-Waxler, C. (2003). The development of psychopathology in females and males: Current progress and future challenges. *Development and Psychopathology*, *15*, 719–742.

Crowe, E. C., Conner, C. M., & Petscher, Y. (2007). Examining the core: Relations among reading curricula, poverty, and first through third grade reading achievement. *Journal of School Psychology*, *47*, 187–214.

Currie, C., Elton, R. A., Todd, J., & Platt, S. (1997). Indicators of socioeconomic status for adolescents: The WHO Health Behaviour in School-Aged Children Survey. *Health Education Research*, *12*, 385–397.

Daniels, S. R., Jacobson, M. S., McCrindle, B. W., Eckel, R. H., & Sanner, B. M. (2009). American Heart Association childhood obesity research summit: Executive summary. *Circulation*, *119*(15), 2114–2123.

De Sousa, S. M. (2008). Body-image and obesity in adolescence: A comparative study of social-demographic, psychological, and behavioral aspects. *Spanish Journal of Psychology*, *11*(2), 551–563.

Eaton, D. K., Kann, L., Kinchen, S., Shanklin, S., Ross, J., Hawkins, J., Wechsler, H. (2010). Youth Risk Behavior Surveillance—United States, 2009. *MMWR Morbidity and Mortality Weekly Report*, *59*(SS-5), 1–142.

Eaton, D. K., Kann, L., Kinchen, S., Shanklin, S., Ross, J., Hawkins, J., Harris, W. A., Wechsler, H. (2008). Youth risk behavior surveillance—United States, 2007. *Morbidity and Mortality Weekly Report: Surveillance Summaries*, *57*(4), 1–131.

Evans, G. W. (2004). The environment of childhood poverty. *American Psychologist*, *59*(2), 77–92.

Federal Interagency Forum on Child and Family Statistics. (2010). America's children in brief: Key national indicators of well-being, 2010. Retrieved from http://www.childstats.gov /americaschildren/famsoc.asp.

Gau, S. S., & Chiang, H. L. (2009). Sleep problems and disorders among adolescents with persistent and subthreshold attention-deficit/hyperactivity disorders. *Sleep, 32*(5), 671–670.

Gillham, J. E., Reivich, K. J., Freres, D. R., Chaplin, T. M., Shatte, A. J., Samuels, B., Sheffeild, J. (2007). School-based prevention of depressive symptoms: A randomized controlled study of the effectiveness and specificity of the Penn Resiliency program. *Journal of Consulting and Clinical Psychology, 75*(1), 9–19.

Goldsmith, S. K., Pellmar, T. C., Kleinman, A. M., & Bunney, W. E. (2002). *Reducing suicide: A national imperative.* Washington, DC: National Academy Press.

Goodman, E., & Whitaker, R. C. (2002). A prospective study of the role of depression in the development and persistence of adolescent obesity. *Pediatrics, 110*(3), 497–504.

Goodman, R. (1997). The Strengths and Difficulties Questionnaire: A research note. *Journal of Child Psychology and Psychiatry, 38,* 581–586.

Gowers, S. G. (2008). Management of eating disorders in children and adolescents. *Archives of Disease in Childhood, 93,* 331–334.

Gruber, R., Laviolette, R., Deluca, P., Monson, E., Cornish, K., & Carrier, J. (2010). Short sleep duration is associated with poor performance on IQ measures in healthy school-age children. *Sleep Medicine, 11,* 289–294.

Hawton, K., & James, A. (2005). ABC of adolescence: Suicide and deliberate self harm in young people. *British Medical Journal, 330,* 891–894.

Herba, C. M., Ferdinand, R., Ende, J., & Verhulst, F. (2007). Long-term associations of childhood suicide ideation. *American Academy of Child & Adolescent Psychiatry, 46*(11), 1473–1481.

Hodges, V. E., Boivin, M., Bukowski, W. M., & Vitaro, F. (1999). The power of friendship: Protection against an escalating cycle of peer victimization. *Developmental Psychology, 35*(1), 94–101.

Horowitz, J. L., Garber, J., Ciesla, J. A., Young, J. F., & Mufson, L. (2007). Prevention of depressive symptoms in adolescents: A randomized trial of cognitive-behavioral and interpersonal prevention programs. *Journal of Consulting and Clinical Psychology, 75*(5), 693–706.

Jasik, C. B., & Lustig, R. H. (2008). Adolescent obesity and puberty: the "perfect storm." *Annals of the New York Academy of Sciences, 1135,* 265–279.

Katzman, D. K. (2005). Medical complications in adolescents with anorexia nervosa: A review of the literature. *International Journal of Eating Disorders, 37,* S52–S59.

Kjelsas, E., Bjornstrom, C., & Gotestam, K. G. (2004). Prevalence of eating disorders in female and male adolescents (14–15 years). *Eating Behaviors, 5,* 13–25.

Kimonis, E. R., & Frick, P. J. (2010). Oppositional defiant disorder and conduct disorder grown-up. *Journal of Developmental & Behavioral Pediatrics, 31*(3), 244–254.

Krug, E. G., Mercy, J. A., Dahlberg, L. L., & Zwi, A. B. (2002). The world report on violence and health. *Lancet, 360,* 1083–1088.

Landa, R. J. (2008). Diagnosis of autism spectrum disorders in the first 3 years of life. *Nature Clinical Practice: Neurology, 4*(3), 138–147.

Lee, J., Grigg, W. S., & Donahue, P. L. (2007). *The nation's report card: Reading 2007.* Washington, DC: National Center for Education Statistics.

Loeber, R., & Stouthamer-Loeber, M. (1997). Development of juvenile aggression and violence: Some common misconceptions and controversies. *American Psychologist, 53,* 242–259.

Luthar, S. S., Cicchetti, D., & Becker, B. (2000). The construct of resilience: A critical evaluation and guidelines for future work. *Child Development, 71*(3), 543–562.

Martin, G., Richardson, A. S., Bergen, H. A., Roeger, L., & Allison, S. (2005). Perceived academic performance, self-esteem and locus of control as indicators of need for assessment of adolescent suicide risk: Implications for teachers. *Journal of Adolescence, 28*, 75–87.

McVey, G., Tweed, S., & Blackmore, E. (2007). Healthy schools-healthy kids: A controlled evaluation of a comprehensive universal eating disorder prevention program. *Body Image, 4*, 115–136.

Merry, S., McDowell, H., Wild, C. J., Bir, J., & Cunliffe, R. (2004). A randomized placebo-controlled trial of a school-based depression prevention program. *Journal of the American Academy of Child and adolescent Psychiatry, 43*(5), 538–547.

Mikami, A. Y., Hinshaw, S.P., Arnold, L. E., Hoza, B., Hechtman, L., Newcorn, J. H. et al. (2010). Bulimia nervosa symptoms in the multimodal treatment study of children with ADHD. *International Journal of Eating Disorders, 43*(3), 248–259.

Mindell, J. A., & Meltzer, L. J. (2008). Behavioural sleep disorders in children and adolescents. *Annals Academy of Medicine of Singapore, 37*, 722–728.

National Sleep Foundation. (2009). How much sleep do we really need? Retrieved from http://www.sleepfoundation.org/article/how-sleep-works/how-much-sleep-do-we-really-need.

Newschaffer, C. J., Croen, L. A., Daniels, J., Giarelli, E., Grether, J. K., Levy, S. E., Windham, G. C. (2007). The epidemiology of autism spectrum disorders. *Annual Review of Public Health, 28*, 21.1–21.24.

Nock, M. K., Kazdin, A. E., Hiripi, E., & Kessler, R. C. (2006). Prevalence, subtypes, and correlates of DSM-IV conduct disorder in the National Comorbidity Survey Replication. *Psychological Medicine, 36*(5), 699–710.

Nock, M. K., Kazdin, A. E., Hiripi, E., & Kessler, R. C. (2007). Lifetime prevalence, correlates, and persistence of oppositional defiant disorder: results from the National Comorbidity Survey Replication. *Journal of Child Psychology and Psychiatry, 48*(7), 703–713.

Ogden, C. L., Carroll, M. D., Curin, L. R., Lamb, M. M., & Flegal K. M. (2010). Prevalence of high body mass index in U.S. children and adolescents, 2007–2008. *Journal of the American Medical Association, 303*(3), 242–249.

Olds, T. S. (2009). One million skinfolds: Secular trends in the fatness of young people 1951–2004. *European Journal of Clinical Nutrition, 63(8)*, 934–946.

Possel, P., Baldus, C., Horn, A. B., Groen, G., & Hautizinger, M. (2005). Influence of general self-efficacy on the effects of a school-based universal primary prevention program of depressive symptoms in adolescents: A randomized and controlled follow-up study. *Journal of Child Psychology and Psychiatry, 46*(9), 982–994.

Pastor, P. N., & Reuben, C. A. (2008). Diagnosed attention deficit hyperactivity disorder and learning disability: United States, 2004–2006. National Center for Health Statistics. *Vital Health Statistics, 10*(237), 1–22.

Presnell, K. (2007). Body dissatisfaction in adolescent females and males: Risk and resilience. *The Prevention Researcher, 14*(3), 3–6.

Ravens-Sieberer, U., Erhart, M., Gosch, A., Wille, N., & the European KIDSCREEN Group. (2008). Mental health of children and adolescents in 12 European countries-results from the European KIDSCREEN study. *Clinical Psychology and Psychotherapy, 15*(3), 154–63.

Ravens-Sieberer, U., Gosch, A., Rajmil, L., Erhart, M., Bruil, J., Duer, W., the European KIDSCREEN Group. (2005). The KIDSCREEN-52 Quality of life measure for children and adolescents: Development and first results from a European survey. *Expert Review of Pharmaco-economics and Outcome Research, 5*, 353–364.

Resnick, M.D., Ireland, M., & Borowsky, I. (2004). Youth violence perpetration: What protects? What predicts? Findings from the National Longitudinal Study of Adolescent Health. *Journal of Adolescent Health, 35*, e1–e10.

Rigby, K. (2003). Consequences of bullying in schools. *Canadian Journal of Psychiatry, 48*(9), 583.

Rubin, K. H., Wojslawowicz, J. C., Rose-Krasnor, L., Booth-LaForce, C., & Burgess, K. B. (2006). The best friendships of shy/withdrawn children: Prevalence, stability, and relationship quality. *Journal of Abnormal Child Psychology, 34*(2), 143–157.

Rubinstein, T. B., McGinn, A. P., Wildman, R. P., & Wylie-Rosett, J. (2010). Disordered eating in adulthood is associated with reported weight loss attempts in childhood. *International Journal of Eating Disorders, 43*(7), 663–666.

Santrock, J. W. (2002). *Life-span development* (8th ed.). New York: McGraw-Hill.

Shain, B., N. (2007). Suicide and suicide attempts in adolescents. *Pediatrics, 120*(3), 669–676.

Sharma, M., & Romas, J. A. (2008). *Theoretical foundations of health education and health promotion* (1st ed.). Sudbury, MA: Jones and Bartlett.

Silenzio, V., Pena, J. B., Duberstein, P. R., Cerel, J., & Knox, K. L. (2007). Sexual orientation and risk factors for suicidal ideation and suicide attempts among adolescents and young adults. *American Journal of Public Health, 97*(11), 2017–2019.

Simons, L. G., & Conger, R. D. (2007). Linking mother–father differences in parenting to a typology of family parenting styles and adolescent outcomes. *Journal of Family Issues, 28*, 212–242.

Spence, S. H., Sheffield, J. K., & Donovan, C. L. (2003). Preventing adolescent depression: An evaluation of the problem solving for life program. *Journal of Consulting and Clinical Psychology, 71*(1), 3–13.

Stallard, P., Simpson, N., Anderson, S., Hibbert, S., & Osborn, C. (2007). The *FRIENDS* emotional health programme: Initial findings from a school-based project. *Child and Adolescent Mental Health, 12*(1), 32–37.

Stith-Prothrow, D. B. (1995). The epidemic of youth violence in America: Using public health prevention strategies to prevent violence. *Journal of Health Care for the Poor and Underserved, 6*(2), 95–101.

Stein, B. D., Joycox, L. H., Kataoka, S. H., Wong, M., T, W., Elliott, M. N., & Fink, A. (2003). A mental health intervention for schoolchildren exposed to violence: A randomized controlled trial. *Journal of the American Medical Association, 290*(5), 603–611.

Strine, T. W., Lesesne, C. A., Okoro, C. A., McGuire, L. C., Chapman, D. P., Balluz, L. S., & Mokdad, A. H. (2006). Emotional and behavioral difficulties and impairments in everyday functioning among children with a history of attention- deficit/hyperactivity disorder. *Preventing Chronic Diseases, 3*(2), 1–10.

Tomba, E., Belaise, C., Ottolini, F., Ruini, C., Brayi, A., Albieri, E., Fava, G. A. (2010). Differential effects of well-being promoting and anxiety-management strategies in a non-clinical school setting. *Journal of Anxiety Disorders, 24*, 326–333.

Touchette, E., Cote, S. M., Petit, D., Liu, X., Boivin, M., Falissard, B., Montplaisir, J., Y. (2009). Short nighttime sleep-duration and hyperactivity trajectories in early childhood. *Pediatrics, 124*, e985–e993.

United Nations General Assembly. (1989). Convention on the Rights of the Child. Retrieved from http://www.hrweb.org/legal/child.html.

Visser, S. N., & Lesesn, C. A. (2005). Mental Health in the United States: Prevalence of diagnosis and medication treatment for Attention-Deficit/Hyperactivity Disorder—United States, 2003. *Morbidity and Mortality Weekly Report: Surveillance Summaries, 54*(34), 842–847.

Ware, J. E., Kosinski, M., & Keller, S. D. (1996). A 12-Item short-form health survey: Construction of scales and preliminary tests of reliability and validity. *Medical Care, 34*, 220–233.

Wehmeier, P. M., Schacht, A., & Barkley, R. A. (2010). Social and emotional impairment in children and adolescents with ADHD and the impact on quality of life. *Journal of Adolescent Health, 46*, 209–217.

Wiggs, L., & France, K. (2000). Behavioural treatments for sleep problems in children and adolescents with physical illness, psychological problems or intellectual disabilities. *Sleep Medicine Review, 4*(3), 299–314.

Wilkinson, K. M. (2008). Increasing obesity in children and adolescents: An alarming epidemic. *Journal of the American Academy of Physician Assistants, 21*(12), 31-6, 38.

Wolraich, M. L., Wibbelsman, C. J., Brown, T. E., Evans, S. W., Gotlieb, E. M., Knight, J. R., Wilens, T. (2005). Attention-deficit/hyperactivity disorder among adolescents: A review of the diagnosis, treatment, and clinical implications. *Pediatrics, 115*(6), 1734–1746.

World Health Organization. (2002). Suicide rates (per 100,000), by gender, USA, 1950–2005. Retrieved from http://www.who.int/mental_health/prevention/suicide/country_reports.

World Health Organization. (2007). Suicide prevention. Retrieved from http://www.searo.who.int/en/section1174/section1199/section1567_6745.htm.

Zahn-Waxler, C., Shirtcliff, E. A., & Marceau, K. (2008). Disorders of childhood and adolescence: Gender and psychopathology. *Annual Review of Clinical Psychology, 4*, 275–303.

CHAPTER 10

Mental Health Promotion for Adults

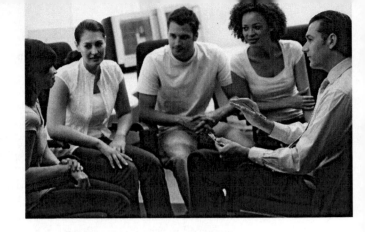

CHAPTER OBJECTIVES

After reading this chapter you should be able to
- Identify various issues in early adulthood, adulthood, and middle age
- Describe the family life cycle
- Identify the benefits of going to college
- Identify different reasons young people stay at home longer than in the past
- Identify the difference between underweight, normal weight, overweight, and obese
- Discuss various community and environmental interventions aimed to prevent mental health problems among adults

ISSUES IN EARLY ADULTHOOD (18–24 YEARS)

The transition from adolescence into adulthood can be a difficult and even scary. There are many questions we ask ourselves during this transition. Should I go to school? How long should I go to school? Should I get married? How long is too long to wait for these milestones? Before we go into these issues, let us first discuss the transition from childhood and adolescence into adulthood. Many cycles have been proposed to describe the process of entering adulthood that center on the principles that we leave home, complete school, enter the workforce, get married, and have children (Settersten & Ray, 2010). One popular model that describes this transition is the Family Life Cycle, which consists of six stages, as summarized in **Table 10.1** (Carter & McGoldrick, 1999). Although these stages appear to be straightforward, the amount of time it takes to transition from stage to stage can vary and overall has increased in recent years. Research has shown three factors that contribute to this delay: the process of becoming an adult is more gradual, families are overburdened by giving support to young adult children, and there is a mismatch between making the transition to adulthood and existing institutional supports from establishments such as universities and community colleges (Settersten & Ray, 2010).

> *The transition from adolescence into adulthood can be difficult and even scary.*

Single Young Adults Leave Home

In this first stage of the family life cycle, youth **launch** from a life of security they receive from their families into a life of greater independence. During this time young adults start to make decisions on future goals for themselves and how they will become self-sufficient. They start to choose what careers interest them, find what careers are available to them, identify what education they need to attain a given career, and consider other options, such as the military.

One important determinant of mental health for this group is educational attainment; however, not all young adults decide to continue their education into college or higher education. Educational attainment among residents of countries is important (i.e., high school and college graduation rates), as such rates indicate how prepared a nation's workforce is for the future and changing economy. In the United States, during the first half of the 20th century each generation's high school graduation rates were higher than the preceding generation, which helped contribute to America's economic growth during this time (Heckman & LaFontaine, 2010). Today, approximately 77% of our young people graduate from high school; however, graduation rates differ across racial groups, with

TABLE 10.1   The Family Life Cycle
Single young adults leave home
Two single adults joining their families through marriage
Families with young children
Families with adolescents
Family at midlife
Family in later life

Source: Data from Carter, B., & McGoldrick, M. (1999). *The expanded family life-cycle: individual, family and social perspectives* (3rd ed.). Needham, MA: Allyn & Bacon.

81% of White, 66% of Black, and 63% of Hispanic adolescents graduating from high school annually (Heckman & LaFontaine, 2010).

Although most youth will graduate from high school, for those who do not, making it in today's society can be challenging. The most obvious reason is economic: those who drop out of high school typically make less money than those who graduate. For example, in 2006 the median annual incomes of men and women without a high school diploma were $22,151 and $13,255, respectively, whereas the median earnings of men and women with a diploma were $31,715 and $20,650, respectively. In today's society it is challenging for those without a high school diploma to attain full-time employment. High school dropouts have higher unemployment rates and work fewer weeks per year, and the estimated life-time earnings of dropouts are $260,000 less than those of high school graduates. Dropouts are also less likely to receive work-related benefits such as health insurance or retirement plans, making it more difficult for them to take care of themselves or a family member when they fall ill. Dropouts also bear a larger social cost for those who are working. For example, high school dropouts make less money and thus the government generates less tax revenues from their smaller salaries. Dropouts pay approximately 42% of what high school graduates pay in federal and state income taxes annually. High school dropouts also rely on greater public spending for public assistance, including health care and other government programs (Tyler & Lofstrom, 2009).

> *Currently, approximately 77% of our young people graduate from high school; however, graduation rates differ across racial groups, with 81% of White, 66% of Black, and 63% of Hispanic adolescents graduating from high school annually.*
>
> —Heckman & LaFontaine (2010)

One popular option for those who do not receive a high school diploma is a **General Educational Diploma** (GED). A GED is a high school equivalency diploma that is accepted by over 98% of colleges and 96% of employers and evaluates an adult's high school level skills and knowledge in five core academic areas (math, reading, writing, science, and social studies) (American Council on Education, 2010). Each year over 700,000 high school dropouts take the GED exam, and over 65% of those are less than 24 years of age. Of all the high school credentials that are awarded each year, those with GEDs account for 15%. The GED program is disproportionately used by racial minorities: Black men are almost twice as likely as White men to apply for and receive a GED. Although the GED program appears to be a promising option for dropouts, those with their GED still face struggles in the job market. First, those with GEDs tend to make less money than those with high school diplomas and typically make the same amount of money as high school dropouts without a GED. Those with GEDs also have a harder time finding and keeping full-time employment compared with high school graduates. Finally, those with GEDs are less likely to go on to postsecondary education, which is increasingly needed in today's job market (Cameron & Heckman, 1993).

For high school graduates the decision to go to college can be very stressful. Higher education was once only considered for elite, higher-class families. As jobs become less secure and careers become more fluid, the need for education is greater. Today's young adults are more educated than any other generation in the nation's history. In 2010, 27.4% of young adults, who are at least 25 years old, have a bachelor's degree or higher. From this 10.1% have a graduate or professional degree (Settersten & Ray, 2010).

In 2010, 18.2 million students were enrolled in college. Of these, 11.6 million were 18 to 24 years old and 6.6 million were older than 25 years. This represents 39% of the entire young adult population aged 18 to 24. College enrollment has been increasing in recent decades due to changes in the job market, which demands higher trained workers. Of those attending college, there are more women (60%) than men (40%). There are also racial disparities for those who attend college. In 2010 there were more White students (64%) than Black (13%), Hispanics (11%), and Asians (7%) combined. Enrollment among older adults is also higher, as these adults wish to finish school or change career paths. This has led to more students attending college part time to be able to pay for the high expense of education: in 2010 66% of students were full time, whereas 34% were part time (National Center for Educational Statistics, 2010).

For young adults attending college can also be a particularly difficult decision due to the large costs associated with higher education. An important question is how much debt should one incur. From 1995 to 2004 the average yearly tuition costs for full-time students increased from $3,800 to $4,700 at public 4-year colleges and from $12,700 to $18,400 at private 4-year colleges. To help pay for their education students can receive loans and/or financial aid from a variety of places, including private businesses and charity organizations. A popular means of financial support for high education is through the federal loan program that issues Stafford loans. **Stafford loans** are a form of needs-based aid and consist of unsubsidized loans, for which the beneficiary pays interest while in college, and subsidized loans, in which the government pays interest while the student is enrolled in college. The use of these loans has increased in the past decade, and now 33% of all undergraduate students use this program. As a result, average total loan debts have increased: in 1995 the average Stafford loan was $11,000 for fourth/fifth-year seniors, but today it is $15,500 for fourth/fifth-year seniors (Wei & Berkner, 2008).

Fewer students can now afford to go to college without some form of assistance. Two-thirds of 4-year undergraduate students (65.6%) graduate with some form of debt, with an average student loan debt among graduating seniors at $23,186 (excluding PLUS Loans but including Stafford, Perkins, state, college, and private loans). Among graduating 4-year undergraduate students who applied for federal student aid, 86.3% borrowed to pay for their education and the average cumulative debt was $24,651. The median cumulative debt among those with a bachelor's degree was $19,999 in 2007–2008. Twenty-five percent also borrowed greater than $30,000, and one-tenth borrowed more than $44,000 (Wei et al., 2009).

Attending college has many private and public advantages, including both economic and social gains. For example, public economic benefits include increased tax revenues for the federal government, greater productivity, increased consumption, increased workforce flexibility, and decreased reliance on government financial support and programs. Public social benefits associated with higher educated groups include reduced crime rates, increased charitable giving and community service, increased quality of civic life/social cohesion, greater appreciation of diversity, and improved ability to adapt to and use technology. Private economic benefits include higher salaries and benefits, higher savings levels, improved working conditions, and professional mobility.

*A*ttending college has many private and public advantages, including both economic and social gains.

Finally, private social benefits include improved health and life expectancy, improved quality of life for offspring, better consumer decision making, increased personal status, and more hobbies and leisure activities (Institute for Higher Education Policy, 2005).

Some high school graduates decide to skip college or come back to college later in life and enter the workforce immediately. However, the labor market is competitive and the number of jobs for high school graduates is lowering, with more jobs requiring greater skills that necessitate some form of special training. As with high school dropouts, the average wage for high school graduates is lower than those with a college education. The average income for a high school graduate is $30,800, whereas the average income for an individual with a bachelor's degree is $49,900, master's degree is $59,500, and doctorate degree is $79,400. Also, children from families with parents who only have high school diplomas will likely be less prepared for school themselves, including college, because opportunities for education are typically less present in their household (Baum & Payea, 2004).

The military is another opportunity for high school graduates, as nearly 175,000 young adults enter some branch annually (Department of Defense, 2010). Most military recruits are high school graduates: 91% are high school graduates, 7% have a GED, and 2% are uncertified dropouts (Heckman & LaFontaine, 2010). The military also appears to be a more attractive option for men than for women. For new recruits 84% are men and 16% are women. Also, more Whites (57%) enter military service than African Americans (15%) and Hispanics (15%).

The U.S. military comprises five major service branches: Army, Navy, Air Force, Marines, and Coast Guard. In 2009 more than 2.4 million people served in the armed forces and more than 1.4 million served on active duty (561,000 in the Army, 327,000 in the Navy, 325,000 in the Air Force, 202,000 in the Marine Corps, and 33,413 in the Coast Guard). Besides full-time service individuals can also serve part time in reserve components of each branch or state National Guard components of the Air Force and Army. More than 1.0 million people served part time in these components (Bureau of Labor Statistics, 2009).

Requirements for military service among adults greatly differ between countries in terms of length and legal requirements. The United States has an all-volunteer military, which indicates civilians are free to choose whether they serve or not. However, other countries such as Norway and Germany require young adults to serve for some short period of time (i.e., 6 months to 2 years).

Military service can be a difficult and stressful life for young adults. Long deployments away from family in unsafe environments can create feelings of anxiety and depression. **Posttraumatic stress disorder (PTSD)** is more common among military service members, as well as those who have experienced hate crimes and other traumatic events. PTSD is an anxiety disorder that develops after an exposure to a traumatizing event, such as physical harm or threat to one's life. Symptoms of PTSD have been categorized into three types: *reexperiencing symptoms*, which includes flashbacks or bad dreams from the experience; *avoidance symptoms*, which includes staying away from places, objects, or situations that remind one of the traumatizing experience; and *hyperarousal symptoms*, which includes being easily startled or constantly on edge (National Institute of Mental Health, 2010). The estimated lifetime prevalence of PTSD has been recorded as 7.8% in the U.S.

population (Kessler, Sonnega, Bromet, Hughes, & Nelson, 1995). Historically, veterans serving in combative areas, such as Vietnam, Iraq, and Afghanistan, experience higher rates than the general population. For example, it was estimated that 10.1% of veterans from the first Gulf War experienced PTSD and 13.8% of veterans from the current wars in Iraq and Afghanistan (Operation Enduring Freedom and Operation Iraqi Freedom) experienced PTSD (Kang, Natelson, Mahan, Lee, & Murphy, 2003; Tanilian & Jaycox, 2008). Also, unlike other jobs in which employees are free to quit at their own will, military service is legally binding.

Military service does, however, offer many advantages. First, the military offers specialized training for its members that can have real-world application, which in turn can prepare them for a life outside of the military in private sector jobs. The military can also be a means for upward social mobility, especially among disadvantaged minority groups (Kleykamp, 2006). The military also offers more steady employment and benefits that are similar to civilian-equivalent jobs. For example, servicemen and women receive free medical care for themselves and their families. Also available is the GI Bill benefit, which can fund postservice higher education. This is an advantage for those who have aspirations for higher education but cannot afford it and serves as another means to attain this goal without going into debt (Kleykamp, 2006).

The **Montgomery GI Bill** (the result of the Servicemen's Readjustment Act of 1944) was started for World War II veterans to provide money to servicemen for college and/or vocational training after military service. This benefit is still around today and requires service members to pay $100.00 per month during their first year of service. After they are honorably discharged they have up to 10 years to use their benefit, which includes 36 months of GI bill benefit payments that can be used for school expenses. The actual amount for this benefit varies by type of training the service member takes and total length of service (U.S. Department of Veteran Affairs, 2009).

This stage of the family life cycle ends when the young adult completely separates him- or herself from the original family unit, without fleeing or cutting off all ties with their families.

FOCUS FEATURE 10.1 A CLOSER LOOK AT THE U.S. AIR FORCE SUICIDE PREVENTION PROGRAM

Joining the military can be stressful, especially in times of war. The U.S. Air Force suicide prevention program was created in 1996 and fully implemented by 1997. The mission of the program is to reduce the number and rate of suicides in the Air Force, advocate a community approach to suicide prevention, provide assistance and guidance to organizations and individuals administering the program, identify risk factors of suicide, and develop a response to reduce the overall prevalence of suicides. This program is guided by 11 initiatives, presented in **Table 10.2**.

Recently a study was published evaluating the program from 1997 through 2008. This time period was especially important, given the important historical conflicts that occurred during this time period, including Operation Enduring Freedom in 2001 and Operation Iraqi Freedom in 2003. Researchers found that suicide rates were much lower during the implementation of this program compared with the time before the implementation (Knox et al., 2010).

TABLE 10.2	Eleven Initiatives of the U.S. Air Force Suicide Prevention Program
1.	*Leadership involvement.* The Air Force involves senior leadership, such as base commanders, to reinforce messages pertaining to suicide prevention.
2.	*Addressing suicide prevention through professional military education.* This includes all forms of military education and training.
3.	*Guidelines for commanders on use of mental health services.* Special training is given to those in leadership pertaining to accessing mental health services.
4.	*Community preventive services.* Focuses on primary prevention efforts rather than treatment efforts.
5.	*Community education and training.* Suicide prevention training is offered on an annual basis.
6.	*Investigative interview policy.* If an airman undergoes an arrest or is under investigation for a crime, leadership at the base is required to assess the airman's risk for suicide.
7.	*Trauma stress response.* This refers to "trauma stress response teams" that are trained to help personnel at any base deal with traumatic events, such as suicide.
8.	*Integrated Delivery System (IDS) and Community Action Information Board (CAIB).* These platforms provide a forum for the cross-organizational evaluation and resolution of individual, family, installation, and community issues that impact the readiness and quality of life for air force members and their families.
9.	*Limited Privilege Suicide Prevention Program.* Airmen who are deemed at risk for suicide are given greater confidentiality with their mental health care provider.
10.	*IDS Consultation Assessment Tool.* This is a needs assessment tools that helps base leadership assess their units strengths and weaknesses, in terms of health and wellness.
11.	*Suicide Event Surveillance System.* This is a centralized database that all information regarding suicides and suicide attempts are entered.

Source: Data from Knox, K. L., Pflanz, S., Talcott, G. W., Campise, R. L., Lavigne, J. E., Bajorska, ... , Caine, E. D. (2010). The US Air Force suicide prevention program: Implications for public health policy. *American Journal of Public Health, 100*(12), 2457–2463.

ISSUES IN ADULTHOOD (25–45 YEARS) AND MIDDLE AGE (45–65 YEARS)

Two Single Adults Joining Their Families Through Marriage

The next stage of the family life cycle is the joining of families through marriage, also known as the **new couple**. This stage entails committing to a partner and realigning your own family to now include a new extended family. The stage typically begins when two individuals get married, which is currently a highly political and debated topic. The United States of American Code of Laws, a compilation of the general and permanent federal laws, defines **marriage** as "only a legal union between one man and one woman as husband and wife." It further defines a **spouse** as "only to a person of the opposite sex who is a husband or a wife" (Office of Law Revision Counsel, U.S. House of Representatives, 2010). Even with this legal definition, however, there is currently much debate over **same-sex marriage**, or a marriage between two people of the same biological sex. Although this type of marriage is not recognized at the federal level, currently five states recognize and conduct same-sex marriages: Connecticut, Iowa, Massachusetts, New

Hampshire, Vermont, and the District of Columbia. Additionally, other states, such as New York, New Jersey, Maryland, and Rhode Island, that do not perform such marriages recognize them as such for state benefits, including health care. Some marriages that are not officiated under legal contract can still be a legal by what is known as a common-law marriage. A **common-law marriage** is a form of interpersonal status that two people enter informally. In some areas these types of marriages are legally binding; however, in others they carry no legal consequences.

Today's young adults take different views about marriage than in previous generations. For example, in the past couples would work toward building a life together from the beginning, whereby the husband would typically take on the role of provider and the wife would take on the role of caregiver. Today, couples are more likely to build separate lives as a single young adult, preparing them for their future careers, and then decide to marry later in life. This has delayed the marriage process. As you can see in **Table 10.3** the median age for marriage has steadily increased for men and women in the past 50 years (U.S. Census Bureau, 2005).

This does not mean, however, young adults are having less sex or are living together less. Whereas 50 years ago it was uncommon for couples to live together before marriage, it is common practice today. Although marriages have been declining in the past half-century, it is still the most common living arrangement. **Table 10.4** shows that whereas marriage has declined over the past 40 years, over half of today's adults still live under this arrangement (Kreider & Elliott, 2007).

Although marriage can be stressful for young adults, John Gottman, cofounder of The Gottman Relationship Institute, has identified seven principles that predict whether a marriage will succeed. The first principle includes *establishing love maps* for one another, which refers to having deep insight into how your partner lives their life and sees the world. The second principle is *nurturing fondness and admiration*, which refers to viewing your partner in a positive manner, respecting and appreciating who they are. The third principle is *turning toward each other instead of away*, or when faced with stressful situations it is important to maintain your connection and not look elsewhere for support. *Let your*

TABLE 10.3   Median Age for Marriage for Men and Women in the Past 50 Years

Year	Men	Women
1950	22.8	20.3
1960	22.8	20.3
1970	23.2	20.8
1980	24.7	22.0
1990	26.1	23.9
2000	26.8	25.1
2005	27.1	25.3

Source: Data from U.S. Census Bureau. (2005). Estimated median age at first marriage, by sex: 1890 to the present. Available at: http://www.census.gov/population/socdemo/hh-fam/ms2.pdf. Accessed August 10, 2011.

TABLE 10.4   Living Arrangements of U.S. Adults

Year	Married	Men Living Alone	Women Living Alone
1970	70.6%	5.6%	11.5%
1980	60.8%	8.6%	14.0%
1990	56.2%	9.7%	14.9%
2000	52.8%	10.7%	14.8%
2007	50.8%	11.7%	15.2%

Source: Kreider, R. M., & Elliott, D. B. (2007). *America's families and living arrangements: 2007.* Current Population Reports, P20–561. Washington, DC: U.S. Census Bureau.

partner influence you is the fourth principle, which refers to allowing your partner to influence your behaviors while maintaining your own identity. The fifth principle is *solving your solvable problems,* which refers to the importance of making compromises in relationships. *Overcoming gridlock* is the sixth principle, which refers to how couples should behave when they are on polar opposites of the spectrum on any issue. For example, one partner is a vegan and the other enjoys eating meat. Or one partner wants to live in the city and the other wants to live in the countryside. When such an event happens, it is important for couples to communicate about the issue, and prevent creating a gridlock. The final principle, *create shared meaning,* refers to how couples should create a new, shared value system that connects them (Gottman & Silver, 2000).

Marriage can also decrease stress for both spouses, because it is a means to provide social support such as problem solving, advice giving, empathic listening, expressions of caring, strategic distraction, and constructive criticism (Story & Bradbury, 2004). This stage of the family life cycle ends when the young couple starts to have children.

Becoming Parents and a Family with Children

This next stage of the family life cycle is met with many difficulties, as young adults now move up a generation to care for the next. As parents, young adults now assume responsibilities such as taking on the new role of being a parent, committing time, money, and resources, all while maintaining a healthy relationship with their spouse. As marriages are now delayed, so too is having children. Although changes in the family system may seem like a recent phenomenon, it is important to note that the family unit and structure have been changing and evolving throughout history. As changes in the economy, demographics, culture, and social institutions occur, families have had to adjust accordingly. This has led to the new term **"postmodern family,"** which includes more women working outside the home, gradual breakdown of the gender-based division of labor within the household, declining birth rate, and rising rates of divorce, cohabitation, and nonmarital childbearing (Furstenberg, 2010).

What forces contributed to the change and delay in this step? Young adults now desire and require jobs that necessitate postsecondary education, which delays having a chance to start a family. Young adults also want to be financially secure when they start a family and therefore may wait longer until they can afford to do so. The idea that young adults are staying home longer and delaying this stage is a new phenomenon is actually false. The proportion of young adults still living at home is similar to that of the early 1900s. During the first decades of the 20th century adolescence was a brief period as by the late teen years most men had started to work and were finished with their education. As the century progressed family formations were beginning to occur earlier in the late teens/early twenties; however, the great depression slowed this down. The next change in the family structure occurred after World War II, when America experienced a postwar boom in the economy and unemployment rates steadily dropped. During this time there was an abundance of good paying jobs with benefits for those with a high school education. From 1949 to 1970 income among lower and middle classes grew 110% and among the higher class grew 85% to 95%. These jobs made it possible for young adults to leave home early, form families, and maintain common gender roles: men defined adulthood as getting a job to support his wife and family, and women defined adulthood as being married and having children (Settersten & Ray, 2010).

The reasons young adults stay home longer in today's society are different from those in the early 1900s. In the past young adults were looked upon to provide support to the family unit and were obliged to stay home and contribute to work and chores. Today, our young adults are quite different, as they now look to their parents for extended material and social support while they finish their education in an attempt to become financially secure (Furstenberg, 2010).

Medical advances have also allowed the family unit to be further delayed. For example, increasing awareness of **family planning** helps young couples plan the number of children they desire and the spacing of time between children. Also, the advent of birth control methods allowed women and men to engage in sexual activity with less fear of the possibility of having children. Having children is also an expensive investment. Parents not only have to invest money into raising their children but also time and energy. Some have even argued that young couples perceive the importance of having fewer "quality" children that can compete in today's workforce rather than having larger families (Furstenberg, 2010).

Another factor that has delayed couples in this stage is unemployment. **Unemployment** refers to those who are currently available to work but have been unable to find work for over 4 weeks. In 2010 1 in 10 Americans (9.8%) were unemployed (U.S. Department of Labor, 2010). Among adults, unemployment increases the risk of depression, and suicide attempts are typically much higher among unemployed young men compared with employed young men (Dorling, 2009; Lerner & Henke, 2008). This stage of the family life cycle ends when the children in the family become adolescents.

Final Stages of the Family Life Cycle

The final stages of the family life cycle entail children growing up and eventually transitioning to repeat the process of their own family life cycle. The fourth stage, the family with adolescents, is a time when children are now becoming more independent and seek to find their own identity. During this stage parents learn to develop which type of parenting style best suits them (see Chapter 9).

The fifth stage of the cycle, the family at midlife, includes the time parents launch their own children, as described in the first stage of the cycle. At this stage individuals can experience a **midlife crisis**, a time in middle adulthood when individuals question their sense of life accomplishments, have an overwhelming sense of self-doubt, and begin to fear their eventual death. Although a midlife crisis is thought to occur between 40 and 60 years of age, research now indicates that such crises are not time driven but event driven. For example, midlife crises are often driven by unemployment, financial problems, illnesses, or a death in the family, which could happen at any stage in an adult's life. Personality type has also been identified as a predisposing factor triggering midlife crises, with more neurotic individuals having a greater risk (Lachman, 2004).

The final stage, the family in later life, includes the family in retirement and becoming grandparents. Details about the later stages of this cycle are presented in Chapter 11.

Deviations from the Family Life Cycle

Although the family life cycle can describe the process that many Americans go through in their adulthood years, it does not describe everybody. One recent phenomenon is couples or single adults deciding not to have children. The percentage of childless women ages 40 to 44 has almost doubled since the 1970s from 10% to presently 19%. Reasons for childlessness include not wanting to have biological children, being unable to have children, and declining marriage rates. There are also differences in women according to their educational status, with higher educated women more likely to be childless. According to the Current Population Survey, 15% of high school dropouts, 17% of high school graduates, 19% with some college, and 24% with a bachelor's degree or higher are childless (Biddlecom & Martin, 2006).

Another deviation from the family life cycle is living together as a homosexual couple. According to 2000 U.S. Census, of the 5.5 million couples living together, unmarried, slightly over 10% were same-sex couples (Kurdek, 2005). The amount of same-sex couples with children are also dramatically increasing, with 34% of lesbian couples and 22% of gay male couples raising children under the age of 18 (Schmieder, 2008). These numbers may be underestimated, however, given the social stigma, such as discrimination or even violence, that some affiliate with homosexuality and therefore do not report.

Homosexual couples differ from heterosexual couples in some ways. For example, as reviewed by Kurdek (2005), when deciding household labor heterosexual couples are more likely to divide chores based on gender roles. Homosexual couples, however, are less likely to assign a "husband" or "wife" figure and more likely to negotiate chores based on interests, skills, and work schedules. Kurdek (2005) also noted that whereas there is limited data comparing hetero- and homosexual couples, studies suggest homosexual couples tend to resolve conflicts more positively and constructively, have equal levels of satisfaction, and perceive lower levels of support from family members but higher levels from friends (Kurdek, 2005).

Compared with heterosexual couples, homosexual couples are less likely to have children (Riskind & Patterson, 2010). There are many possible explanations for this, including lack of desire or interest. One study comparing hetero- and homosexual couples found that gay and lesbian couples had lower desires for parenthood. In addition, gay men who expressed desire for children were less likely to express intentions for becoming a parent; however, this was not true among lesbians. Another issue homosexual couples face that may deter their choice for having children is criticism that their sexual orientation may impact their child's social or psychological development. As Patterson (2006) reviewed, however, studies published over the last decade suggest no evidence that sexual orientation impacts child and adolescent development, and qualities such as daily interactions and the strength of family relationships may be more important (Patterson, 2006).

DETERMINANTS AND INFLUENCES ON MENTAL HEALTH OF ADULTS

Divorce

Although marriage rates have been declining in recent decades, it is important to note the many benefits to marriage. Studies based on longitudinal data have found that getting married is associated with having better mental health outcomes, including overall emotional well-being and happiness. Married couples also tend to make more money than nonmarried couples, with one study showing married men earn 11% more than men who have never been married (Waite & Lehrer, 2003). Given these benefits, however, many marriages end in divorce.

Divorce is a legal dissolution of a marriage by a court or other authoritative body. Divorce rates have increased dramatically in past decades; however, rates have been relatively stable in the last few years. In 2000 the divorce rate in the United States was 4.0 (per 1,000), whereas in 2007 the divorce rate was 3.6 (per 1,000) (Centers for Disease Control and Prevention, 2009a). Previous research has shown that divorce can significantly increase levels of psychological distress and the likelihood of developing anxiety and depression and decrease levels of happiness and mental health (Hewitt, Turrell, & Giskes, 2010).

Divorce can be a stressful time for adults and especially stressful among children, if any are involved. Previous research has shown that children with divorced parents have an increased risk of social and mental health problems during childhood that follows into early adulthood. For example, young adults with divorced parents are more likely to have a lower socioeconomic status, have weaker ties with their parents, and show greater symptoms of depression and relationship instability (Sobolewski & Amato, 2007). One difficulty that arises is teaching children how to live in a new living arrangement. When parents separate they either come to an agreement or allow the courts to decide which parent retains what type of custody. Typically, there are two types of custody, with two types of arrangements. **Legal custody** refers to custody that allows a parent to make any decision regarding the needs of the child, for example, decisions about education, health care, and religion. **Physical custody** refers to the amount of time children live with one parent or the amount of visitation one parent is allowed. Both types of custody can be either **sole**, which allows one parent to make all legal and physical decisions, or **joint**, which allows both parents to share legal and physical decisions. Typically, women retain more custody rights than men. Research has shown that mothers who seek sole physical custody were successful 80% to 85% of the time, whereas fathers seeking sole physical custody were only successful 10% to 15% of the time. Whatever living situation occurs, it is important for parents not to have parental conflict, especially around their children.

One study showed parental divorce with marital conflict increased the odds that children were not close to either parent in adulthood (Sobolewski & Amato, 2007).

Although women typically retain a majority of the custody, the idea of the "absent" father has started to subside. For example, the percentage of children having no contact with their fathers 2 or 3 years after divorce was 50% in the early 1980s but only 18% to 26% in the mid to late 1990s (Kelly, 2006). Reasons fathers rarely see their children can be described by the three Rs: fathers *repartner* and make new lives with a new family, fathers *relocate* or move away from their children, or fathers retain *residual bad feelings* toward their former spouse (Smyth, 2005).

Obesity

Overweight and obesity rates in the United States and other countries are high. According to the most recent National Health and Nutrition Examination Survey (2007–2008), 68% of U.S. adults are either overweight or obese and 33.8% are obese, with slight differences reported among gender: 32.2% of adult men and 35.5% of adult women were reported as obese. There are also differences for obesity prevalence among states, with Colorado having the lowest prevalence rate of 18.6% and Mississippi having the highest prevalence rate of 34.4% (Flegal, Carroll, Ogden, & Curtin, 2010). Obesity is commonly defined using an indicator called **body mass index,** which is a ratio of an individual's height and weight. **Table 10.5** describes the classifications of body mass index. A BMI less than 18.5 indicates that an individual is **underweight** for his or her height. BMIs ranging from 18.5 to 24.9 indicate a **normal weight** for height. A BMI greater than 25 but less than 30 indicates that an individual is **overweight** for his or her height. BMIs greater than 30 indicate **obesity**. Body mass index can be calculated by taking an individual's weight in kilograms and dividing it by his or her height in meters squared:

$$\text{BMI} = \frac{\text{kg}}{\text{m}^2} = \frac{\text{lb} \times 703}{\text{in}^2} = \frac{\text{lb} \times 4.88}{\text{ft}^2}$$

Metabolic consequences of obesity that can decrease an individual's life expectancy include type 2 diabetes, cardiovascular disease, and metabolic syndrome; however, obesity has also been associated with mental health problems. One study found that obesity, physical activity, and daily caloric consumption were significantly associated with depression among middle-aged women (Simon et al., 2008). Another study found that obesity

TABLE 10.5 Classifications Used for Body Mass Index

Category	Body Mass Index Range
Underweight	<18.5
Normal weight	18.5 to 24.9
Overweight	25 to 29.9
Obese class 1	30 to 34.9
Obese class 2	35 to 39.9
Obese class 3	>40

significantly increased the odds for both men and women to develop major depression, bipolar disorder, and panic disorder but significantly lowered the lifetime risk of engaging in substance abuse (Simon et al., 2006).

Obese individuals are also discriminated against in a variety of settings. Work-related stereotypes attributed to obese workers often include lack of self-discipline, laziness, incompetence, sloppiness, bad temperament, emotional instability, slowness, poor attendance, and poor role modeling. Obese managers are also judged more harshly for undesirable behaviors (i.e., taking underserved credit) than were average weight managers (Puhl & Brownell, 2001).

Discrimination can occur in the health care setting (Brownell & Puhl, 2001). One study with nurses found they commonly agreed that obesity can be prevented by self-control and their obese patients were overindulgent and lazy and experience unresolved anger. The nurses felt uncomfortable caring for obese patients to the point that 31% reported they would prefer not to care for obese patients altogether (Maroney & Golub, 1992). Finally, a study from the U.S. Preventive Services Task Force evaluating how obesity affects health-related quality of life showed that after adjustment, health-related quality of life scores decreased as level of obesity increased, and compared with normal weight participants, persons with severe obesity had significantly lower scores for many measures of health, including physical, mental, and overall health (Jia & Lubertkin, 2005).

Socioeconomic Status

Socioeconomic status is a measure of an individual's economic and social position in society. Studies reporting on poverty status are often reporting a status determined by comparing an individual's annual income with a set of dollar values (or thresholds) that vary by family size, number of children, and age of householder. When a family's pretax money income is less than the dollar value of the given threshold, then that family and every individual in it are considered to be in **poverty**. According to the U.S. Census Bureau, in 2009 14.3% of the U.S. population (or 42.9 million people) lived in poverty (DeNavas-Walt, Proctor, & Smith, 2010). Poverty rates also differ by states, to as low as 8.5% in New Hampshire to a high of 21.9% in Mississippi. Poverty rates also appear to be increasing across the United States. From 2008 to 2009 alone, 31 states saw an increase in the percentage and total amount of people living in poverty (U.S. Census Bureau, 2010b).

Poverty has been associated with many adverse mental health outcomes. Poverty is also associated with other psychosocial stressors, such as violence, unemployment, and insecurity, which in turn have all been correlated with the onset of many adult mental disorders (Saxena, Thornicroft, Knapp, & Whiteford, 2007). Epidemiological data from five studies in four low-income and middle-income countries (Zimbabwe, India, Brazil, and Chile) showed that individuals with the lowest education and income levels were most vulnerable to mental disorders (Patel, Araya, de Lima, Ludermir, & Todd, 1999). One study found that among young adults in Australia, living in poverty in childhood was the strongest predictor of having anxiety and depression in adolescence and young adulthood. Researchers also reported a dose effect in that the more exposure to poverty in childhood years increased the risk of having depression or anxiety (Najman et al., 2010). Another study showed that among African American women, after controlling for childhood sexual abuse,

TABLE 10.6 Ten Most and Least Stressful Jobs of 2010	
Top 10 Most Stressful Jobs	**Top 10 Least Stressful Jobs**
1. Firefighter	1. Musical instrument repairer
2. Senior corporate executive	2. Medical records technician
3. Taxi driver	3. Actuary
4. Surgeon	4. Forklift operator
5. Police officer	5. Appliance repairer
6. Commercial pilot	6. Medical secretary
7. Highway patrol officer	7. Librarian
8. Public relations officer	8. Bookkeeper
9. Advertising account executive	9. Piano tuner
10. Real estate agent	10. Janitor

Source: Strieber, A. (2010). The 10 most stressful jobs of 2010. Available at: http://www.careercast.com/jobs-rated /10-most-and-least-stressful-jobs-2010. Accessed August 10, 2011.

poverty was positively associated with mental health outcomes of depression, PTSD, illicit drug use, and suicidal ideation (Byant-Davis, Ullman, Tsong, Tillman, & Smith, 2010).

Work-Related Stress

In the past few decades there has been a growing interest in how stress from work relates to overall mental health. **Work-related stress**, or stress that results from work, has contributed to increasing individual psychosomatic and psychosocial distress, turnover and productivity losses as well as tension, anger, anxiety, depression, mood disorders, mental fatigue, and sleep disturbances (Fortes-Ferreira, Peiro, Gonzalez-Morales, & Martin, 2006). Societal costs include those due to absenteeism, loss of productivity, and health care consumption. For example, in Britain it is estimated that 40 million workdays are lost due to mental and emotional problems (Van der Klink, Blonk, Schene, & Van Dijk, 2001). In some settings workers are exposed to violence. Research has shown that in occupations such as medicine and psychology, a profession at higher risk for working with violent patients, work-related violence and threats are positively associated with psychological distress, depression, anxiety, fatigue, job dissatisfaction, and absenteeism (Wieclaw et al., 2005). **Table 10.6** shows the 10 most and 10 least stressful jobs of 2010 (Strieber, 2010).

FOCUS FEATURE 10.2 EXAMINING THE ASSOCIATION OF DEPRESSION AND ANXIETY WITH SMOKING, OBESITY, PHYSICAL INACTIVITY, AND ALCOHOL CONSUMPTION AMONG U.S. ADULTS

Advances in medicine and public health have reduced the burden of disease and death and increased life expectancy in the United States. However, whereas in the early 1900s communicable (or infectious)

(continued)

diseases were the leading causes of mortality, in today's society noncommunicable (or chronic) diseases, such as heart disease, obesity, and diabetes, now account for most deaths. Lifestyle behaviors attributed to these leading causes of death include tobacco use, poor diet, physical inactivity, and alcohol consumption. In one study researchers used a sample of the U.S. population to determine the extent that depression and anxiety were associated with smoking, physical inactivity, obesity, and alcohol consumption. This was the first large population-based study to examine these risk factors for depression and anxiety in nearly a quarter of a million U.S. adults. Researchers used data from the Behavioral Risk Factor Surveillance System, a state-based system of health surveys conducted by phone that collects information on health risk behaviors, preventive health practices, and health care access primarily related to chronic disease and injury (Centers for Disease Control and Prevention, 2009a). Researchers could only use data from 38 states, the District of Columbia, Puerto Rico, and the U.S. Virgin Islands for this study. To evaluate depressive disorders, researchers used the Patient Health Questionaire-8 (PHQ-8), a widely used, multipurpose, clinically validated questionnaire for screening, diagnosing, monitoring, and measuring eight of nine criteria for depressive disorders (Center for Quality Assessment and Improvement in Mental Health, 1999). The criteria missing from the PHQ-8 was suicidal or self-injurious ideation, which researchers noted would be difficult to evaluate over the phone.

Researchers found that after adjusting for sociodemographic characteristics, adults with a current or lifetime diagnosis for depression or anxiety were significantly more likely than adults without such a diagnosis to be a current smoker, obese, physically inactive, a binge drinker, or a heavy drinker. All associations were also significant among women; however, among men none of these mental health conditions was significantly associated with binge drinking, a lifetime diagnosis of anxiety was not significantly associated with physical inactivity, and a lifetime diagnosis of depression was not significantly associated with heavy drinking. Researchers also found a significant dose–response relationship between depression and smoking, obesity, and physical inactivity; that is, severity of depression was associated with higher smoking rates, severity of obesity, and higher rates of physical inactivity.

MENTAL HEALTH INTERVENTIONS FOR ADULTS

Many interventions have been implemented in the community and other settings that target mental health issues among adults. The first study evaluated two interventions designed to reduce negative body image and eating disordered behaviors. Researchers randomized female college sorority members into one of two different intervention conditions. The first intervention was based on cognitive dissonance (CD), which aims to help participants resolve inconsistencies between their beliefs and actions to ultimately reject the notion that "thin" is ideal. The second intervention was a healthy weight (HW) intervention that aimed to promote balanced eating and exercise to attain a healthy body weight. Both interventions were delivered by peer sorority members who had previously participated in an eating disorders prevention intervention. At the end of the interventions sorority members in the CD group significantly decreased negative affect, thin ideal internalization, and bulimic pathology compared with those in the HW group; however, both groups reported significantly lower negative affect, internalization, body dissatisfaction, dietary restraint, and bulimic pathology after a 14-month follow-up (Becker et al., 2010).

Another intervention was a pilot study implemented in Canada to evaluate the acceptability and efficacy of a multifaith spiritually based intervention (SBI) for generalized anxiety disorder. Participants were recruited and screened for generalized anxiety disorder according to the *Diagnostic and Statistical Manual of Mental Disorders* (4th ed., text revision) and then randomized to receive either a 12-week SBI intervention or 12-week cognitive behavioral therapy intervention (CBT). For both groups sessions lasted 50 minutes, and the SBI intervention was implemented by an ordained minister, who also held a doctoral degree in the psychology of religion. The intervention followed the book *Essential Spirituality* (Walsh, 1999), which draws from seven religious traditions (Buddhism, Christianity, Confucianism, Hinduism, Islam, Judaism, and Taoism) and was designed to promote overall positive mental health. Participants in the other group received a standard CBT intervention implemented by an experienced CBT therapist. Researchers reported that participants in both groups significantly reduced symptoms of generalized anxiety disorder, including pathological worrying, indicating the SBI intervention appeared to be just as effective as the CBT intervention. There was also low attrition in the SBI group, indicating the intervention was received well by the participants (Koszycki, Raab, Aldosary, & Bradwein, 2010).

The next study evaluated an intervention aimed to improve mental health and job performance among blue collar workers in Japan. Workers were randomized into a team-based, problem-solving intervention, which aimed to help workers (1) build on what they were already practicing, (2) focus on achievement, (3) link working conditions with management goals, (4) share and exchange their experiences, (5) become more involved with their work, and (6) use experiential-based learning, or a control condition, which provided no intervention. The intervention was successful for improving overall health among workers in the intervention group. Researchers reported that emotional distress remained stable in the intervention group, whereas it worsened in the control group. Also, overall job performance improved in the intervention group, whereas performance worsened in the control group. Finally, during a follow-up period emotional distress decreased for the intervention group but increased for the control group (Tsutsumi, Nagami, Yoshikawa, Kogi, & Kawakami, 2009).

Another study evaluated an Internet-based intervention to reduce depressive symptoms among overweight and obese women. Women were either randomized to a patient-centered assessment and counseling for exercise and nutrition via the Internet (PACEi) intervention, consisting of a computer-tailored treatment plan with 12 modules, or an "enhanced" standard care comparison group, which consisted of receiving standard advice from a health care provider regarding health lifestyle behaviors, and were provided take-home materials. Researchers reported a significantly greater decrease in depression scores in the PACEi group, as measured by the 10-item short version of the Center for Epidemiological Studies Depression Scale. Researchers also found that those who participated in the intervention more readily were also more likely to reduce their depression scores (Kerr et al., 2008).

The next study evaluated a brief intervention (BIC) compared with normal treatment (NORM) to prevent future suicide among suicide attempters in an emergency room setting in five international sites in Brazil, India, Iran, China, and Sri Lanka. The BIC intervention consisted of a 1-hour, one-on-one session with a health care provider (i.e., doctor, nurse, or psychologist) at the time of discharge from the emergency room and nine follow-up contacts via phone call or hospital visits periodically throughout the proceeding 18 months. The NORM treatment consisted of the standard protocol for each given country. After an 18-month follow-up period researchers reported that significantly fewer suicides were found in the BIC group compared with the NORM group (Fleischmann et al., 2008).

Another study evaluated an intervention aimed to reduce anxiety and depression and enhance coping skills for active duty military personnel deployed in Okinawa, Japan. The Outpatient Crisis Prevention Program was a comprehensive program that integrated information from various types of theories, including cognitive behavioral therapy, dialectical behavior theory, and crisis counseling, and emphasized four core skills: self-awareness and relaxation, emotion regulation, interpersonal effectiveness, and motivation and resilience. The program was implemented to troops over a week of all-day training periods and included short lectures, group exercises, individual activities, and discussion of film clips from popular movies. The intervention was successful for reducing depression and anxiety and at promoting self-reported healthy coping behaviors immediately after the intervention and at a 1-month follow-up period (Jones, Perkins, Cook, & Ong, 2008).

One study evaluated a yoga-based intervention to reduce overall stress among community residents in South Australia. Participants either participated in a 10-session yoga class, based on Hatha yoga, a form of yoga based on breathing and mediation, or a 10-session progressive muscle relaxation (PMR) intervention, which is traditionally designed to relax the body by participating in successive tensing and relaxation of major and minor body muscle groups. At the end of both interventions both groups were successful for reducing stress and anxiety; however, the yoga intervention appeared to be more effective at improving overall mental health. By the end of a 6-week follow-up period stress and anxiety were similar between both groups; however, the PMR intervention appeared to be more effective at improving vitality and social function (Smith, Hancock, Blake-Mortimer, & Eckert, 2007).

A community-based intervention for suicide prevention in Japan was evaluated. Researchers chose six rural towns in Akita Prefecture, Japan to receive an intervention lasting for 3 years. Six similar towns located nearby were used as controls, which received no intervention. This primary prevention intervention consisted of many phases implemented in order. During the first phase of the intervention residents were asked to complete a survey screening for depression, daily stressors, stress coping behaviors, mental health literacy, and attitudes toward suicide prevention. Next, leaflets were distributed to each household in the community, and lecture meetings given by university instructors, local medical practitioners, and public health nurses were held three to five times per year to increase awareness about suicide and empower the citizens. The third phase consisted of implementing special trainings on suicide prevention to public health workers to give mental health consultations to town residents. Next, residents were encouraged to create their own suicide prevention measures. For example, town residents created their own mental health lectures and performed theatrical performances to raise awareness. Next, residents were made aware of a list of counseling centers that provided access to psychological counseling as needed. Finally, special programs were created for senior citizens to promote them feeling a sense of community. Researchers concluded that as a result of these efforts, suicide rates appeared to have decreased. From 1999 to 2004 the suicide rate in the intervention towns decreased from 70.8 (per 100,000) to 34.1 annually, whereas the suicide rate increased in control towns from 47.8 to 49.1 annually (Motohashi, Kaneko, Sasaki, & Yamaji, 2007).

Another study evaluated an eating disorder prevention program among undergraduate college women. Participants attended a 1.5-hour seminar on eating disorders biweekly for an entire 15-week semester. During the semester the seminar series covered topics such as the pathology of anorexia nervosa, bulimia nervosa, binge eating disorder, and obesity;

the epidemiology of such disorders; and an overview of prevention and treatment efforts for eating disorders. Students also engaged in extended classroom discussions pertaining to topics about eating disorders, in which the course attempted to correct misperceptions of body shape/image norms. Students were required to write a 10-page report that represented a critical review of an area of their choice regarding to eating disorders. Compared with a control group of students, students in this intervention reported a greater reduction in thin ideal internalization, body dissatisfaction, and dieting and eating disordered symptoms and significantly gained less weight during the intervention period. These behaviors were also sustained after a 6-month follow-up period (Stice, Orjada, & Tristan, 2006).

Another example is the Campus Bodies intervention, a campus-based intervention aimed at the prevention and control of emotional disorders among college women. The cognitive behavior–based intervention was implemented over the Internet during an 8-week period. Program goals included reducing weight and shape concerns, enhancing body image, promote healthy weight control methods, reducing binge eating, and increasing knowledge about the risks associated with eating disorders. After the intervention female college students in the intervention reported significantly less weight concerns and concerns regarding thinness and bulimia compared with a wait-listed control group, and these changes were sustained after a 1-year follow-up (Taylor et al., 2006).

An autogenic training (AT) intervention to reduce anxiety in college nursing students in the United Kingdom was evaluated. AT consists of six exercises that aim for muscle relaxation and is expected to create an overall feeling of calmness among participants. Nurses in the study were randomized into one of three groups: a group receiving an 8-week AT intervention, a group receiving an 8-week "laughter" therapy intervention, and a group receiving no intervention but offered the AT intervention after the study. Overall, the AT group experienced an immediate postintervention significant reduction in state and trait anxiety, pulse, and blood pressure compared with the other two groups; however, there were no reported differences between groups for emotional exhaustion, depersonalization, or personal accomplishment (Kanji, White, & Ernst, 2006).

The next study evaluated the effects of four aerobic regimens on reducing depressive symptoms. Participants were randomized into a combination of either low-dose exercise (LD) or higher dose exercise (HD) and lower frequency (3 days/week) or higher frequency (5 days/week) (LD-3 days, LF-5 days, HD-3 days, or HD-5 days). An exercise placebo control group was also used whereby participants engaged in 15 to 20 minutes of stretching for 3 days a week. Overall, there were no differences in depression scores across treatment groups; however, depression scores decreased among all treatment groups, with the lowest scores reported for the HD-3 days group and the highest scores reported for the placebo group (Dunn, Trivedi, Kampert, Clark, & Chambliss, 2005).

A yoga-based pilot study was investigated that examined the effects of a 5-week yoga class on the symptoms of depression in mildly depressed young adults. Participants participated in a type of yoga called Iyengar yoga, a form of yoga based on the teachings of yoga master B.K.S. Iyengar, which focuses on specific sequences of *asanas* (or body positions) thought to reduce depression. Participants were compared with a wait-listed control group. Researchers reported that those in the yoga group showed significant reductions in depression and trait anxiety, compared with the control group. Researchers also measured participants' cortisol levels, which have been associated with depression, and noted a trend for higher morning cortisol levels in the yoga group compared with the control group (Woolery, Myers, Sternlieb, & Zeltzer, 2004).

Finally, one study investigated the effects of an exercise and social support intervention on depressive symptoms of new mothers in Australia. Women who had given birth in the past 12 months were recruited for this study and randomized into an experimental intervention group, consisting of a 12-week intervention promoting physical activity and offering social support, or a nonintervention group. The experimental intervention consisted of three group-walking sessions lasting 30 to 40 minutes, pre- and poststretching exercises, and a weekly informal "chat and play" session, encouraging mothers to socialize with each other and concurrently play with their children. Results indicated that when compared with the nonintervention group, mothers in the intervention group significantly improved their fitness levels and depressive symptoms. However, there did not appear to be any difference between groups for social support levels (Armstrong & Edwards, 2003).

FOCUS FEATURE 10.3 SOUTH AFRICAN STRESS AND HEALTH STUDY

The role of stressful life events in the development of mental disorders is not well understood; however, such events can initiate or exacerbate mental health problems, such as depression. Stressful life events can be characterized as proximal (or recent) events, such as a death in the family or birth of a child, or distal (or older) events, such as childhood adversities or abuse. Few studies have reported nationally representative data, especially among low and middle income countries, describing the distribution of proximal and distal life events in the population and how these events relate to psychological distress. The purpose of the South African Stress and Health (SASH) study was to determine how such life events were associated with anxiety, mood, substance use, and impulse control in citizens of South Africa.

The SASH study included 4,351 adults. Mental disorders were assessed using the World Health Organization Composite International Diagnostic Interview version 3.0 and included a wide variety of disorders from depression and anxiety disorders to substance abuse disorders and intermittent explosive disorder. Concurrently, several stressful life events were evaluated, including *global negative life events* (i.e., recent experiences with illness or injury), *relationship stress, domestic violence or physical partner violence, social strain* (i.e., demands friends and family put on the individual), and *early life stress* (i.e., childhood adversities).

Researchers found that women, those of Indian decent, ages 35 through 49, and married were more likely to be victims of domestic violence. There were no other differences among gender for types of stress; however, Blacks were significantly much more likely to experience global life events or early life economic strain compared with any other racial group. Physical partner violence was also predicted by all other lifetime disorders. Finally, a single marital status was the strongest demographic predictor of any 12-month and lifetime disorder. This study provides evidence that stressful life events, both distal and proximal, significantly contribute to major psychiatric disorders among citizens of South Africa (Seedat et al., 2009).

SKILL-BUILDING ACTIVITY

Imagine you have been asked to work with a group at young adults. How would you go about assessing their risk for mental health problems? What factors would you look for? What would be the key topics for your program? What would be the duration of your program? You can take the help of an existing program from this chapter to help you in your task.

SUMMARY

The transition into adulthood can be a difficult and even scary one from adolescence. Common questions are asked at this stage: Should I go to school? How long should I go to school? Should I get married? How long is too long to wait for these milestones? Regardless of how we define the life cycle process, many cycles focus on the principle that we leave home, complete school, enter the workforce, get married, and have children. One popular model that describes this transition is the Family Life Cycle, which consists of six stages.

The first stage of this cycle is leaving home and becoming a single young adult. During this stage young adults launch from the security of their childhood into a life of independence and self-sustainability. Questions young adults answer for themselves in this stage include will I finish high school? If not, will I get a GED? Will I go to college? How long will I go to college? Should I join the military? What holds true for each of these decisions is that higher education is typically related to higher salaries and less life stress. High school graduates make more money than high school dropouts, and the higher the postsecondary education (bachelor's, master's or doctorate degree), the higher the salary.

The next stage of the family life cycle is the joining of families through marriage, whereby a new couple joins together for marriage. Marriage is social union or legal contract between a man and woman, and rules and regulations regarding marriage differ between countries and cultures. Some recognize marriage as an act that can only occur between a man and women; however, others and some states now recognize marriage as an act that can be done between members of the same sex. Although marriage remains the popular choice for a living arrangement among adults, the trend toward marriage has been declining in recent years, as the median age of marriage for men and women increases.

The next stage of the cycle is becoming parents with young children. With advances in family planning and the advent of various birth control methods, this stage has been delayed in recent decades among young adults. The final stages of the family life cycle entail children growing up and eventually transitioning to repeat the process of their own family life cycle. The fourth stage of the cycle is called the family with adolescents. This stage entails a time period when children are now becoming more independent and seek to find their own identity. During this stage parents learn to develop which type of parenting style best suits them. The fifth stage of the cycle is the family at midlife. This stage includes the time parents launch their own children, as described in the first stage of the cycle. The final stage of the cycle is the family in later life. This includes the family in retirement and becoming grandparents.

There are many important determinants to mental health among adults as mentioned in previous chapters. This chapter focuses on divorce, obesity, socioeconomic status or poverty, and work-related stress. There have been many reported mental health benefits of marriage; however, when marriages end couples go through a process called divorce. Divorce has increased dramatically in recent decades; however, rates have stabilized in the past few years. If children are involved when couples divorce, parents must decide important matters such as who retains legal and physical custody of the children and whether one parent should have sole custody or both parents should retain joint custody. Marital conflict and divorce have been shown to cause distress among both parents and children.

Obesity is another important determinant of mental health among adults. Obesity is often defined by an individuals body mass index, with an index less than 18.5 considered underweight, an index of 18.5 to 24.9 considered normal weight, an index of 25 to 29.9 considered overweight, and an index greater than 30 considered obese. Obesity has been found to be associated with major depression, bipolar disorder, and panic disorder. Obese adults are also often unfairly discriminated against in a variety of settings, including their workplace and health care settings.

Socioeconomic status is another determinant, usually described as level of poverty, which refers to a status that is determined by comparing an individual's annual income to a set of dollar values (or thresholds) that vary by family size, number of children, and age of householder. This is an important issue, as poverty rates have increased across the nation. Poverty rates also differ by states, to as low as 8.5% in New Hampshire to a high of 21.9% in Mississippi. Poverty has been associated with many adverse mental health outcomes, including depression and anxiety, as well as violence, unemployment, and insecurity, which in turn have all been correlated with the onset of many adult mental disorders.

Finally, work-related stress is an important determinant of mental health among adults, as it has been attributable to individual psychosomatic and psychosocial distress; absenteeism; turnover and productivity losses; tension, anger, anxiety, depression, mood disorders, mental fatigue, and sleep disturbances; and societal costs including absenteeism, loss of productivity, and health care consumption.

Primary interventions that aim for the prevention of mental heath issues and promoting overall good health are typically implemented in the community or college setting. Many of these interventions are based on cognitive behavior therapy, enhancing problem-solving skills, dialectical behavior theory, and crisis counseling. Some even implemented environmental changes and enacted policies to prevent and make mental health awareness. Interventions ranged from brief participation to as long as 3 years and were implemented in a variety of ways, including sororities, through churches, worksite wellness, colleges, over the Internet, in the emergency room, military bases, yoga groups, and entire rural towns. Overall, these interventions were found to be effective for preventing the onset of mental issues and reducing current mental health issues.

REVIEW QUESTIONS

1. Summarize the six stages of the Family Life Cycle.
2. Describe what factors attribute to the delayed launching today's young adults face.
3. Explain the benefits and barriers of going to college in adulthood.
4. Differentiate between federal Stafford loans and the Montgomery GI Bill.
5. Discuss the current trends in marriage and living as a single adult.
6. Describe various types of custody that divorced couples have, pertaining to their children.
7. Differentiate between underweight, normal weight, overweight, and obese.
8. Define poverty and discuss why rates may be different across the United States.

WEBSITES TO EXPLORE

Network on Transitions to Adulthood

http://transad.pop.upenn.edu/

This is the official website of the Network on the Transitions to Adulthood, an organization that examines the changing nature of early adulthood (ages 18–34). This network consists of experts in many fields, including pediatrics, public health, and sociology, with research interests focusing on six major areas: education, labor economics, social history, changing attitudes and norms, developmental changes, and ethnography. *Locate the "Trends and Profiles" link on this website and read through the information. What surprised you the most?*

National Suicide Prevention Lifeline (1-800–273-TALK (8255))

http://www.suicidepreventionlifeline.org/

This is the official website of the National Suicide Prevention Lifeline, which is a 24-hour, toll-free, confidential helpline for any individual at risk for suicide. Upon calling the number individuals are connected to 1 of 140 crisis centers located in each state, including the District of Columbia. The helpline provides crisis counseling and mental health referrals. *Review the various links on this website. Review the various educational materials on the "Materials" link. What are your impressions?*

Job Stress Network

http://www.workhealth.org/

This is the official homepage of the Center for Social Epidemiology, a private/nonprofit foundation with a purpose to promote the awareness of the role of environmental and occupational stress in the development of cardiovascular disease. The purpose of this website is to provide a platform for new and innovative research regarding work-related stress, to help facilitate communication among researchers and the public. This organization is also involved with the STEP program (Surveillance, Training, and Early Prevention) and aims to improve workers psychosocial well-being and cardiovascular health. *Review the "Risk Factors" links on this website. Write a reflection for which risk factors you currently have or foresee you having in the future. Also write on what you believe you could do to prevent these risk factors from happening.*

Young Families Program, Children's Inc.

http://www.childreninc.org/young-families-program.html

This is the official website of the Young Families program provided by Children's Inc., an organization that aims to advance the success of young children by partnering with families, professionals, and the community. This organization runs many programs, but this specific program provides free home visitation sessions for first-time parents of Kenton County, Kentucky, until the child is 3 and a half. The goals of the program are to ensure a healthy pregnancy, encourage positive parent–child interactions, increase indices of child health, ensure that children are on target developmentally, and assist families to become self-sufficient. *Review this program at the website listed above. Write out your impressions about this program. Is there a similar program in your area? If not, do you believe first-time parents in your area would benefit from such a program?*

Reaching Out About Depression (ROAD)

http://www.reachingoutaboutdepression.org/

This is the official website of the Reaching Out About Depression (ROAD) program, an innovative program for women in poverty suffering from depression. ROAD's four main mission objectives are (1) creating a network of support for low-income women experiencing stress or depression, (2) offering strategies and resources for individuals and communities, (3) creating leadership opportunities for ROAD participants, and (4) educating mental health and social service providers and advocates for women and families in the ROADS program. *Locate the "Our Stories" link on this website and read through two or three stories. Write your impressions about the story that touched you the most.*

REFERENCES AND FURTHER READINGS

American Council on Education. (2010). GED testing services. Retrieved from http://www.acenet .edu/AM/Template.cfm?Section=GED_TS.

Armstrong, K., & Edwards, H. (2003). The effects of exercise and social support on mothers reporting depressive symptoms: A pilot randomized controlled trial. *International Journal of Mental Health Nursing, 12*(2), 130–138.

Baum, S., & Payea, K. (2004). *Education pays 2004.* New York: The College Board.

Becker, C. B., Wilson, C., Williams, A., Kelly, M., McDaniel, L., & Elmquist, J. (2010). Peer-facilitated cognitive dissonance versus healthy weight eating disorders prevention: A randomized comparison. *Body Image, 7,* 280–288.

Biddlecom, A., & Martin, S. (2006). Childless in America. *Contexts, 5*(4), 54.

Puhl, R., & Brownell, K. D. (2001). Bias, discrimination, and obesity. *Obesity Research, 9*(12), 788–805.

Byant-Davis, T., Ullman, S. E., Tsong, Y., Tillman, S., & Smith, K. (2010). Struggling to survive: Sexual assault, poverty, and mental health outcomes of African American women. *American Journal of Orthopsychiatry, 80*(1), 61–70.

Bureau of Labor Statistics. (2009). Job opportunities in the armed forces. Retrieved from http:// www.bls.gov/oco/ocos249.htm.

Cameron, S. V., & Heckman, J. J. (1993). The nonequivalence of high school equivalents. *Journal of Labor Economics, 11*(1), 1–47.

Carter, B., & McGoldrick, M. (1999). *The expanded family life-cycle: individual, family and social perspectives* (3rd ed.). Needham, MA: Allyn & Bacon.

Centers for Disease Control and Prevention. (2009a). About the BRFSS: Turning information into public health. Retrieved from http://www.cdc.gov/brfss/about.htm.

Centers for Disease Control and Prevention. (2009b). National marriage and divorce rate trends. Retrieved from http://www.cdc.gov/nchs/nvss/marriage_divorce_tables.htm.

Center for Quality Assessment and Improvement in Mental Health. (1999). The Patient Health Questionnaire (PHQ-9)—Overview. Retrieved from http://www.cqaimh.org/pdf/tool_phq9.pdf.

Department of Defense. (2010). *Population representation in the military services, fiscal year 2008 report.* Washington, DC: Office of the Assistant Secretary of Defense (Force Management and Personnel).

DeNavas-Walt, C., Proctor, B. D., Smith, J. C. (2010). *Income, poverty, and health insurance coverage in the United States: 2009.* Washington, DC: U.S. Government Printing Office.

Dorling, D. (2009). Unemployment and health: Health benefits vary according to the method of reducing unemployment. *British Medical Journal, 338,* 829.

Dunn, A. L., Trivedi, M. H., Kampert, J. B., Clark, C., & Chambliss, H. O. (2005). Exercise treatment for depression: Efficacy and dose response. *American Journal of Preventive Medicine, 28*(1), 1–8.

Fleischmann, A., Bertolote, J. M., Wasserman, D., Leo, D. D., Bolhari, J., Botega, N. J., …, & Than, H. T. T. (2008). Effectiveness of brief intervention and contact for suicide attempters: A randomized controlled trial in five countries. *Bulletin of the World Health Organization, 86,* 703–709.

Flegal, K. M., Carroll, M. D., Ogden, C. L., & Curtin, L. R. (2010). Prevalence and trends in obesity among US adults, 1999–2008. *Journal of the American Medical Association, 303*(3), 235–241.

Fortes-Ferreira, L., Peiro, J. M., Gonzalez-Morales, M. G., & Martin, I. (2006). Work-related stress and well-being: The roles of direct action coping and palliative coping. *Scandinavian Journal of Psychology, 47,* 293–302.

Furstenberg, F. F. (2010). On a new schedule: Transitions to adulthood and family change. *Future of children, 20*(1), 67–87.

Gottman, R. M., & Silver, N. (2000). *The seven principles for making marriages work: A practical guide from the country's foremost relationship expert* (1st ed.). New York: Three Rivers Press.

Heckman, J. J., & LaFontaine, P. A. (2010). The American high school graduation rate: Trends and levels. *Review of Economics and Statistics, 92*(2), 244–262.

Hewitt, B., Turrell, G., & Giskes, K. (2010). Marital loss, mental health and the role of perceived social support: Findings from six waves of an Australian population based panel study. *Journal of Epidemiology and Mental Health,* 1–7. Retrieved from http://jech.bmj.com.proxy.libraries.uc.edu/content/early/2010/10/21/jech.2009.104893.abstract?sid=c87e578d-fd8e-48a2-813e-463256495d40.

Institute for Higher Education Policy. (2005). The investment payoff: A 50 state analysis of the public and private benefits of higher education. Retrieved from http://www.ihep.org/Pubs/PDF/InvestmentPayoff2005.pdf.

Jia, H., & Lubetkin, E. I. (2005). The impact of obesity on health-related quality-of-life in the general adult US population. *Journal of Public Health, 27,* 156–164.

Jones, D. E., Perkins, K., Cook, J. H., & Ong, A. L. (2008). Intensive coping skills training to reduce anxiety and depression for forward-deployed troops. *Military Medicine, 173,* 241–246.

Kang, H. K., Natelson, B. H., Mahan, C. M., Lee, K. Y., & Murphy, F. M. (2003). Post-traumatic stress disorder and chronic fatigue syndrome-like illness among Gulf War Veterans: A population-based survey of 30,000 veterans. *American Journal of Epidemiology, 157*(2), 141–148.

Kanji, N., White, A., & Ernst, E. (2006). Autogenic training to reduce anxiety in nursing students: Randomized controlled trial. *Journal of Advanced Nursing, 53*(6), 729–735.

Kelly, J. B. (2006). Children's living arrangements following separation and divorce: Insights from empirical and clinical research. *Family Process, 46*(1), 35–52.

Kerr, J., Patrick, K., Norman, G., Stein, M. B., Calfas, K., Zabinski, M., & Robinson, A. (2008). Randomized control trial of a behavioral intervention for overweight women: Impact on depressive symptoms. *Depression and Anxiety, 25,* 555–558.

Kessler, R. C., Sonnega, A., Bromet, E., Hughes, M., & Nelson, C. B. (1995). Posttraumatic stress disorder in the national comorbidity survey. *Archives of General Psychiatry, 52*(12), 1048–1060.

Kleykamp, M. A. (2006). College, jobs, or the military? Enlistment during a time of war. *Social Science Quarterly, 87*(2), 272–290.

Knox, K. L., Pflanz, S., Talcott, G. W., Campise, R. L., Lavigne, J. E., Bajorska, …, Caine, E. D. (2010). The US Air Force suicide prevention program: Implications for public health policy. *American Journal of Public Health, 100*(12), 2457–2463.

Koszycki, D., Raab, K., Aldosary, F., & Bradwein, J. (2010). A multifaith spiritually based intervention for generalized anxiety disorder: A pilot randomized trial. *Journal of Clinical Psychology, 66*(4), 430–441.

Kreider, R. M., & Elliott, D. B. (2007). *America's families and living arrangements: 2007.* Current Population Reports, P20-561. Washington, DC: U.S. Census Bureau.

Kurdek, L. A. (2005). What do we know about gay and lesbian couples? *Current Directions in Psychological Science, 14*(5), 251–254.

Lachman, M. E. (2004). Development in midlife. *Annual Review of Psychology, 55,* 305–331.

Lerner, D., & Henke, R. M. (2008). What does research tell us about depression, job performance, and work productivity? *Journal of Occupational and Environmental Medicine, 50*(4), 401–410.

Maroney, D., & Golub, S. (1992). Nurses' attitudes toward obese persons and certain ethnic groups. *Perceptual & Motor Skills, 75,* 387–391.

Motohashi, Y., Kaneko, Y., Sasaki, H., & Yamaji, M. (2007). A decrease in suicide rates in Japanese rural towns after community-based intervention by the health promotion approach. *Suicide and Life-Threatening Behavior, 37*(5), 593–599.

Najman, J. M., Hayatbakhsh, M. H., Clavarino, A., Bor, W., O'Callaghan, M. J., & Williams, G. M. (2010). Family poverty over the early life course and recurrent adolescent and young adult anxiety and depression: A longitudinal study. *American Journal of Public Health, 100*(9), 1719–1723.

National Center for Educational Statistics. (2010). Fast facts. Retrieved from http://nces.ed.gov /fastfacts/display.asp?id=98.

National Institute of Mental Health. (2010). Post traumatic stress disorder (PTSD). Retrieved from http://www.nimh.nih.gov/health/topics/post-traumatic-stress-disorder-ptsd/index.shtml.

Office of Law Revision Counsel, U.S. House of Representatives. (2010). Definition of "marriage" and "spouse." Retrieved from http://uscode.house.gov/uscode-cgi/fastweb.exe?getdoc+uscview +t01t04+10555+3++%28Marriage%29%20%20%20%20%20%20%20%20%20%20%20.

Patel, V., Araya, R., de Lima, M., Ludermir, A., & Todd, C. (1999). Women, poverty, and common mental disorders in four restructuring societies. *Social Science & Medicine, 49,* 1461–1471.

Patterson, C J. (2006). Children of lesbian and gay parents. *Current Directions in Psychological Science, 15*(5), 241–244.

Riskind, R. G., & Patterson, C. J. (2010). Parenting intentions and desires among childless lesbian, gay, and heterosexual individuals. *Journal of Family Psychology, 24*(1), 78–81.

Saxena, S., Thornicroft, G., Knapp, M., & Whiteford, H. (2007). Resources for mental health: Scarcity, inequity, and inefficiency. *Lancet, 370,* 879–889.

Schmieder, A. M. (2008). Best interests and parental presumptions: Bringing same-sex custody agreements. *William & Mary Bill of Rights Journal, 17,* 293–318.

Seedat, S., Stein, D. J., Jackson, P. B., Heeringa, S. G., Williams, D. R., & Myer, L. (2009). Life stress and mental disorders in the South African stress and health study. *South African Medical Journal, 99*(5), 375–382.

Settersten, R. A., Jr., & Ray, B. (2010). What's going on with young people today? The long and twisting path to adulthood. *Future of Children, 20*(1), 19–41.

Simon, G. E., Ludman, E. J., Linde, J. A., Operskalski, B. H., Ichikawa, L., Rohde, P., . . . , Jeffery, R. W. (2008). Association between obesity and depression in middle aged women. *General Hospital Psychiatry, 30*(1), 32–39.

Simon, G. E., Von Korff, M., Saunders, K., Miglioretti, D. L., Crane, P. K., van Belle, G., & Kessler, R. C. (2006). Association between obesity and psychiatric disorders in the US adult population. *Achieves of General Psychiatry, 63*(7), 824–830.

Smith, C., Hancock, H., Blake-Mortimer, J., & Eckert, K. (2007). A randomised comparative trial of yoga and relaxation to reduce stress and anxiety. *Complementary Therapies in Medicine, 15*, 77—83.

Smyth, B. (2005). Time to rethink time? The experience of time with children after divorce. *Family Matters, 71*, 4–10.

Sobolewski, J. M., & Amato, P. R. (2007). Parents' discord and divorce, parent-child relationships and subjective well-being in early adulthood: Is feeling close to two Parents always better than feeling close to one? *Social Forces, 85*(3), 1105–1124.

Stice, E., Orjada, K., & Tristan, J. (2006). Trial of a psychoeducational eating disturbance intervention for college women: A replication and extension. *International Journal of Eating Disorders, 39*(3), 233–239.

Story, L. B., & Bradbury, T. N. (2004). Understanding marriage and stress: Essential questions and challenges. *Clinical Psychology Review, 23*, 1139–1162.

Strieber, A. (2010). The 10 most stressful jobs of 2010. Retrieved from http://www.careercast.com /jobs/content/ten-most-stressful-jobs-2010-jobs-rated-9#slide.

Tanilian, T., & Jaycox, L. (2008). *Invisible wounds of war: Psychological and cognitive injuries, their consequences, and services to assist recovery* (1st ed.). Santa Monica, CA: RAND Publishing.

Taylor, C. B., Bryson, S., Luce, K. H., Cunning, D., Doyle, A. C., Abascal, L. B., . . . , & Wilfley, D. E. (2006). Prevention of eating disorders in at-risk college-age women. *Archives of General Psychiatry, 63*, 881–888.

Tsutsumi, A., Nagami, M., Yoshikawa, T., Kogi, K., & Kawakami, N. (2009). Participatory intervention for workplace improvements on mental health and job performance among blue-collar workers: A cluster randomized controlled trial. *Journal of Occupational & Environmental Medicine, 51*, 554–563.

Tyler, J. H., & Lofstrom, M. (2009). Finishing high school: Alternative pathways and dropout recovery. *Future of Children, 19*(1), 77–103.

U.S. Census Bureau. (2005). Estimated median age at first marriage, by sex: 1890 to the present. Retrieved from http://www.census.gov/population/socdemo/hh-fam/ms2.pdf.

U.S. Census Bureau. (2010a). 2006–2008 American community survey. Retrieved from http:// factfinder.census.gov/.

U.S. Census Bureau. (2010b). Poverty: 2008 and 2009 American Community Survey. Retrieved from http://www.census.gov/hhes/www/poverty/poverty.html.

U.S. Department of Labor. (2010). Labor force statistics from the current population survey. Retrieved from http://www.bls.gov/cps/lfcharacteristics.htm#unemp.

U.S. Department of Veteran Affairs. (2009). Montgomery GI bill active duty (Mgib-Ad). Retrieved from http://www.gibill.va.gov/.

Van der Klink, J. J. L., Blonk, R. W. B., Schene, A. H., & Van Dijk, F. J. H. (2001). The benefits of interventions for work-related stress. *American Journal of Public Health, 91*, 270–276.

Waite, L. J., & Lehrer, E. L. (2003). The benefits from marriage and religion in the United States: A comparative analysis. *Population and Development Review, 29*(2), 255–276.

Walsh, R. (1999). *Essential spirituality: The 7 central practices to awaken heart and mind.* New York: John Wiley & Sons, Inc.

Wei, C. C., & Berkner, L. (2008). Trends in undergraduate borrowing. II. Federal student loans in 1995–96, 1999–2000, and 2003–04 (NCES 2008–179 rev). Washington, DC: National Center for Education Statistics, Institute of Education Sciences, U.S. Department of Education.

Wei, C. C., Berkner, L., He, S., Lew, S., Cominole, M., & Siegel, P. (2009). 2007–08 National Postsecondary Student Aid Study (NPSAS:08): Student financial aid estimates for 2007–08: First look (NCES 2009-166). Washington, DC: National Center for Education Statistics, Institute of Education Sciences, U.S. Department of Education.

Wieclaw, J., Agerbo, E., Mortensen, P. B., Burr, H., Tüchsen, F., & Bonde, J. P. (2005). Work related violence and threats and the risk of depression and stress disorders. *Journal of Epidemiology and Community Health, 60*, 771–775.

Woolery, A., Myers, H., Sternlieb, B., & Zeltzer, L. (2004). A yoga intervention for young adults with elevated symptoms of depression. *Alternative Therapies, 10*(2), 60–63.

CHAPTER 11

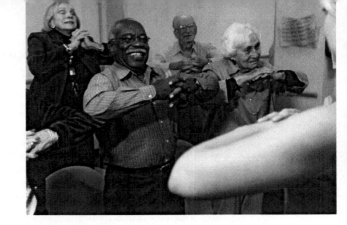

Mental Health
for Older Adults

CHAPTER OBJECTIVES

After reading this chapter you should be able to
- Identify various issues among older adults
- Identify differences between young-old, middle-old, and old-old adults
- Describe the demography of older adults
- Identify reasons why older adults are living longer
- Identify various types of social support for older adults
- Differentiate between the types of elder abuse and maltreatment
- Describe spirituality and how it can affect the mental health of older adults
- Discuss various community and environmental interventions aimed to prevent mental health problems among older adults

ISSUES IN OLDER ADULTS

Demography of Older Adults

The U.S. population is growing older. In many countries the term *old* refers to those who are 65 years of age or older. However, in an attempt to further classify this group, researchers typically divide older adults into three strata: **young-old** refers to adults between the ages of 65 and 74 years, **middle-old** refers to adults between the ages of 75 and 84 years, and **old-old** refers to adults 85 years and older. In 2008 39 million older adults were living in the United States, accounting for 12.8% of the population. This number is expected to dramatically grow in upcoming years. By 2040 the older adult population is expected to almost double to 72 million, which would be nearly 20%, or one-fifth, of the U.S. population (Federal Interagency Forum on Aging-Related Statistics, 2010). The growth of the older population comes mostly from two sources: life expectancy has increased, with

> *By 2030 the older adult population is expected to almost double to 72 million, which would be nearly 20% of the U.S. population.*

advances in medicine and technology; and the aging **baby boomer generation**, a generation of children born during the post World War II era from 1946 to 1964, will begin to turn 65 in 2011. **Table 11.1** shows the changes in the proportion of older adults from 1900 and projected changes until 2050.

This population differs from the younger and middle adult population in many ways. Women tend to outnumber men in this group, especially as they age. In 2008 women accounted for 58% of the population age 65 and over and for 67% of the population 85 and over. The older population is also expected to become more racially diverse in coming years. In 2008 non-Hispanic Whites represented 80.4% of older adults, whereas African Americans (8.5%), Hispanics (7%), Asians (3.3%), and all other races combined (1.3%) represented

TABLE 11.1   Reported Percentage and Projections of U.S. Population 65 and Older and 85 and Older

Year	65 and Older	85 and Older
1900	4.1%	0.2%
1920	4.7%	0.2%
1940	6.8%	0.3%
1960	9.0%	0.5%
1980	11.3%	1.0%
2000	12.4%	1.5%
2010*	13.0%	1.9%
2020*	16.1%	1.9%
2030*	19.3%	2.3%
2050*	20.2%	4.3%

*Represents projected statistics.
Source: Federal Interagency Forum on Aging-Related Statistics. (2010). Older Americans 2010: Key indicators of well-being. Washington, DC: U.S. Government Printing Office.

TABLE 11.2 Marital Trends Among the Young-Old, Middle-Old, and Old-Old								
	Young-Old 65–74 years			**Middle-Old** 75–84 years			**Old-Old** 85 and Older		
	Total	**Men**	**Women**	**Total**	**Men**	**Women**	**Total**	**Men**	**Women**
Married	67% / 79% / 57%			51% / 72% / 37%			29% / 55% / 15%		
Widowed	17% / 7% / 25%			39% / 19% / 53%			63% / 38% / 76%		
Divorced	12% / 10% / 14%			7% / 6% / 7%			4% / 3% / 5%		
Never married	4% / 4% / 4%			4% / 4% / 4%			4% / 5% / 4%		

Source: Federal Interagency Forum on Aging-Related Statistics. (2010). Older Americans 2010: Key indicators of well-being. Washington, DC: U.S. Government Printing Office.

a much smaller portion. However, by 2050 it is projected that non-Hispanic Whites will represent 58.5% of older adults, and Hispanics (20%), African Americans (11.9%), Asians (8.5%), and all other races combined (2.7%) will represent a much larger portion of the population (Federal Interagency Forum on Aging-Related Statistics, 2010). Older adults also reside in some states more so than others. States with the highest proportion of older adults include Florida (17.4%), West Virginia (15.7%), and Pennsylvania (15.3%), and states with the lowest proportion of older adults include Alaska (7.3%), Utah (9.0%), and Georgia (10.1%) (Federal Interagency Forum on Aging-Related Statistics, 2010).

Marital status can greatly impact an individual's mental health status. Marriage is still the preferred living arranging among older adults, as 57% are married; however, there are great disparities between men and women. For example, among adults 65 years and older 74.5% of men are married, whereas only 43.9% of women are married. As they age this disparity gets even wider. Overall, 51.2% of adults aged 74 to 85 years are married; however, 72.2% of men are married and only 36.6% of women are married. One factor that contributes to this divide is widowhood. **Widowhood** refers to a time for women (who are referred to as a widow) or men (who are referred to as a widower) when their spouse has died and they have not remarried. Widowhood is much more common among women. **Table 11.2** shows marital trends for this group (Federal Interagency Forum on Aging-Related Statistics, 2010).

Because men are more likely to have a spouse compared with women, they are also less likely to live alone. In 2008 only 19% of older men lived alone, whereas 40% of older women lived alone. Besides living with a spouse, other living arrangements included living with other relatives (7% for men and 17% for women) and living with nonrelatives (3% for men and 2% for women) (Federal Interagency Forum on Aging-Related Statistics, 2010). Most older adults live in homes they own. According to data from the Health and Retirement Study (HRS), a nationally representative study of the U.S. older population (U.S. Department of Health and Human Services [DHHS], 2009), 79% of older adults live in a home they own, whereas very few live in nursing homes or assisted living facilities. The number of older adults living in nursing homes is generally low until they reach old-old status. By that time almost 20% live in this setting (USDHHS, 2009).

FOCUS FEATURE 11.1 USE OF TAI CHI TO IMPROVE MENTAL HEALTH IN OLDER ADULTS

There appears to be a strong association between the engagement in physical activities and mental health among older adults. Although physical activity is recommended to older adults for its cognitive and physical benefits, it can be difficult for some to engage in such activities, especially those experiencing chronic pain or conditions such as arthritis. Therefore, exercise such as *Tai Chi* may be suitable because it is easily adapted for all body types and activity levels. Tai Chi is considered a "mind–body" exercise that is based on Taoism philosophy of balancing *chi*, or an individuals personal bioelectric energy. This type of exercise has also been shown to improve muscle strengthening, aerobic endurance, and flexibility. Tai Chi begins with breathing exercises that help the participant relax major muscle groups and joints and improve their posture. This is followed by a series of small-alternating circular movements with the hands and arms, followed by shifting the participant's body weight between legs. During the movements participants are encouraged to respect their personal limitations instead of attempting to exert themselves beyond what they are capable. Through practice, Tai Chi movements become easier, more fluid, and faster.

The proposed mechanism behind the effects of Tai Chi has been described in terms of *impairments*, *functional limitations*, and *disability*. For impairments, Tai Chi reduces pain by strengthening muscles and joints. It also reduces depression and anxiety by stimulating the relaxation response (i.e., increased cortisol levels and possibly endorphin secretion). For functional limitations Tai Chi improves an individual's *gait*, or the way in which they walk and support their bodies. This improves balance and decreases physical and mental pain. Finally, for disability, because Tai Chi improves impairments and functional limitations, individuals can engage in activities of daily living with greater ease.

Older adults who are interested in this activity should first ask their primary care physician or other health professionals to ensure they are physically able. It is important to take Tai Chi training from a qualified trainer and understand that this type of exercise takes time and patience to learn. Unlike other martial arts, Tai Chi does not have a belt system that indicates skill level. Older adults can access Tai Chi training in a variety of methods. Classes are typically available at senior centers or community adult education programs but can also be accessed on the Internet, from video rental stores, and/or libraries (Adler & Roberts, 2006). Yoga is another form of physical activity that is similar to Tai Chi and has similar beneficial effects.

Health Status

The life expectancy of older adults has increased in recent years. **Life expectancy** refers to the average number of years an individual is expected to live beyond his or her current age, as long as death rates remain constant. In 2006 life expectancy for older adults at age 65 was 18.5 years and for older adults aged 85 was 6.4 years (Federal Interagency Forum on Aging-Related Statistics, 2010). There are also noted disparities by gender and race, as women typically have longer life expectancies than men and Whites typically have longer life expectancies than African Americans and Hispanics (Federal Interagency Forum on Aging-Related Statistics, 2010). Many other industrialized countries also have longer life expectancies for their older adults compared with the United States. For example, older men and women (aged 65) in Switzerland, Japan, Australia, and Canada can all expect to live approximately 2 to 4 years longer than their American counterparts. With improved life expectancies overall death rates in the United States have declined in past decades. For example, deaths from heart disease and stroke have declined 50% since the early 1980s. However, some causes of death, including Alzheimer's disease, diabetes, and chronic lower respiratory diseases, have increased since then. In 2006 the leading causes of death among older adults, irrespective of race and gender, were heart disease (1,297 deaths per 100,000), cancer (1,025 per 100,000), and stroke (297 per 100,000) (Federal Interagency Forum on Aging-Related Statistics, 2010).

As we grow older the risk of diseases, most notably chronic diseases, and other health problems increases. The leading causes of death among older adults are from chronic diseases. A **chronic disease** is a type of disease that occurs over a long period of time. Chronic illnesses account for many of the conditions from which older adults suffer and can lead to premature death, disability, lower quality of life, and higher health care costs. In fact, 75% of the health care money spent in the United States is spent on conditions related to chronic diseases (National Center for Chronic Disease Prevention and Health Promotion, 2009). There are also disparities for chronic diseases among racial groups and genders. For example, heart disease affects more men (28.2%) than women (27.1%), but asthma tends to affect more women (11.5%) than men (8.9%). Cancer tends to affect more Whites (24.8%) than African Americans (13.3%), but hypertension tends to affect more African Americans (71.1%) than Whites (54.3%) (Federal Interagency Forum on Aging-Related Statistics, 2010).

The leading causes of death among older adults are from chronic diseases.

Our mental health also declines as we age. According to the HRS (USDHHS, 2009), researchers found that overall 10% of the older adult population (70 years and older) had moderate to severe cognitive impairments. Cognitive impairments are also the leading causes for institutionalizing older adults. Depression is the most prevalent mental health condition in the older population and a leading cause of disability. Overall, 14% of older adults suffer from severe depression; however, women are more likely to report depressive symptoms than men. Depression also increases with age, with old-old adults reporting higher depression rates for men and women (Federal Interagency Forum on Aging-Related Statistics, 2010; National Center for Chronic Disease Prevention and Health Promotion, 2009). Less older adults suffer from anxiety disorders. Overall, 11.6% of older adults suffer from some form of anxiety disorder, including panic disorders (1.3%), specific phobias (6.5%), social phobias (3.5%), generalized anxiety disorder (2.0%), and post-traumatic stress disorder (2.1%). As with depression, anxiety rates are significantly higher among women than men; however, unlike depression, anxiety rates appear to decline with age (Byers, Yaffe, Covinsky, Friedman, & Bruce, 2010).

Older adults also suffer from dementia and Alzheimer's disease in greater numbers than in the past. Historically when older adults' cognitive abilities would begin to diminish, we would label them as *senile*; however, that term is no longer used. Instead, the proper name for this disease is **dementia**, which is a progressive brain impairment that hinders memory and other cognitive functions that can interfere with normal daily living activities (Plassman et al., 2007). The most common form of dementia (approximately 70%) among older adults is **Alzheimer's disease**, which is a chronic condition that involves parts of the brain that control thought, memory, and language (Centers for Disease Control and Prevention, 2010a). Other forms of dementia include *vascular dementia*, which develops from impaired blood flow to certain regions of the brain; *Lewy body dementia*, which develops from abnormal protein deposits inside brain nerve cells; *Huntington's disease*, which develops from genetic abnormalities leading to the destruction of nerve cells in certain regions of the brain; and *Creutzfeldt-Jakob disease*, a rare (affecting 1 in 1 million people per year) disease affecting mostly younger adults (Alzheimer's Association, 2010).

Alzheimer's disease is the seventh leading cause of death among Americans and the fifth leading cause among older adults (Centers for Disease Control and Prevention, 2010a). Using data from the Aging, Demographics, and Memory Study (ADAMS), the first population-based study of dementia, researchers found that 13.9% (or 3.4 million) of adults 71 years and older have dementia and 9.7% have Alzheimer's disease (Plassman et al., 2007). Researchers found important predictors of dementia and Alzheimer's disease to be older age, lower education levels, and African American race (Plassman et al., 2007). Older adults with dementia or Alzheimer's disease also experience greater mental and physical health problems. In a study using community-dwelling older adults with and without Alzheimer's disease, researchers found older adults with the disease were more likely to have higher rates of bone fractures, to have other urgent medical conditions such as cardiovascular disease or diabetes, and to be hospitalized (Malone et al., 2009). Older adults with Alzheimer's disease also reported significantly higher rates of anxiety and depression (Malone et al., 2009). Depression among those with Alzheimer's disease and dementia has also been asso-

Depression is the most prevalent mental health condition in the older population and a leading cause of disability.

ciated with a lower quality of life, increased disability in activities of daily living, faster cognitive declines, higher rates of nursing home placements, relatively higher mortality, and a higher frequency of depression and burden on the caregivers (Starkstein, Mizrahi, & Power, 2008).

Death and Related Issues

Death is a natural part of life. There are several questions one should consider before death: Who do I want to make health care decisions in case I cannot? What medical treatments do I want or not want? What kind of funeral service do I prefer? How do I want my remains to be handled? How do I want my estate handled? All these questions can be outlined in advance directives. An **advance directive** is a document that specifies what actions should be taken for an individual's health in case they can no longer make such decisions due to sickness or incapacity and appoints a person to make such decisions on that individual's behalf. **Living wills** are one type of advance directives in which an individual's instructions for health care and medical emergencies are formally stated. Another type of an advance directive is a **power of attorney**, for which someone is appointed by the individual to make decisions on his or her behalf when he or she is unable. It is also important for individuals to write a formal will. This can help to ease family tension or conflict in situations when it is difficult for family members to agree on the requisition of assets. A **will** is a legal document by which a **testator**, or individual who leaves a will upon his or her death, names one or more individuals to manage his or her estate and outlines who receives which properties of the testator. In cases when an individual dies without a will, his or her property will be inherited typically to the next of kin; however, state laws can differ for this process. In cases when next of kin cannot be found, properties can be transferred to the government.

Employment and Retirement

In 2009 approximately 70% of men and 60% of women in their 50s worked full time (USDHHS, 2009). For these Americans many see their older years as a time to eventually stop working and retire. **Retirement** has historically been known as the act of leaving a job and ceasing to work, which typically happened around the age of 65. Attitudes, expectations, and behaviors related to work and retirement have changed in recent decades. For example, from the 1950s to the 1980s the average retirement age dropped, as many opted to retire before the age of 65. However, this trend appears to have subsided since then, as the average age for retirement has steadily increased. The baby boomer generation is also expected to work longer, and many are expected to work past the age of 65. Retirement rates first begin to sharply increase at the age of 62, which is the age adults first qualify for social security benefits (USDHHS, 2009).

Social Security refers to a federal entitlement program paid through worker payroll taxes. Benefits are paid out to individuals who already have retired, are disabled, are survivors of workers who have died, or are dependents of beneficiaries. The basic premise of this program is that current taxpayers pay money into a trust and benefits are paid out to beneficiaries, for which are mostly older adults. Historically, this meant a much larger taxpaying population that could support a smaller older adult population; however, as the baby boomer generation enters into the years they are eligible to receive social security benefits, this system will become stressed. For example, by 2037 it is projected that the amount of money set aside to pay social security benefits will become exhausted, and given the current tax structure the government will only be able to pay 76% of scheduled benefits (Goss, 2010). Because Social Security benefits are the most common source of income for older adults, this will likely create more financial stress for them in years to come. Older adults might also have to rely more on other sources of income such as pensions, annuities, income from assets, earnings from continued employment, and savings.

By the time adults turn 65, full-time employment rates reduce to approximately half of what they are for adults aged 50, and many of the older adults are still working work part time rather than full time. According to the HRS (USDHHS, 2009) many older adults report being happy and active in their retirement. Of those surveyed, 61% of retirees reported the retirement transition as "very satisfying" and only 7% reported it as "not satisfying." The HRS also asked retirees which factors motivated their choice for retirement. Among those aged 65 to 69 years 34% reported the desire to have "more time with family" as being very important, 28% reported they "wanted to do other things," 28% reported it was due to "poor health," and 7% reported they "didn't like work" (USDHHS, 2009).

FOCUS FEATURE 11.2 USE OF COMPLEMENTARY AND ALTERNATIVE THERAPIES IN COMMUNITY-DWELLING OLDER ADULTS

Complementary and alternative medicine (CAM) and therapy are defined as a group of diverse medical and health care systems, practices, and products that are not generally considered part of conventional medicine. The National Center for Complementary and Alternative Medicine (2010) categorizes CAM into four basic groups: natural products (i.e., dietary supplements, herbal products, probiotics, etc.), mind–body medicine (meditation, yoga, acupuncture, etc.), manipulative and body-based practices (i.e., spinal manipulation, massage), and other CAM practices (i.e., magnet therapy, light therapy). CAM and therapy are becoming increasing popular in today's society and are used frequently for aging-related conditions such as back pain, arthritis, anxiety, depression, and cancer. Researchers were interested in describing the current

(continued)

prevalence and patterns of CAM use among older adults, describing the characteristics of older CAM users, and identifying factors associated with older CAM use/nonuse (Cheung, Wyman, & Halcon, 2007).

Researchers surveyed 1,200 community-dwelling older adults (>65 years old) by mailing surveys to their households. The framework of the Health Belief Model conceptually guided the development of the survey questions. On average, respondents were 74.4 years old (standard deviation = 6.4 years), and most were women (55%), White (98%), married (65%), and educated (57% had greater than a high school education). Overall, 62.9% reported using at least one CAM and therapy, 10% reported using six or more CAMs and therapies, and on average participants reported using 3.0 (± 1.9) CAMs and therapies. The most widely used CAMs and therapies were nutritional supplements (44.3%) and spiritual healing/prayer (29.7%) and the least widely used were folk medicine (1.6%) and homeopathy (2.5%). Overall, women were more likely to use CAM and therapy than men, especially aromatherapy, massage therapy, healing touch, therapeutic touch, spiritual healing, yoga, and Tai Chi. CAM users reported a greater number of physically unhealthy days, combined physically and mentally unhealthy days, and number of clinical visits within the past year, compared with non-CAM users. CAM users also reported significantly more regular exercise than non-CAM users, and non-CAM users reported more tobacco use than CAM users. Older adults reported the most influential factors for using CAMs and therapies were perceived symptoms of health problems, greater personal control over their own health, and recommendations from family and friends. Older adults reported the most influential reasons for not using CAMs and therapies were lack of knowledge about their use and not believing they were effective (Cheung et al., 2007).

DETERMINANTS AND INFLUENCES ON MENTAL HEALTH OF OLDER ADULTS

Several factors influence mental health in older adults. These are shown in **Figure 11.1**.

Sleep and Sleep Patterns

Adequate sleep is essential for mental health. As we age physical changes happen to our bodies that affect our sleeping patterns. Healthy sleep progresses through several stages in a systematic manner that includes non-REM (non–rapid eye movement) sleep and REM

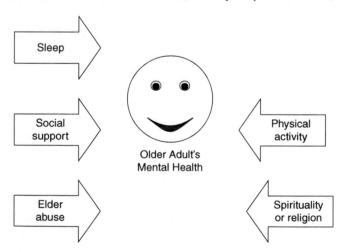

FIGURE 11.1   Determinants of older adult's mental health.

(rapid eye movement) sleep. Non-REM sleep is further divided into four stages, which starts with light sleep in stage 1 and progresses to heavier sleep in stages 3 and 4. As we age disturbances occur in this process and stages are interrupted, resulting in a tendency to go to bed earlier in the evenings and awaken earlier in the mornings (Wolkove, Elkholy, Baltzan, & Palayew, 2007).

Studies have consistently shown that sleep complaints increase as we get older, and 40% to 50% of older adults experience some type of sleep disturbance on a regular basis (Vitiello, 2009). A common complaint among older adults includes frequent and repeated interruptions during sleep, which are followed by long periods of wakefulness. Older adults are also awakened more easily by environmental stimuli or sounds at nighttime, resulting in less quality sleep. Other common problems are less total sleep and poor sleep efficiency, or the percentage of time in bed spent asleep. To compensate for these problems and lost sleep, older adults engage in more naps throughout the day (Vitiello, 2009). The need for sleep, however, does not actually change as we get older. According to the National Sleep Foundation (2009) our sleep needs remain constant throughout adulthood, with young, middle, and older adults all needing 7 to 9 hours of sleep per night.

Epidemiological evidence shows that sleep disturbances are more common among older adults with existing chronic diseases and poor physical and mental health. In a study using a nationally representative sample (from the 2003 National Sleep Foundation's annual Sleep in America poll), sleep disturbances were compared with 11 medical conditions: heart disease, hypertension, arthritis, diabetes, cancer, stroke, lung disease, depression, osteoporosis, memory problems/forgetfulness, and enlarged prostate (men only). Overall, 84% of respondents reported at least one medical condition, with hypertension (47%), arthritis (46%), and heart disease (18%) as the most common conditions and stroke (6%) and memory problems (11%) as the least common conditions (Foley, Ancoli-Israel, Britz, & Walsh, 2004).

The prevalence of many of these conditions also significantly increases with age. Quality of sleep was significantly associated with the presence of medical conditions, except hypertension, cancer, and an enlarged prostate. Among older adults memory loss has been associated with being awake frequently during the night and difficulty falling asleep, and depression has been associated with waking up too early, waking up feeling tired, daytime sleepiness, and unpleasant feelings in the legs (Foley, et al., 2004).

Another study using community-dwelling older adults (aged 65–80 years) compared *good sleepers* with *bad sleepers* (as measured by the Pittsburgh Sleep Quality Index) with measures of information-processing speed, working memory, inhibitory function, attention shifting, episodic memory, and abstract reasoning, all aspects of cognition that are expected to decline with age. Researchers found that good sleepers performed significantly better than bad sleepers on tests of working memory, attention shifting, and abstract problem solving, even when controlling for confounding variables that might affect sleep (i.e., depression or medication usage). However, no differences were found for processing speed, inhibitory function, or episodic memory between groups (Nebes, Buysse, Halligan, Houck, & Monk, 2009).

Poor sleep also appears to be related to increased risk of depression in older adults. In a 2-year longitudinal study of community-dwelling older adults, sleep disturbances significantly predicted prior depression and depression recurrence.

> *Currently 40% to 50% of older adults experience some type of sleep disturbance.*
>
> —Vitiello, 2009

These relationships were also independent of other depressive symptoms, chronic medical diseases, and antidepressant usage (Cho et al., 2008).

Social Support

Epidemiological evidence indicates that social support and relationships have a positive impact on mental health as well as mortality risk and physical health benefits, including improved cardiovascular, neuroendocrine, and immune system functioning (Fiori, Antonucci, & Cortina, 2006; Uchino, 2006). **Social support** has been described as "real or perceived resources provided by others that enable a person to feel cared for, valued, and part of a network of communication and mutual obligation" (Keyes, Kobau, Zahran, Zack, & Simoes, 2005, p. 433). Social support can include perceived emotional support, instrumental support, appraisal support, and informational support. **Perceived emotional support** includes any emotional support an individual believes he or she has available, whether it is needed or not. **Instrumental support** includes any support an individual receives directly from someone else, such as transportation or help with daily living activities. **Informational support** includes any support an individual receives regarding sharing knowledge that could benefit him or her, such as information about resources that are available (Keyes et al., 2005). Finally, **appraisal support** includes support from people who have given useful feedback for self-evaluation (House, 1981).

Older adults can be at higher risk of receiving inadequate social support, which in turn can impact their mental health. According to a survey using a nationally representative sample of community-dwelling older adults, researchers found more than 7 million older adults (or 17% of the studied population) were dissatisfied with the extent of emotional support available to them, and more than 2 million (or 5%) had no source of emotional support (White, Philogene, Fine, & Sinha, 2009). In the same study researchers found that older adults' perception of having adequate emotional support was associated with having a better health status, with those with perceived lower social support reporting a poorer health status (White et al., 2009).

In another study using a nationally representative sample of older adults (>54 years old) from the HRS, levels of loneliness were positively associated with depressive symptoms (Cacioppo, Hughes, Waite, Hawkley, & Thisted, 2006). In a study among community-dwelling older adults, those who were rarely visited by friends and family members reported more mentally unhealthy days, depressed days, worried, tense or anxious days, and fewer vitality days than those who were visited by friends and family members several times within the previous week (Keyes, et al., 2005). Also, older adults who reported having no close friends for emotional support also reported more physically unhealthy days, mentally unhealthy days, days with depressive symptoms, days with symptoms of anxiety, and significantly fewer days with vitality than those with three or more friends. Finally, those who perceived that help was available, although only for a short time, had fewer physically unhealthy days, depressed days, or worried, tense, or anxious days than those who perceived no help was available (Keyes et al., 2005).

In addition to receiving social and emotional support, giving such support through opportunities such as volunteering has been shown to enhance mental health and longevity. For example, using data from the Changing Lives of Older Couples survey, researchers found mortality was significantly lower among older adults who provided instrumental support to friends, relatives, and neighbors (Brown, Nesse, Vinokur, & Smith, 2003). Another study found that older adults who volunteered more frequently also measured significantly higher with regards to three measures of well-being, including functional dependency, self-rated health, and depression, compared with those who had not volunteered frequently (Morrow-Howell, Hinterlong, Rozario, & Tang, 2003).

Elder Abuse and Maltreatment

Elder abuse is also a determinant of the mental health of older adults, with an estimated overall prevalence 3% to 4% within this group (Lachs & Pillemer, 2004; Lindbloom, Brandt, Hough, & Meadows, 2007). Specific types of abuse also differ in prevalence. In the National Social Life, Health and Aging Project, the first population-based, nationally representative study evaluating mistreatment among older adults, it was found that overall 9% of older adults reported verbal mistreatment, 3.5% financial mistreatment, and 0.2% physical mistreatment (Laumann, Leitsch, & Waite, 2008). Results from the National Elder Mistreatment Study were similar, as researchers found a prevalence of 4.6% for emotional abuse, 1.6% for physical abuse, 0.6% for sexual abuse, 5.1% for potential neglect, and 5.2% for current financial abuse among older adults (Acierno et al., 2010).

Elder abuse has been defined by the U.S. National Academy of Sciences as "intentional actions that cause harm or create a serious risk of harm (whether or not harm is intended), to a vulnerable elder by a caregiver or other person who stands in a trust relationship to the elder," or "failure by a caregiver to satisfy the elder's basic needs or to protect the elder from harm" (Lachs, & Pillemer, 2004, p. 1264). According to the National Center of Elder Abuse (2007) there are seven types of elder abuse: physical abuse, sexual abuse, emotional or psychological abuse, neglect, abandonment, financial or material exploitation, and self-neglect. **Physical abuse** is the use of any physical force that may result in bodily injury, physical pain, or impairment, such as hitting, beating, pushing, and shoving. **Sexual abuse** is the nonconsensual sexual contact with an older person, such as unwanted touching, rape, sodomy, and coerced nudity. **Emotional or psychological abuse** includes severe mental or physical pain suffered through verbal or nonverbal acts, such as verbal assaults, threats, intimidation, or harassment. **Neglect** is an act committed by any individual who refuses or fails to fulfill any part of his or her obligation or duty to serving an older person. **Abandonment** is an act of desertion of an older person by the individual taking responsibility for providing his or her care. **Financial or material exploitation** includes any illegal or improper use of an older person's money, property, or other asset, including unauthorized credit card purchases or stealing money from an older person's account. Finally, **self-neglect** includes any behavior an older person exhibits that threatens his or her own life, health, or safety, including refusal or failure to provide him- or herself with adequate food, water, clothing, or shelter (National Center of Elder Abuse, 2007).

Elder abuse can occur in a variety of settings, including households, hospitals, assisted living arrangements, and nursing homes. There have been many reported risk factors for elder abuse and neglect. Paveza, Vande Weerd, and Laumann (2008) described these risk factors as being either *vulnerabilities*, which are internal factors that place an individual at risk, or *risks*, which are external factors that place an individual at risk. Reported vulnerabilities for older adults include such demographic characteristics as age, sex, and ethnicity; level of cognition; depression; ability to perform basic living activities; the presence of comorbid conditions; alcohol use; childhood trauma; psychological status; self-esteem; behavioral acculturation; and coping style. Reported risks for older adults include demographic characteristics, such as living arrangement, social support, history of other forms of abuse, having an unmet need for care such as transportation, and characteristics of their surrounding neighborhood (Paveza et al., 2008).

Elder abuse has also been associated with lowered mortality and morbidity. Using data from the Chicago Health and Aging Project, a longitudinal, population-based study of community-dwelling residents aged 65 years and older, researchers found that both elder self-neglect and abuse were significantly associated with an increased risk of mortality (Dong et al., 2010). Using the same cohort of older adults, researchers also found self-neglect was significantly associated with declines in cognitive functioning (Dong et al., 2010), and lower levels of physical functioning (Dong, Mendes de Leon, & Evans, 2009). In a study conducted in India, mistreated or abused older adults were more depressed and less satisfied with their life than those who were not mistreated or abused (Chokkanathan & Lee, 2005). Finally, in a study conducted in China, feelings of dissatisfaction with life, often being bored, often feeling helpless, and feeling worthless were all associated with increased risk of abuse and neglect among older adults (Dong, Simon, Odwazny, & Gorbien, 2008).

Physical Activity

The Dietary Guidelines for Americans, 2005 defines **physical activity** as "any bodily movement produced by skeletal muscles resulting in energy expenditure" (USDHHS & U.S. Department of Agriculture, 2005, p. 19). This is distinct from **physical fitness**, which is "a multi-component trait related to the ability to perform physical activity" (USDHHS & U.S. Department of Agriculture, 2005, p. 19). Engaging in physical activities is important because it helps build and maintain muscle mass, which in turn can help older adults with daily living activities. As we age we tend to increase our body fat percentage and reduce our muscle mass, making it more difficult to engage in physical activities. Compared with young and middle-aged adults, older adults (>65 years) are least likely to be physically active, with national statistics reporting in 2007 that 32.7% participated in no leisure-time physical activity, 23.7% were inactive, 36.9% were insufficient, and only 39.3% met current recommendations for physical activity (Centers for Disease Control and Prevention, 2010b). In one study with older adults, researchers found 11 barriers reported by older adults to participating in leisure time physical activities: lack of interest, lack of daily access to a car, shortness of breath, joint pain, dislike of going out alone, dislike of going out in the evening, perceived lack of fitness, lack of energy, doubting that exercise can lengthen life, not belonging to a group, and doubting that meeting new people is beneficial (Crombie et al., 2004).

Recommendations for physical activities in adults are approximately 60 minutes of activity per day most days of the week. Older adults are also recommended to participate in regular physical activities to reduce functional declines that are associated with aging (USDHHS & U.S. Department of Agriculture, 2005). Physical activity is another determinant of mental health among older adults. In one study using community-dwelling older adults, researchers found that the engagement in physical activity was a protective factor from depression (Strawbridge, Deleger, Roberts, & Kaplan, 2002). In another study researchers found that regular exercise among an older adult population was associated with a delay in onset of dementia and Alzheimer's disease (Larson et al., 2006). Another study found similar results with a Canadian elderly population, as high levels of physical activity were associated with reduced risks for cognitive impairments and the development of Alzheimer's disease and dementia (Laurin, Verreault, Lindsay, MacPherson, & Rockwood, 2001). Researchers studying older men from Finland, Italy, and the Netherlands found that participation in at least medium- to low-intensity activities postponed cognitive declines with age, compared with participation in the lowest intensity physical activities (Gelder et al., 2004). Similar results have been found with women. In a study on older women, researchers found that higher levels of physical activity were associated with higher levels of cognitive functioning and regular physical activity was associated with less cognitive declines (Weuve et al., 2004).

Spirituality and Religion

Previous studies reported spirituality and religion plays an important role in older people's lives, as participation in such activities has been positively linked with measures of mental health such as higher rates of overall well-being and physical health such as lower likelihood of hypertension and mortality (Kirby, Coleman, & Dalay, 2004). Studies also suggest that spirituality and religion can play an important role in illness recovery, which is especially important among older adults. **Spirituality** refers to an individual's connection to self, family members, and their surrounding community and does not necessary imply the involvement of organized or other types of religions. Researchers who study spirituality do not suggest that "prayer heals illnesses"; rather, theories, such as Jeffrey Levin's on "How Religion influences Morbidity and Health" (1996), suggest dimensions of religion and religious activities, such as religious commitment and religious faith, can act as mediating factors to improve health and well-being. Examples of these dimensions and how they act as mediating factors can be found in **Table 11.3**.

TABLE 11.3   Dimensions of Religion and Proposed Mediating Factors of Health

Religious Dimension	Mediating Factor(s)	Health Implication
Religious devotion	Avoidance of unhealthy lifestyle behaviors such as smoking, drinking, and drug use	Lowers risk for chronic disease and improves overall health
Participation in religious activities and associations with other religious individuals	Increases social support, networks, and enhances relationship with family and friends	Reduces stress and improves coping mechanisms
Religious worship, prayer, and meditation	Increases relaxation, forgiveness, and positive emotions and lowers stress	Supports immune function

Source: Levin, J. S. (1996). How religion influences morbidity and health: Reflections on natural history, salutogenesis and host resistance. *Social Science and Medicine, 43*(5), 849–864.

Spiritual and religious beliefs and activities can play a central role in older adults' attempts to cope with stressful life events, especially from life-threatening chronic diseases. The use of religion has also been noted as a preferred coping strategy among older adults who are confronted with negative life events, such as a death of a spouse (Siegel & Schrimshaw, 2002). In one study using a racially diverse group of community-dwelling older adults researchers found that higher levels of spiritual experiences (i.e., "I feel God's presence") were associated with lower levels of depressive symptoms (Mofidi et al., 2006). Another study found among older Mexican Americans religious attendance, or attending church monthly, weekly, or more than weekly, was associated with slower rates of decline for cognitive functioning, compared with those who did not attend church (Hill, Burdette, Angel, & Angel, 2006).

Siegel and Schrimshaw (2002) interviewed community-dwelling older adults with HIV/AIDS on their perceived benefits of participating in spiritual or religious activities, and participants reported nine benefits: (1) evokes comforting emotions and feelings; (2) offers strength, empowerment, and control; (3) eases the emotional burden of the illness; (4) offers social support and a sense of belonging; (5) offers spiritual support through a personal relationship with God; (6) facilitates meaning and acceptance of the illness; (7) helps preserve health; (8) relieves the fear and uncertainty of death; and (9) facilitates self-acceptance and reduces self-blame. Finally, in a small study with older African American survivors of Hurricane Katrina who were relocated after the event, researchers found that the most common method of coping with the traumatic event was reliance on a Higher Power (Lawson & Thomas, 2007).

FOCUS FEATURE 11.3 SEXUALITY AND HEALTH AMONG OLDER ADULTS IN THE UNITED STATES

Despite the growth of the aging population, relatively little is known about older adults' sexuality or engagement in sexual behaviors. Sexuality includes a spectrum of behaviors such as having partnerships, sexual activity, attitudes toward sex, and adequate sexual functioning. As we age sexual functioning appears to decline; however, no study until the National Social Life, Health, and Aging Project evaluated such behaviors across a nationally representative sample of community-dwelling older adults.

The primary and secondary objectives of the National Social Life, Health, and Aging Project were to obtain estimates for the prevalence of sexual activity, behaviors, and problems for older adults and to describe the relationship between sexuality and various health conditions. Researchers sampled 3,005 U.S. adults (1,550 women and 1,455 men) between the ages of 57 and 85. Sex or sexual activity was defined as "any mutually voluntary activity with another person that involves sexual contact, whether or not intercourse or orgasm occurs" (Lindau et al., 2007, p. 2). Older adults who had sex within the previous year with at least one partner were considered "sexually active." The most commonly preferred sexual activity was vaginal intercourse for men and women; however, many more men engaged in masturbation compared with women.

Overall, sexual activity also appeared to decrease with age, as 73% of respondents between the ages of 57 and 64 reported engaging in sexual activity, 53% between the ages of 65 and 74 reported sexual activity, and only 26% between the ages of 75 and 85 reported sexual activity. Across all age groups women were more likely to have less sexual activity than men. Reasons women reported less sexual activity included low desire, difficulty with vaginal lubrication, and inability to climax. Women were also less likely to have a spouse or intimate partner and more likely to report sexual activity was "not at all important," which likely contributed to this finding.

For men, the most prevalent sexual problem was erectile difficulties. Men were also more likely to use medications or supplements to enhance their sexual performance. Fourteen percent of men and only 1% of women reported using such products to improve sexual function. Finally, sexuality did not appear to be an important topic older adults spoke of during visits to their physicians. Among men, 38% reported discussing sex with their physician recently and 22% of women reported discussing it with their physician (Lindau et al., 2007).

MENTAL HEALTH INTERVENTIONS FOR OLDER ADULTS

Many interventions have been implemented in the community and other settings that target mental health issues among older adults. The first study was conducted on nursing home residents in Canada. Researchers randomly assigned nursing home residents to either an experimental intervention called HOPE or a comparison intervention, which consisted of weekly friendly meetings with research assistants. The HOPE program consisted of a 4-week intervention that aimed to reduce depression by engaging residents in a variety of activities, such as goal setting. At the end of the intervention period the HOPE program was not found to be effective at reducing depression or increasing hope; however, this is likely due to the small sample size for both groups (Wilson et al., 2010).

The next study evaluated the effectiveness of an intervention designed to reduce depressive symptoms among older adults with depression and executive dysfunction, a group likely to be resistant to antidepressant medications. Researchers randomized participants into one of two intervention groups. The first intervention was a problem-solving intervention that consisted of 12 weekly sessions aimed to teach problem-solving skills using a five-step model: participants set treatment goals, discussed and evaluated different ways to reach set goals, created action plans, evaluated their effectiveness in reaching set goals, and created a relapse prevention plan. The second group was assigned to a supportive therapy intervention. This intervention was also 12 weeks and was similar to person-centered psychotherapy. Participants in both groups were evaluated at weeks 3, 6, 9, and 12 of the intervention. Both groups were similar in outcome measures at weeks 3 and 6; however, at weeks 9 and 12 the problem-solving therapy group had a significantly greater reduction in symptom severity of depression, response rate, and remission rate than the supportive therapy group (Areán et al., 2010).

Another study evaluated the efficacy of an intervention designed to reduce depressive symptoms among older women in Portugal. Researchers randomized participants into either the Life Review intervention that focused on reminiscence to help them remember and cover life themes or a control group that did not receive an intervention. The Life Review intervention consisted of four sessions implemented over 2 weeks, and in each session a life period was addressed: session one covered infancy, session two covered adolescence, session three covered adulthood, and session four covered the present and future. A total of 14 questions were also asked to help women recall specific and positive memories. For example, "Do you remember receiving a present, being a child or an adolescent, which made you extremely happy?" and "Do you remember achieving an important goal when you were an adult?" were asked. After 1 week of completing the intervention women in the Life Review group reported significant improvements in depressive symptoms, life satisfaction, and specificity and positivity toward autobiographical memories, whereas in the control condition no significant improvements were made for any measure (Gonçalves, Albuquerque, & Paul, 2009).

The effects of a group-based Turkish folkloric dance intervention were evaluated among older adults in Turkey. Participants were randomly assigned to either an 8-week, age-tailored dance intervention based on traditional Turkish folk music rhythms or a control group that received no program. The dance intervention consisted of three, 1-hour sessions per week, with each lesson consisting of a warm-up period, a special folklore dance stepping period, and a stretching and a cool-down period. Participants were also asked to walk at least two times per week for 30 minutes on their own. Compared with the control group, after the intervention period participants in the Turkish dance group reported significant improvements for most of the physical performance tests, a measure of balance and various measures of quality of life, including physical functioning, general health, and mental health; however, there were no differences in either group for depressive symptoms (Eyigor, Karapolat, Durmaz, Ibisoglu, & Cakir, 2009).

The next study evaluated a silver yoga exercise intervention for older community-dwelling women in Taiwan. Participants participated in 12 yoga classes (three sessions per week for 4 weeks) led by a certified yoga instructor. Yoga sessions were 70-minutes in length and included four phases: warm-up, engagement in *Hatha* yoga, relaxation, and guided-imagery meditation. At the end of the interventions participants reported significant improvements for body fat percentage, systolic blood pressure, balance and range of motion on shoulder flexion and abduction, and sleep disturbances; however, there was no significant change in measures of mental health, such as depressive state or mental health actualization (Chen & Tseng, 2008).

A day-care program in India designed to enhance quality of life and reduce psychiatric morbidity and cognitive impairments among low socioeconomic status older adults was evaluated. Participants attended a day-care program that provided recreational activities, occupational therapy, counseling services, medical services, and a meal. Forty-one older adults were asked to participate in the intervention; however, only 20 agreed to participate. Therefore, the remaining 21 older adults were treated as a control group. Three months after the intervention there appeared to be a significant reduction for psychiatric morbidity and improvement in quality of life for the intervention group, compared with the control group. The costs for the program were also generally low, suggesting this program is likely sustainable (Jacob, Abraham, Abraham, & Jacob, 2007).

The next study evaluated the Improving Mood-Promoting Access to Collaborative (IMPACT) intervention designed to reduce depressive symptoms among older adults with diabetes. Researchers randomized participants into the IMPACT intervention or usual care, which consisted of normal care by their primary care physician. The IMPACT intervention consisted of a stepped collaborative program of six to eight sessions, which were delivered by a depression care manager (i.e., nurse) who provided a behavioral activation intervention, such as active engagement in physical activities, and a problem-solving activity. Participants were also able to take antidepressant medication during the intervention. Compared with participants from the usual care group, those in the IMPACT intervention had on average 115 more depression-free days 24-months after the intervention period. Total outpatient costs were slightly higher for the IMPACT group (+$25.00; 95% confidence interval: –1,638 to 1,689) during this same period; however, when inpatient costs were taken into account, the usual care group ended up spending much more money for treatment (–$896.00; 95% confidence interval: –4,549 to 2,755) (Katon et al., 2006).

Another study evaluated a yoga-based intervention for generally healthy older men and women. Participants were randomized into one of three groups: a 6-month yoga class, a 6-month walking exercise class, or a wait-list control group. The yoga intervention was designed and based on a type of yoga called *Iyengar yoga*. Yoga classes were implemented for one, 90-minute class session per week along with home practice. On average 7 to 8 yoga poses were covered each week, and in all 18 poses were taught. Each session ended with a 10-minute deep relaxation period, which consisted of progressive relaxation, visualization, and meditation techniques. The walking intervention, just as the yoga intervention, consisted of one class session per week along with home exercises. The aerobic exercise consisted of walking on an outdoor 400-meter track for 1 hour. No intervention was provided for the wait-list control participants. Neither of the exercise interventions produced an effect for any of the cognitive and alertness outcome measures evaluated in this study; however, the participants in the yoga intervention group reported significant improvements in physical measures (i.e., timed one-legged standing, forward flexibility), psychosocial measures of quality of life (i.e., social functioning, vitality), and fatigue compared with control subjects (Oken et al., 2006).

An intervention designed to reduce depression and improve self-esteem and life satisfaction was evaluated among older adults in Taiwan. Researchers implemented a reminiscence group therapy (RGT) intervention to nursing home residents in one section of a hospital, whereas residents of another section served as control subjects (CON). Participants in the RGT group met for 9 weeks of therapy sessions, lasting 1 hour per week. Each weekly activity covered a topic that was designed to avoid threatening or irritating residents, such as "that's how I grew up" and "the home I created." Researchers also encouraged both the residents and their family members to gather old photos, magazine articles, albums, or news clippings from the past that might never have been shared with others. After the intervention levels of depression, self-esteem, and the degree of life satisfaction improved in the experimental group (Chao et al., 2006).

The next study evaluated a chorale intervention designed to promote mental and physical health among older adults. Participants were randomized into either a chorale group, consisting of weekly singing rehearsals for 30 weeks, or a control group that did not receive any intervention. The chorale group also gave public performances several times during the intervention period. After the intervention the chorale group reported higher overall ratings for physical health, including fewer doctor visits, less medication use, fewer instances of falls, and fewer other health problems than the comparison group. The chorale group also improved their mental health, as evidenced by higher levels of morale, lower levels of depression, and less reported loneliness than the comparison group (Cohen et al., 2006).

Two interventions were evaluated aimed at increasing physical activity and mental health measures among older adults. The first intervention, Active Choices, was a 6-month program delivered by an initial face-to-face meeting, which was then followed up with telephone counseling biweekly for the first 2 months and monthly for the last 4 months. Counseling was tailored to the participant's readiness for change, and the intervention operationalized constructs of social cognitive theory including social support, self-regulation, and self-efficacy. The second intervention, Active Living Every Day, was a program implemented over 20 weeks. This intervention was also based on constructs of social cognitive theory and the transtheoretical model. Compared with participants that dropped out of the intervention, research participants reported statistically significant improvements in body mass index, moderate-to-vigorous physical activity, total physical activity, depressive symptoms, stress, and body appearance and function (Wilcox et al., 2006).

Another study evaluated a community-based intervention for suicide prevention among older adults in Yuri Town, Japan. A committee for suicide prevention consisting of general practitioners, public health nurses, welfare commissioners, and the people's old club members implemented this intervention, which consisted of three main components implemented over an 8-year period. The first component consisted of a series of mental health workshops implemented by psychiatrists or public health nurses. Workshops consisted of psychoeducational programming in small groups, which provided information regarding depression with suicide risks. The next component consisted of a series of group activity programs implemented in community centers. During the activity programs elderly residents were given the opportunity to (1) engage in volunteer services, such as taking care of young children; (2) participate in indoor activities, such as arts and crafts and cooking: and (3) participate in physical activities. As a result of the intervention reductions for suicide risk significantly decreased in older female residents; however, there was no change for risk among older male residents (Oyama et al., 2005).

The effects of exercise on depression among older adults in Australia were evaluated. Participants were randomly assigned to one of three 8-week interventions: a high-intensity progressive resistance training (PRT) program (HIGH), a low-intensity PRT program (LOW), or standard general practitioner care (GP). Both HIGH and LOW groups participated in a 3-day per week regimen of exercises, using weight resistant machines that included chest press, upright row, shoulder press, leg press, knee extension, and knee flexion. The HIGH group used resistance set at 80% of the maximal load participants could lift at one time, whereas the LOW group used resistance set at 20% of their maximal load. At the end of the study significant improvements were made in overall depression, quality of life, and sleep for both intervention groups; however, the HIGH PRT group experienced greater improvements than the LOW PRT and GP groups (Singh et al., 2005).

The next study evaluated the effects of a treatment initiation program (TIP) among older adults to target their attitudes about depression and treatment to reduce barriers and increase treatment acceptance. Participants were first screened for major depression, and those with a confirmed diagnosis were randomly assigned to either a pharmacotherapy-only group or a pharmacotherapy with the TIP intervention. The TIP intervention started with an assessment to identify patients' specific barriers to care, with common barriers reported as (1) misconceptions about depression and treatment, (2) perceived need for care, (3) perceived stigma, (4) cognitive distortions associated with depression, and (5) logistical barriers. After barriers were identified they became the focus of the intervention. The TIP implementation staff used cognitive behavior and nonspecific therapeutic techniques (e.g., empathy, support) to address barriers, activate older adults, and increase depression treatment self-efficacy. After the intervention period participants in the TIP group had a greater decrease in depression severity and reported less hopelessness than those receiving usual care. TIP participants were also more likely to remain in treatment after seeking care (Sirey, Bruce, & Alexopoulos, 2005).

The final study evaluated a community-based intervention for suicide prevention among older adults in Japan. Researchers used the town of Joboji, Japan to implement the program, and two surrounding communities acted as a control group. This intervention consisted of three main steps, implemented over a 15-year period. The first step (1985–1989) was the *preparation step* in which researchers studied the town's suicide epidemiology, organized the management of the intervention, set local planning goals, and pilot tested programs. The next step (1990–1994), the *intention step*, and the third step (1995–1999), the *maintenance step*, included suicide screenings, follow-up screenings, and targeted health education strategies, such as a workshop that educated participants on the signs and symptoms of suicidal behaviors. As a result of the intervention a 73% reduced risk of suicidal mortality among men and a 76% reduced risk of suicidal mortality among women was observed in the intervention community, whereas there was no significant change for either gender in the control areas (Oyama, Koida, Sakashita, & Kudo, 2004).

SKILL-BUILDING ACTIVITY

Imagine you have been asked to work with a group of older adults. How would you go about assessing their risk for mental health problems? What factors would you look for? What would be the key topics for your program? What would be the duration of your program? You can take the help of an existing program from this chapter to help you in your task.

SUMMARY

The U.S. population is growing older. In many counties the term *old* refers to those who are 65 years of age or older; however, we can further classify older adults as young-old (ages 65–74 years), middle-old (ages 75–84 years), and old-old (85 years and older). In 2008 there were 39 million older adults living in the United States, accounting for 13% of the population; however, by 2030 the older adult population is expected to almost double to 72 million, nearly 20% of the U.S. population (Federal Interagency Forum on Aging-Related Statistics, 2010). The growth of the older population comes mostly from two sources: life expectancy has increased with advances in medicine and technology and the aging baby boomer generation.

The demographics of the older adult population differ from the young and middle adult populations, with greater disparities between genders and racial groups. Women tend to live longer, accounting for a much greater percentage of the older population than men. Today, 80.4% of older adults are White; however, the diversity of this group is expected to change dramatically in upcoming years, and by 2050 it is projected that Whites will represent slightly over half of older adults (58.5%) with other groups growing. Marriage also appears to be the preferred living arranging among older adults, as 57% are married. However, rates of widowhood increase as adults age, especially among women.

The life expectancy of older adults has increased in recent years. Life expectancy refers to the average number of years an individual is expected to live beyond his or her current age, as long as death rates remain constant. The overall life expectancy for older adults at age 65 is 18.5 years and for older adults at age 85 is 6.4 years. Death rates in the United States have also declined. The leading causes of death among older adults, irrespective of race and gender, are from chronic diseases and include heart disease, cancer, and stroke. Depression is also the most prevalent mental health problem among this group and a leading cause of disability. Depression increases with age, with old-old adults reporting higher depression rates for men and women.

Finally, employment and retirement are two major issues that affect the older population. Approximately 70% of men and 60% of women in their 50s work full time; however, once Americans enter their 60s retirement rates increase. In recent decades the average retirement age for workers has fallen; however, this decline has subsided since the 1990s. Older adults today are expected to work longer than those in recent years.

There are many important determinants to mental health among older adults: sleep and sleep patterns, social support, elder abuse and maltreatment, physical activity, and spirituality and religion. Adequate sleep is essential for mental health among older adults, but as we age our sleeping patterns change. Common sleep disturbances reported by older adults include frequent and repeated interruptions during sleep and long periods of wakefulness, which lead to less overall sleep and poor sleep efficiency. Poor sleep can also affect problems such as memory loss and depression. Social support and relationships are also vital to maintaining mental health. Benefits of social support include lower levels of depression and higher reported mentally healthy days, which includes having feelings free of depression, worry, or anxiety. In addition to receiving social and emotional support, giving such support through opportunities such as volunteering has also been shown to enhance mental health and longevity. Elder abuse is also detrimental to the mental health of older adults. Elder abuse comes in many different forms, including physical abuse, sexual abuse, emotional or psychological abuse, neglect, abandonment, financial or material exploitation, and self-neglect. Studies of elder abuse have shown it to be linked with declines in cognitive functioning, depression, lower life satisfaction, and feelings of helplessness and worthlessness.

The engagement of physical activities is also important because it helps older adults maintain adequate mental and physical health. Participating in physical activity has been found to be associated with lower rates of depression and less cognitive declines. It has also been shown to delay the onset of dementia and Alzheimer's disease and to reduce the risks for cognitive impairments. Finally, spirituality and religion have been shown to be an important determinant for the mental health and overall well-being of older adults. Theories suggest that participation in religious activities, such as religious commitment and religious faith, can act as mediating factors to improve health and well-being. Spirituality and religion have been associated with lower levels of depressive symptoms, slower rates of decline for cognitive functioning, and linked with numerous benefits.

Primary interventions that aim to prevent mental heath issues and promote overall good health are typically implemented in the community setting or nursing homes. Many of these interventions are based on goal setting, problem solving, supportive therapy, reminiscence group therapy, physical activities, yoga, social cognitive theory, and the transtheoretical model. Some even implemented environmental changes and enacted policies to prevent and make mental health awareness a priority in the community, such as suicide prevention. Interventions ranged from brief programs lasting 1 or 2 weeks to longer programs lasting 15 years and were implemented in a variety of settings, such as churches, elder day-care centers, nursing homes, the Internet, gyms, and entire rural towns. Overall, these interventions were found to be effective for preventing the onset of mental issues and reducing current mental health issues.

REVIEW QUESTIONS

1. Summarize the demographics of older adults in terms of gender, race, and marital status.
2. Explain why older adults are living longer.
3. Define life expectancy, and explain why it is a relative term.
4. Describe the living arrangements of most older adults.
5. Describe the consequences older adults may face if they do not receive adequate sleep.
6. Define social support, and describe the three main types of support outlined in this chapter.
7. Discuss physical abuse about older adults, and differentiate between the various types covered in this chapter.
8. Describe the theoretical basis behind how spirituality enhances health outcomes among older adults.

WEBSITES TO EXPLORE

Geriatric Mental Health Foundation

http://www.gmhfonline.org/gmhf/

This is the official website of the Geriatric Mental Health Foundation, a not-for-profit organization established by the American Association for Geriatric Psychiatry. This foundation raises awareness for psychiatric and mental health disorders affecting the elderly, strives to eliminate the stigma of mental illness and treatment, promotes healthy aging strategies, and helps the elderly access quality mental health care. This is done through the development and dissemination of consumer information; partnerships with government, private, community, and consumer organizations; public information campaigns; and the development of evidence-based tool kits. *Identify and review the various resources under the "Consumer/Patient Information" tab. On a separate piece of paper, write your impressions.*

Alzheimer's Association

http://www.alz.org/index.asp

This is the website for the Alzheimer's Association, a national, nonprofit group that is the leading voluntary organization for Alzheimer care and support. This organization supports their own mission by enhancing care and support for Alzheimer's patients and their families and supports research to accelerate progress for new treatments and preventions to ultimately find a cure for Alzheimer's disease. This organization also has local organizations in every state and holds an international annual meeting annually, called the Alzheimer's Association International Conference on Alzheimer's Disease. *Using this website locate an organization near you. Try to attend a local meeting or the annual national meeting and write a reflection for what you learned.*

National Institute of Aging (NIA)

http://www.nia.nih.gov/

This is the government website for the National Institute of Aging (NIA), 1 of 27 institutes of the National Institutes of Health. The NIA's mission is to improve the health and well-being of older Americans by supporting research in aging-related topics, training and developing scientists who work with this group, and disseminating the most up-to-date research for practice. On this website there is also a link to NIHSeniorHealth, a website with basic health and wellness information for older adults. *Click through the topic areas on this webpage. Select one or two from the 49 topics, and write a one-page reflection.*

American Geriatrics Society (AGS) Foundation for Health in Aging

http://www.healthinaging.org/about/index.php

This is the official website for the American Geriatrics Society (AGS) Foundation for Health in Aging, a nonprofit organization that aims to help translate research into current practice and advocate for older adults so they receive adequate health care. Each year this organization also gives the Lifetime of Caring Award to an individual who continually adds to the current state of knowledge of how to take better care of the elderly. *Click on the "Public Education" tab on the website and read through some of the resources provided. Write a one-page paper on your reflections.*

National Center on Elder Abuse (NCEA)

http://www.ncea.aoa.gov/NCEAroot/Main_Site/Index.aspx

The National Center on Elder Abuse is a government-run center to prevent elder mistreatment and abuse. It is currently directed by the U.S. Administration on Aging and is committed to helping national, state, and local partners to ensure the elderly live with dignity, integrity, and independence and without abuse, neglect, or exploitation. The website contains a state directory of help lines, hotlines, and elder abuse prevention resources. *Explore the website, and click on the "Find State Resources" tab. Write a brief summary of what resources you have access to in your state. Are you surprised that you have access to certain resources or you do not have resources to others?*

REFERENCES AND FURTHER READINGS

Acierno, R., Hernandez, M. A., Amstadter, A. B., Resnick, H. S., Steve, K., Muzzy, W., & Kilpatrick, D. G. (2010). Prevalence and correlates of emotional, physical, sexual, and financial abuse and potential neglect in the United States: The national elder mistreatment study. *American Journal of Public Health, 100*(2), 292–297.

Adler, P. A., & Roberts, B. L. (2006). The use of Tai Chi to improve health in older adults. *Orthopaedic Nursing, 25*(2), 122–126.

Alzheimer's Association. (2010). Related dementias. Retrieved from http://www.alz.org/alzheimers_disease_related_diseases.asp.

Areán, P. A., Raue, P., Mackin, R. S., Kanellopoulos, D., McCulloch, C., & Alexopoulos, G. S. (2010). Problem-solving therapy and supportive therapy in older adults with major depression and executive dysfunction. *American Journal of Psychiatry, 167,* 1391–1398.

Brown, S. L., Nesse, R. M., Vinokur, A. D., & Smith, D. M. (2003). Providing social support may be more beneficial than receiving it: Results from a prospective study of mortality. *Psychological Science, 14*(4), 320–327.

Byers, A. L., Yaffe, K., Covinsky, K. E., Friedman, M. B., & Bruce, M. L. (2010). High occurrence of mood and anxiety disorders among older adults: The national comorbidity survey replication. *Archives of General Psychiatry, 67*(5), 489–496.

Cacioppo, J. T., Hughes, M. E., Waite, L. J., Hawkley, L. C., & Thisted, R. A. (2006). Loneliness as a specific risk factor for depressive symptoms: Cross-sectional and longitudinal analyses. *Psychology and Aging, 21*(1), 140–151.

Centers for Disease Control and Prevention. (2010a). Alzheimer's disease. Retrieved from http://www.cdc.gov/aging/aginginfo/alzheimers.htm.

Centers for Disease Control and Prevention. (2010b). U.S. Physical Activity Statistics. Retrieved from http://apps.nccd.cdc.gov/PASurveillance/DemoCompareResultV.asp#result.

Chao, S. Y., Liu, H. Y., Wu, C. Y., Jin, S. F., Chu, T. L., Huang, T. S., & Clark, M. J. (2006). The effects of group reminiscence therapy on depression, self esteem, and life satisfaction of elderly nursing home residents. *Journal of Nursing Research, 14*(1), 36–44.

Chen, K. M., & Tseng, W. S. (2008). Pilot-testing the effects of a newly-developed silver yoga exercise program for female seniors. *Journal of Nursing Research, 16*(1), 37–45.

Cheung, C. K., Wyman, J. F., & Halcon, L. L. (2007). Use of complementary and alternative therapies in community-dwelling older adults. *Journal of Alternative and Complementary Medicine, 13*(9), 997–1006.

Cho, H. J., Lavretsky, H., Olmstead, R., Levin, M. J., Oxman, M. N., & Irwin, M. R. (2008). Sleep disturbance and depression recurrence in community-dwelling older adults: A prospective study. *American Journal of Psychiatry, 165*(12), 543–1550.

Chokkanathan, S., & Lee, A. E. Y. (2005). Elder mistreatment in urban India: A community based study. *Journal of Elder Abuse & Neglect, 17*(2), 45–61.

Cohen, G. D., Perlstein, S., Chapline, J., Kelly, J., Firth, K. M., & Simmens, S. (2006). The impact of professionally conducted cultural programs on the physical health, mental health, and social functioning of older adults. *Gerontologist, 46*(6), 726–734.

Crombie, I. K., Irvine, L., Williams, B., McGinnis, A. R., Slane, P. W., Alder, E. M., & McMurdo, M. E. T. (2004). Why older people do not participate in leisure time physical activity: A survey of activity levels, beliefs and deterrents. *Age and Aging, 33,* 287–292.

Dong, X., Mendes de Leon, C. F., & Evans, D. A. (2009). Is greater self-neglect severity associated with lower levels of physical function? *Journal of Aging and Health, 21*(4), 596–610.

Dong, X. D., Simon, M. A., Odwazny, R., & Gorbien, M. (2008). Depression and elder abuse and neglect among a community-dwelling Chinese elderly population. *Journal of Elder Abuse & Neglect, 20*(1), 25–41.

Dong, X. Q., Simon, M. A., Wilson, R. S., Mendes de Leon, C. F., Rajan, K. B., & Evans, D. A. (2010). Decline in cognitive function and risk of elder self- neglect: Finding from the Chicago health aging project. *Journal of the American Geriatrics Society, 58,* 2292–2299.

Eyigor, S., Karapolat, H., Durmaz, B., Ibisoglu, U., & Cakir, S. (2009). A randomized controlled trial of Turkish folklore dance on the physical performance, balance, depression and quality of life in older women. *Archives of Gerontology and Geriatrics, 48,* 84–88.

Federal Interagency Forum on Aging-Related Statistics. (2010). Older Americans 2010: Key indicators of well-being. Washington, DC: U.S. Government Printing Office.

Fiori, K. L., Antonucci, T. C., & Cortina, K. A. (2006). Social network typologies and mental health among older adults. *Journals of Gerontology, 61B*(1), P25–P32.

Foleya, D., Ancoli-Israelb, S., Britzc, P., & Walsh, J. (2004). Sleep disturbances and chronic disease in older adults: Results of the 2003 National Sleep Foundation Sleep in America survey. *Journal of Psychosomatic Research, 56,* 497–502.

Gelder, B. M., Tijhuis, M. A. R., Kalmijn, S., Giampaoli, S., Nissinen, A., & Kromhout, D. (2004). Physical activity in relation to cognitive decline in elderly men: The FINE study. *Neurology, 63,* 2316–2321.

Gonçalves, D. C., Albuquerque, P. B., & Paul, C. (2009). Life review with older women: An intervention to reduce depression and improve autobiographical memory. *Aging Clinical and Experimental Research, 21,* 369–371.

Goss, S. C. (2010). The future financial status of the social security program. *Social Security Bulletin, 70*(3), 111–125.

Hill, T. D., Burdette, A. M., Angel, J. L., & Angel, R. J. (2006). Religious attendance and cognitive functioning among older Mexican Americans. *Journals of Gerontology, 61B*(1), P3–P9.

House, J. S. (1981). *Work, stress, and social support.* Reading, MA: Addison-Wesley.

Jacob, M. E., Abraham, V. J., Abraham, S., & Jacob, K. S. (2007). The effect of community based daycare on mental health and quality of life of elderly in rural south India: A community intervention study. *International Journal of Geriatric Psychiatry, 22,* 445–447.

Katon, W., Unutzer, J., Fan, M. Y., Williams Jr., J. W., Schoenbaum, M., Lin, E. H. B., & Hunkeler, E. M. (2006). Cost-effectiveness and net benefit of enhanced treatment of depression for older adults with diabetes and depression. *Diabetes Care, 29,* 265–270.

Keyes, C. L., Kobau, R., Zahran, H., Zack, M. M., & Simoes, E. J. (2005). Social support and health-related quality of life among older adults-Missouri, 2000. *MMWR Morbidity and Mortality Weekly Report, 54*(17), 433–437.

Kirby, S. E., Coleman, P. G., & Dalay, D. (2004). Spirituality and well-being in frail and nonfrail older adults. *Journals of Gerontology, 59B*(3), P123–P129.

Lachs, M. S., & Pillemer, K. (2004). Elder abuse. *Lancet, 364,* 1263–1272.

Larson, E. B., Wang, L., Bowen, J. D., McCormick, W. C., Teri, L., Crane, P., & Kukull, W. (2006). Exercise is associated with reduced risk for incident dementia among persons 65 years of age and older. *Annals of Internal Medicine, 144,* 73–81.

Laumann, E. O., Leitsch, S. A., & Waite, L. J. (2008). Elder mistreatment in the United States: Prevalence estimates from a nationally representative study. *Journals of Gerontology, 63*(4), S248–S254.

Laurin, D., Verreault, R., Lindsay, J., MacPherson, K., & Rockwood, K. (2001). Physical activity and risk of cognitive impairment and dementia in elderly persons. *Archives of Neurology, 58,* 498–504.

Lawson, E. J., & Thomas, C. (2007). Wading in the waters: Spirituality and older black Katrina survivors. *Journal of Health Care for the Poor and Underserved, 18,* 341–354.

Levin, J. S. (1996). How religion influences morbidity and health: Reflections on natural history, salutogenesis and host resistance. *Social Science and Medicine, 43*(5), 849–864.

Lindau, S. T., Schumm, L. P., Laumann, E. O., Levinson, W., O'Muircheartaigh, C. A., & Waite, L. J. (2007). A study of sexuality and health among older adults in the United States. *New England Journal of Medicine, 357*(8), 762–774.

Lindbloom, E. J., Brandt, J., Hough, L. D., & Meadows, S. E. (2007). Elder mistreatment in the nursing home: A systematic review. *Journal of the American Medical Directors Association, 8*, 610–616.

Malone, D. C., McLaughlin, T. P., Wahl, P. M., Leibman, C., Arrighi, M., Cziraky, M. J., & Mucha, L. M. (2009). Burden of Alzheimer's disease and association with negative health outcomes. *American Journal of Managed Care, 15*(8), 481–488.

Mofidi, M., DeVellis, R. F., Blazer, D. G., DeVellis, B. M., Panter, A. T., & Jordan, J. M. (2006). Spirituality and depressive symptoms in a racially diverse US sample of community-dwelling adults. *Journal of Nervous and Mental Disease, 194*(12), 975–977.

Morrow-Howell, N., Hinterlong, J., Rozario, P. A., & Tang, F. (2003). Effects of volunteering on the well-being of older adults. *Journal of Gerontology, 58B*(3), S137–S145.

National Center for Chronic Disease Prevention and Health Promotion. (2009). *The power of prevention: Chronic disease...the public health challenge of the 21st century.* Washington, DC: U.S. Government Printing Office.

National Center for Complementary and Alternative Medicine. (2010). What is complementary and alternative medicine? Retrieved from http://nccam.nih.gov/health/whatiscam/#natural.

National Center of Elder Abuse. (2007). Major types of elder abuse. Retrieved from http://www.ncea.aoa.gov/NCEAroot/Main_Site/FAQ/Basics/Types_Of_Abuse.aspx.

National Sleep Foundation. (2009). How much sleep do we really need? Retrieved from http://www.sleepfoundation.org/article/how-sleep-works/how-much-sleep-do-we-really-need.

Nebes, R. D., Buysse, D. J., Halligan, E. M., Houck, P. R., & Monk, T. H. (2009). Self-reported sleep quality predicts poor cognitive performance in healthy older adults. *Journal of Gerontology: Psychological Sciences, 64B*(2), 180–187.

Oken, B. A., Zajdel, D., Kishiyama, S., Flegal, K., Dehen, C., Haas, M., ..., Leyva, J. (2006). Randomized, controlled, six-month trial of yoga in health seniors: Effects on cognition and quality of life. *Alternative Therapies in Health and Medicine, 12*(1), 40–47.

Oyama, H., Koida, J., Sakashita, T., & Kudo, K. (2004). Community-based prevention for suicide in elderly by depression screening and follow-up. *Community Mental Health Journal, 40*(3), 249–263.

Oyama, H., Watanabe, N., Ono, Y., Sakashita, T., Takenoshita, Y., Taguchi, M., ..., Kumaga, K. (2005). Community-based suicide prevention through group activity for the elderly successfully reduced the high suicide rate for females. *Psychiatry and Clinical Neurosciences, 59*, 337–344.

Paveza, G., Vande Weerd, C., & Laumann, E. (2008). Elder self-neglect: A discussion of a social typology. *Journal of the American Geriatric Society, 56*, S271–S275.

Plassman, B. L., Langa, K. M., Fisher, G. G., Heeringa, S. G., Weir, D. R., Ofstedal, M. B., ..., Wallace, R. B. (2007). Prevalence of dementia in the United States: The aging, demographics, and memory study. *Neuroepidemiology, 29*, 125–132.

Siegel, K., & Schrimshaw, E. W. (2002). The perceived benefits of religious and spiritual coping among older adults living with HIV/AIDS. *Journal for the Scientific Study of Religion, 41*(1), 91–102.

Singh, N. A., Stavrinos, T. M., Scarbek, Y., Galambos, G., Liber, C., & Fiatarone Singh, M. A. (2005). A randomized controlled trial of high versus low intensity weight training versus general practitioner care for clinical depression in older adults. *Journal of Gerontology, 60A*(6), 768–776.

Sirey, J. A., Bruce, M. L., & Alexopoulos, G. S. (2005). The treatment initiation program: An intervention to improve depression outcomes in older adults. *American Journal of Psychiatry, 162,* 184–186.

Starkstein, S. E., Mizrahi, R., & Power, B. D. (2008). Depression in Alzheimer's disease: Phenomenology, clinical correlates and treatment. *International Review of Psychiatry, 20*(4), 382–388.

Strawbridge, W. J., Deleger, S., Roberts, R. E., & Kaplan, G. A. (2002). Physical activity reduces the risk of subsequent depression for older adults. *American Journal of Epidemiology, 156*(4), 328–334.

Uchino, B. N. (2006). Social support and health: A review of physiological processes potentially underlying links to disease outcomes. *Journal of Behavioral Medicine, 29*(4), 377–387.

U.S. Department of Health and Human Services (DHHS). (2009). *Growing older in America: The Health and Retirement Study.* Washington, DC: U.S. Government Printing Office.

U.S. Department of Health and Human Services (DHHS), & U.S. Department of Agriculture. (2005). *Dietary guidelines for Americans* (6th ed.). Washington, DC: U.S. Government Printing Office.

Vitiello, M. V. (2009). Recent advances in understanding sleep and sleep disturbances in older adults: Growing older does not mean sleeping poorly. *Current Directions in Psychological Science, 18*(6), 316–320.

Weuve, J., Kang, J. H., Manson, J. E., Breteler, M. M. B., Ware, J. H., & Grodstein, F. (2004). Physical activity, including walking, and cognitive function in older women. *Journal of the American Medical Association, 292*(12), 1454–1461.

White, A. M., Philogene, G. S., Fine, L., & Sinha, S. (2009). Social support and self- reported health status of older adults in the United States. *American Journal of Public Health, 99,* 1872–1878.

Wilcox, S., Dowda, M., Griffin, S. F., Rheaume, C., Ory, M. G., Leviton, L., ..., Mockenhaupt, R. (2006). Results of the first year of active for life: Translation of 2 evidence-based physical activity programs for older adults into community settings. *American Journal of Public Health, 96*(7), 1201–1209.

Wilson, D. M., Marin, A., Bhardwaj, P., Lichlyter, B., Thurston, A., & Mohankumar, D. (2010). A Hope intervention compared to friendly visitors as a technique to reduce depression among older nursing home residents. *Nursing Research and Practice, 2010,* 1–6.

Wolkove, N., Elkholy, O., Baltzan, M., & Palayew, M. (2007). Sleep and aging. 1. Sleep disorders commonly found in older people. *Canadian Medical Association Journal, 176*(9), 1299–1304.

CHAPTER 12

Mental Health Organizations

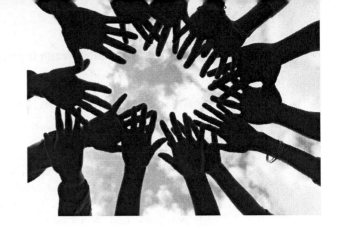

CHAPTER OBJECTIVES

After reading this chapter you should be able to
- Discuss the mission, vision, and organizational structure of the American Psychological Association
- Describe the mission, vision, and organizational structure of the American Psychiatric Association
- Summarize the mission, vision, and organizational structure of the National Institute of Mental Health
- Identify the mission, vision, and organizational structure of the National Alliance on Mental Illness
- Describe the mission, vision, and organizational structure of the World Federation for Mental Health
- Explain the mission, vision, and organizational structure of the American Psychotherapy Association
- Describe the mission, vision, and organizational structure of the American Academy of Psychotherapists
- Explain the mission, vision, and organizational structure of the American Public Health Association–Mental Health Section

In this chapter we discuss the various mental health organizations. There are several types of mental health organizations: Some are professional associations, others are governmental agencies, whereas others are community-based organizations. In this chapter we discuss each organization's history, mission, vision, organizational structure, and other details.

AMERICAN PSYCHOLOGICAL ASSOCIATION

Website: http://www.apa.org/

Founded: 1892

History: The **American Psychological Association** (APA) was formed in 1892 with 31 members at Clark University and G. Stanley Hall as its first President (American Psychological Association, 2010a). The first constitution was adopted in 1894 (Fernberger, 1932). It was governed by a Council and an Executive Committee. By 1940 it had 664 members. The field of psychology grew after World War II as the National Institute of Mental Health was formed and many returning servicemen saw the need for psychological services during the war. In 1945 there were 4,183 members, which grew to 30,839 by 1970. In 1944 there were 19 divisions that slowly grew to its present number of 54 (Dewsbury, 1997). Detailed history of the organization can be found in the book, *The American Psychological Association: A Historical Perspective,* edited by Evans, Sexton, and Cadwallader (1992).

Current membership: 148,000 members

Mission: The mission of the APA is "to advance the creation, communication and application of psychological knowledge to benefit society and improve people's lives" (APA, 2010b). They accomplish this mission by (American Psychological Association, 2010b)

- "Encouraging the development and application of psychology in the broadest manner.
- Promoting research in psychology, the improvement of research methods and conditions, and the application of research findings.
- Improving the qualifications and usefulness of psychologists by establishing high standards of ethics, conduct, education, and achievement.
- Increasing and disseminating psychological knowledge through meetings, professional contacts, reports, papers, discussions, and publications."

Vision: The vision of the APA (2010b) is that it "aspires to excel as a valuable, effective and influential organization advancing psychology as a science, serving as:

- A uniting force for the discipline
- The major catalyst for the stimulation, growth and dissemination of psychological science and practice
- The primary resource for all psychologists
- The premier innovator in the education, development, and training of psychological scientists, practitioners and educators

> *The American Psychological Association is a membership-based national professional organization of psychologists with the aims of advancing the creation, communication, and application of psychological knowledge to benefit society and improve people's lives.*

- The leading advocate for psychological knowledge and practice informing policy makers and the public to improve public policy and daily living
- A principal leader and global partner promoting psychological knowledge and methods to facilitate the resolution of personal, societal and global challenges in diverse, multicultural and international contexts
- An effective champion of the application of psychology to promote human rights, health, well being and dignity."

Organizational structure: At the top of the organization is the *President*. The President is elected by the entire membership. The President chairs the *Board of Directors* and the *Council of Representatives*. The *Board of Directors* consists of six members-at-large and six officers. The six officers are the (1) President-Elect, (2) President, (3) Past President, (4) Treasurer, (5) Recording Secretary, and (6) Chief Executive Officer (CEO). The Board of Directors also has an additional member in the form of the chair of the American Psychological Association of Graduate Students. In 2010 the President was Carol Goodheart, the President-Elect was Melba Vasquez, Past President was James Bray, and CEO was Norman Anderson.

The Board of Directors is the administrative agent of the Association, supervises the work of the CEO and exercises general supervision over the affairs of the Association. The *Council of Representatives* is the legislative body of the Association that sets policies and appropriates annual budget. According to its website, the APA has a current annual income of about $60 million per year. The Council of Representatives is composed of elected members from state/provincial/territorial psychological associations, APA divisions, and the APA Board of Directors.

The Association also has several committees and boards to carry out its functions. Some examples of these are as follows: (1) *Committee on Structure and Function of Council*, which reviews recommendations, suggestions, and complaints about Council functions and operations and maintains rules adopted by the Council; (2) *Policy and Planning Board*, which reviews current and long-range policy and appraises the structure and function of APA as a whole; (3) *Board for the Advancement of Psychology in the Public Interest*, which is responsible for fostering empowerment of underrepresented groups and improving educational and training opportunities through use of culturally sensitive models; (4) *Board of Convention Affairs*, which recommends policies and procedures and arranges programs for the Annual Convention; (5) *Board of Educational Affairs*, which recommends educational policy for the APA; (6) *Board of Professional Affairs*, which recommends and implements APA policy, standards, and guidelines for psychology as a profession, develops relationships with other professional organizations, and gives awards and honors in psychology; (7) *Board of Scientific Affairs*, which collaborates with agencies giving financial support to scientific projects; (8) *Election Committee*, which is responsible for conducting elections; (9) *Ethics Committee*, which investigates complaints of unethical conduct and other ethical issues; (10) *Finance Committee*, which deals with all the financial issues of the association; (11) *Membership Board*, which deals with recruitment and retention of members; and (12) *Publications and Communications Board*, which deals with publications.

The Association has 54 divisions or interest groups that its members can choose. Each division elects its own officers and has its own website, publications, listservs, awards, convention activities, own meetings.

Other details: The Association also has some related organizations: (1) *APA practice organization*, which fosters the professional development of psychologists through provision of continuing education and legislative and legal advocacy; (2) *APA Insurance Trust* which provides various types of insurances to its members; (3) *American Psychological Foundation*, which provides financial support for research projects; (4) *International Psychological Organizations*, which maintains a directory of international psychology organizations;

(5) *Psi Chi*, the national honor society in psychology which provides academic recognitions to students who meet academic criteria; and (6) *Psi Beta*, the national honor society in psychology for community and junior colleges which recognizes excellence in scholarship, leadership, research, and community service in community and junior colleges.

AMERICAN PSYCHIATRIC ASSOCIATION

Website: http://www.psych.org/

Founded: 1844

History: The earlier name of the **American Psychiatric Association** was the Association of Medical Superintendents of the American Institutions for the Insane, which was founded by 13 asylum directors in 1844 (Grob, 1973; Hirschbein, 2004; Kirkbride, 1845). The Association's objectives were "to communicate their experiences to each other, to cooperate in collecting statistical information relating to insanity and assisting each other in improving the treatment of the insane" (American Psychiatric Association, 2003). During the early years (1844–1921) there were annual meetings and the members worked on committee assignments, visited local asylums, and listened to presentations of papers (Hirschbein, 2004). Dorothea Dix, who is mentioned in Chapter 1, played an important role in shaping the Association of Medical Superintendents of American Institutions for the Insane (Brown, 1998). In 1882 the association members formalized the presidential office and mandated an address by the outgoing president. This tradition is a regular feature of American Psychiatric Association since 1883. During this period institution-based psychiatric care was common and the name of the journal of the organization was the *American Journal of Insanity.*

In 1892 the Association's name was changed to The American Medico-Psychological Association, and physicians working in mental hospitals or private offices became eligible for membership (American Psychiatric Association, 2003). In 1921 the organization changed its name to the American Psychiatric Association. The journal also changed its name to the *American Journal of Psychiatry*, which is published to date. In 1946 the APA established the first standards for psychiatric hospitals and outpatient clinics (American Psychiatric Association, 2003). In 1948 Daniel Blain became the first Medical Director of the APA and served 10 years. He was followed by Matthew Ross (4 years), Walter Barton (11 years), Melvin Sabshin (23 years), Steven Mirin (5 years), and James Scully, Jr. (current Medical Director) (American Psychiatric Association, 2003). In 1952 the American Psychiatric Association published the first edition of the *Diagnostic and Statistical Manual of Mental Disorders*, which is now in its 4th edition.

The Association has at present several district branches. The first meeting of the Assembly of District Branches of the American Psychiatric Association was held in Los Angeles on May 5, 1953 with participation of 16 district branches that had formed at that time (American Psychiatric Association, 2007).

Current membership: 38,000 U.S. and international member physicians

Mission: The mission of the American Psychiatric Association (2010a) is to

- "promote the highest quality care for individuals with mental disorders (including mental retardation and substance-related disorders) and their families;
- promote psychiatric education and research;
- advance and represent the profession of psychiatry; and
- serve the professional needs of its membership."

Vision: "The American Psychiatric Association is an organization of psychiatrists working together to ensure humane care and effective treatment for all persons with mental disorders, including mental retardation and substance-related disorders. It is the voice and conscience of modern psychiatry. Its vision is a society that has available, accessible quality psychiatric diagnosis and treatment" (American Psychiatric Association, 2010a)

The American Psychiatric Association is a membership-based national professional organization of psychiatrists with the aims of promoting the highest quality care for individuals with mental disorders and their families, promoting psychiatric education and research, advancing and representing the profession of psychiatry, and serving the professional needs of its membership.

Organizational structure: The organization includes as members only those medical specialists who are either qualified or in the process of being qualified as psychiatrists. The eligibility requirement is completion of a residency program in psychiatry that is accredited by the Residency Review Committee for Psychiatry of the Accreditation Council for Graduate Medical Education, the Royal College of Physicians and Surgeons of Canada, or the American Osteopathic Association. Members must also hold a valid medical license (with the exception of medical students and residents) and include one reference who is a member of the American Psychiatric Association.

The structure of the American Psychiatric Association includes (1) a legislative branch of elected representatives called the *Assembly*, (2) a group of appointed experts in a particular area called the *Components* (councils and committees), and (3) the executive branch called the *Board of Trustees* (American Psychiatric Association, 2010b). The Assembly meets twice a year and comprises individual members of the Association, as well as elected members from district branches of the Association. It deliberates in the areas of government relations, legislation, membership, issues pertaining to district branches, managed care, education, and research. The Components are like the Cabinet of the U.S. President and comprise the councils, committees, and task forces. Members are appointed by the President-Elect. The *Board of Trustees* comprises American Psychiatric Association's chief officers, elected trustees, three trustees at large, and a member in training. The Board is the final decision-making body of the American Psychiatric Association.

Other details: The American Psychiatric Association has an affiliated organization called the *American Psychiatric Institute for Research and Education.* It implements and supports projects designed to "conduct clinical and health services research to bridge the gap between research and practice, and to inform health policy; enhance educational and research capacities to improve the quality of psychiatric care; foster careers in psychiatric research, focusing on all levels of career development; identify scientific opportunities and stimulate research to refine national and international classifications of mental and behavioral disorders across the life span; inform health policy by providing fellowship and visiting scholar opportunities in a range of areas related to psychiatric research, training, and practice" (American Psychiatric Association, 2010c).

NATIONAL INSTITUTE OF MENTAL HEALTH

Website: http://www.nimh.nih.gov/index.shtml

Founded: 1949

History: During World War II it was recognized that due to conflict mental illnesses were more pervasive and serious than previously thought (Grob, 1996). It was also found that community-based treatment models were superior to hospital-based approaches. After World War II there was growing interest in a federal role in mental health. In 1946 the National Mental Health Act was signed into law. This Act was designed to support the research, prevention, and treatment of mental illnesses and mandated the establishment of a National Mental Health Advisory Council to provide advice and to recommend grants and the establishment of the **National Institute of Mental Health (NIMH)** to carry out an intramural research program. The NIMH was formally established on April 15, 1949, with Robert Felix as its first director. The initial allocation was $30 million per year for state programs and $7.5 million for physical infrastructure. By 1959 appropriation to NIMH was $50 million, and that increased to $189 million in 1964 (Grob, 1996). In 2011 the appropriation was approximately $1.5 billion (National Institute of Mental Health, 2010a).

Mission: "The mission of NIMH is to transform the understanding and treatment of mental illnesses through basic and clinical research, paving the way for prevention, recovery and cure. For the Institute to continue fulfilling this vital public health mission, it must foster innovative thinking and ensure that a full array of novel scientific perspectives are used to further discovery in the evolving science of brain, behavior, and experience. In this way, breakthroughs in science can become breakthroughs for all people with mental illnesses. In support of this mission, NIMH will generate research and promote research training to fulfill the following four objectives:

- Promote discovery in the brain and behavioral sciences to fuel research on the causes of mental disorders
- Chart mental illness trajectories to determine when, where, and how to intervene
- Develop new and better interventions that incorporate the diverse needs and circumstances of people with mental illnesses
- Strengthen the public health impact of NIMH-supported research

To reach these goals, the NIMH divisions and programs are designed to emphasize translational research spanning bench, to bedside, to practice" (National Institute of Mental Health, 2010b).

Vision: "NIMH envisions a world in which mental illnesses are prevented and cured" (National Institute of Mental Health, 2010b).

Organizational structure: NIMH funds research of scientists spread all over the country and also houses approximately 500 scientists at its office. The organization has seven divisions along with the Office of the Director:

National Institute of Mental Health (NIMH) is a federal organization with the aim of preventing and treating mental illnesses through basic and clinical research.

1. Division of Neuroscience and Basic Behavioral Science, which supports research programs in basic neurosciences, basic behavioral sciences, genetics, technology development, drug discovery, and research dissemination
2. Division of Adult Translational Research and Treatment Development, which focuses on research pertaining to pathophysiology of mental illnesses and increasing the translation of advances in behavioral sciences and neurosciences as innovations in clinical care
3. Division of Developmental Translational Research, which deals with research pertaining to prevention and treatment of mental disorders such as mood disorders, schizophrenia, etc.
4. Division of AIDS Research, concerned with research and training related to HIV/AIDS
5. Division of Services and Intervention Research, which deals with mental health services research and intervention research
6. Division of Extramural activities, responsible for extramural programs and policies
7. Division of Intramural Research Programs, which conducts direct basic and applied research on mental health and mental disorders

Other details: For the fiscal year 2011 the budget of NIMH was around 1.5 billion dollars. The organization has several advisory boards and groups. One of these is the National Advisory Mental Health Council, which is the advising body for the Secretary of Health and Human Services, Director of National Institutes of Health, and the Director of NIMH on matters relating to mental health research, research training, and other programs of NIMH. The strategic plan of NIMH includes four objectives: (1) to promote discovery in the brain and behavioral sciences to fuel research on the causes of mental disorders; (2) to chart mental illness trajectories to determine when, where, and how to intervene; (3) to develop new and better interventions for mental disorders that incorporate the diverse needs and circumstances of people with mental illness; and (4) to strengthen the public health impact of NIMH-supported research.

NATIONAL ALLIANCE ON MENTAL ILLNESS

Website: http://www.nami.org/

Founded: 1979

History: The **National Alliance on Mental Illness (NAMI)** was founded in 1979 as a grassroots organization devoted to improving the lives of individuals and families affected by mental illnesses. Six independent support groups of parents of adults with severe and persistent mental illnesses from all over the United States came together in Madison, Wisconsin to organize the first conference of the National Alliance for the Mentally

Ill in April 1979 (National Alliance on Mental Illness South West, n.d.). This meeting was attended by 284 people and led to the formation of NAMI. It is now linked to state organizations and local affiliates in approximately 1,100 communities around the country (National Alliance on Mental Illness, 2010a).

Current membership: Approximately 200,000 members

Mission: NAMI has a three-pronged mission that focuses on (1) awareness and support, (2) education, and (3) advocacy related to mental illnesses (National Alliance on Mental Illness, 2010a). For awareness and support NAMI focuses on educating about mental illnesses, removing stigma associated with mental illnesses, providing resources to those suffering from mental illnesses, and working toward making mental illnesses a high national priority. For education NAMI provides a variety of peer education and training programs for those suffering from mental illnesses, their family members, health care providers, and the general public. These programs are based on experiences of individuals who have coped effectively with mental illnesses as well as mental health professionals and educators. For advocacy NAMI fights for improving mental illness care and promoting its treatment and research at par with other illnesses at all levels.

According to its bylaws (National Alliance on Mental Illness, 2010b, p.3), "NAMI will accomplish its mission through the following:

- Coordination of activities of state and local advocacy groups.
- Serving as an information collection and dissemination center.
- Monitoring existing health care facilities, staff, and programming for adequacy and accountability, influencing the pre-professional and continuing education of mental health service providers.
- Promotion of new and remedial legislation.
- Fostering public education.
- Insisting upon, and advocating for, high quality Recovery and Resiliency-oriented services and care. Services must be designed to meet the individual needs of the person—and family—living with mental illness. These services must be freely available to all persons when and where they need them, regardless of the individual's setting or status—homeless, residential, extended care, outpatient, inpatient, independent living, schools or criminal justice settings
- Promotion of community support programs, including appropriate living arrangements linked with supportive social, vocational rehabilitation and employment programs.
- Improvement of private and governmental funding for mental health facilities and services, care and treatment, and residential and research programs.
- Collaboration with other national and international mental health and substance abuse organizations and advocacy groups.
- Delineation and enforcement of rights of persons with serious mental illness and their families.
- Soliciting and receiving funds in support of all of the above.
- Advocate forcefully for additional research into mental illness, with a goal of developing treatments and cures for all these disorders."

Vision: The vision of NAMI is to improve the lives of individuals and families affected by mental illness.

Organizational structure: The organization has three types of members: members, local affiliates, and state organizations. A member includes (1) a person with a mental illness, or (2) a relative of a person with a mental illness, or (3) a friend of a person with a mental illness. The members elect a 16-member *Board of Directors* to provide strategic guidance to accomplish the mission of the organization. The organization has four Councils. The first one is the *Consumer Council* comprising of people who have or have had a mental illness and serves as an advisory body to the Board of Directors. The purpose of the Consumer Council is to move forward the activities and participation of the consumers (people with mental illness) at the local, state, and national levels by active involvement in advocacy issues and development of programs. The second organization of the Council is the *State Presidents' Council*, which comprises the current state president of each state organization and the immediate past president of each state organization. This Council also serves as an advisory body to the Board of Directors. The third Council is the *Veterans Council*, which comprises persons with mental illnesses, relatives of persons with mental illnesses, or friends with mental illnesses who have an involvement and/or interest in issues impacting and veterans and active personnel who suffer from severe and persistent mental illness. This Council advocates for improved care for veterans and active military and dependents with severe and persistent mental illness. The fourth Council is the *Executive Director's Council*, which provides advice to the Executive Director's office.

Other details: NAMI operates at the local, state, and national levels. At the local level NAMI has more than 1,100 affiliates in all 50 states, the District of Columbia, Puerto Rico, the Virgin Islands, and Canada. Local affiliates usually start as a small group of people who come together to provide mutual support. Some of these support groups have just five or six members, whereas others are larger. The state organizations operate at a larger level, and NAMI has state organizations in all 50 states. Finally, NAMI has a national office in Arlington, Virginia. In 2009 the total assets of the national office of NAMI were $11,285,825 (National Alliance on Mental Illness, 2009). Of these, $1,620,516 were in cash and cash equivalents, $2,732,338 were in accounts receivable, $103,643 was in inventory, $5,551,053 were in investments, $246,111 were in prepaid expenses, $985,264 were in property and equipment, and $46,900 were in deposits.

> *The National Alliance on Mental Illness (NAMI) is a grassroots membership-based organization devoted to improving the lives of individuals and families affected by mental illnesses.*

WORLD FEDERATION FOR MENTAL HEALTH

Website: http://www.wfmh.org/

Founded: 1948

History: **World Federation for Mental Health (WFMH)** was founded in 1948 as an international organization composed of members all over the world to prevent mental disorders, ensure proper treatment of mental disorders, and promote mental health (World Federation for Mental Health, 2007). The World Health Organization first suggested the need for such an organization. George Brock Chisholm, a Canadian psychiatrist, conceived this organization as an international, nongovernmental entity that would serve as a link between "grassroots" mental health organizations and United Nations agencies. An organization, the International Committee for Mental Hygiene, had been founded in 1919 by Clifford Beers (see Chapter 1). Chisholm and John Rawlings Rees, a British military psychiatrist, convinced the International Committee for Mental Hygiene to reorganize as WFMH in 1948 with a new purpose, "to promote among all peoples and nations the highest possible level of mental health in its broadest biological, medical, educational, and social aspects."

Mission: The mission of WFMH is "to promote the advancement of mental health awareness, prevention of mental disorders, advocacy, and best practice recovery focused interventions worldwide" (World Federation for Mental Health, 2007). To accomplish this mission the WFMH has three goals (World Federation for Mental Health, 2007):

- "To heighten public awareness about the importance of mental health, and to gain understanding and improve attitudes about mental disorders.
- To promote mental health and prevent mental disorders.
- To improve the care, treatment and recovery of people with mental disorders."

The World Federation for Mental Health (WFMH) is an international membership-based organization composed of members all over the world to prevent mental disorders, ensure proper treatment of mental disorders, and promote mental health.

Vision: The vision of WFMH is "a world in which mental health is a priority for all people. Public policies and programs reflect the crucial importance of mental health in the lives of individuals" (World Federation for Mental Health, 2007).

Organizational structure: The organization has an *Executive Committee*, which is elected every 2 years and consists of President, Past President, President Elect, Treasurer, Secretary, Vice-President Constituency Development, and Vice-President Program Development. The organization has seven regional Vice-Presidents in the regions of Africa, Asia Pacific, Eastern Mediterranean, Europe, Latin America, North America, and Oceania. WFMH has developed a set of principles to guide them (World Federation for Mental Health, 2007):

- "Adults and children in all communities shall be made aware of the importance of mental health, and of the recognition and response to treatment of mental illness and disability.
- Users/consumers and families/carers will participate in all the health and social service departments and committees of member countries.
- Local services for mental illness and disability shall be given equal consideration for resource allocation to those of physical illness in every country.
- Mental illness and disability shall be equally represented with physical illness in the proceedings and resolutions of the United Nations, the World Bank and the World Health Organization, and through them of governments.
- Human rights abuse, malpractice or discrimination, or bad living or working conditions for users/consumers and those who care for them, including families/

carers, professional and voluntary workers, shall be widely reported and governments held accountable.

- There will be mental health associations in all countries to advocate for improvements in mental health, better provision of services for those with mental illness and disability, and to provide voluntary services.
- There will be adequate and affordable access to appropriate mental health treatment and recovery services for all those who need them.
- There will be an efficient means of communicating and disseminating policy, educational, technological and scientific information on mental health from those who have it to those who do not.
- There will be an effective program for encouraging advocacy and research in the prevention of mental illness and disability and in the promotion of mental health.
- There will be no race, age, gender, religious or cultural discrimination in the provision of mental health services."

WFMH has its secretariat in Woodbridge, Virginia. The secretariat houses the Secretary General and CEO, Director of Office for Promotion of Mental Health and Prevention in Mental Disorders, Director of Mental Health Awareness and Information Services, Executive Assistant in charge of membership services, and a financial and administrative assistant.

Other details: The organization has adopted the following values for its functioning (World Federation for Mental Health, 2007):

- "Organizational representation, transparency and accountability.
- Proactive interventions, such as advocacy and education, to promote human rights, self-development and self-management.
- Respect for cultural diversity.
- Mental health promotion and prevention of mental disorders compliment treatment and recovery.
- Inclusive, user and family centered, recovery-oriented mental health treatment and rehabilitation services.
- Compassion and selflessness in all human endeavors.
- Balancing self-sufficiency and inter-dependence as a principle of personal mental health.
- Responsiveness to change as a principle of effective mental health treatment."

AMERICAN PSYCHOTHERAPY ASSOCIATION

Website: http://www.americanpsychotherapy.com/

Founded: Year not known

History: The **American Psychotherapy Association** was founded by Robert O'Block to provide credentialing, build professional identity, develop standards of practice, and provide self-regulation for the profession of psychotherapy. The organization aims at credentialing psychotherapists that are well trained, well educated, and ethical.

Current membership: Approximately 6,000

Mission: The mission of the American Psychotherapy Association is to assume a leadership role in advancing the profession of psychotherapy (American Psychotherapy Association, 2010a). The organization helps members to assist their clients and to increase their professional practice. The organization establishes guidelines, promotes education and training, confirms the professional identity of its members, educates the public about benefits of psychotherapy, and provides networking and resource development.

> *The American Psychotherapy Association is a membership-based national professional organization of psychotherapists that credentials psychotherapists and advances the profession of psychotherapy.*

Vision: Among the goals of the organization as listed on their website, the best one that describes the vision is as follows: "To be the pre-eminent national association for psychotherapists of various disciplines: counseling, social work, marriage and family therapy, psychology, nurse psychotherapy, pastoral counseling, psychiatry, psychoanalysis, psychotherapy, and related fields" (American Psychotherapy Association, 2010b).

Organizational structure: It is a membership organization with members spread all over the country. There is an Executive Board with 19 members, including a Chair and a Vice Chair.

Other details: The organization coordinates a national conference every year. It also publishes a journal, *Annals of American Psychotherapy Association*, which is published quarterly and is peer reviewed and indexed in PsycINFO and other databases. The organization also offers online courses.

AMERICAN ACADEMY OF PSYCHOTHERAPISTS

Website: http://www.aapweb.com/

Founded: 1955

History: The founders of **American Academy of Psychotherapists** included Jules Barron, Henry Guze, and Albert Ellis (Brown, 1989). There are three purposes of the American Academy of Psychotherapists: (1) to enhance the person of the psychotherapist, (2) to challenge the experienced practitioner to professional excellence, and (3) to explore the relationship of person and process to psychotherapy (American Academy of Psychotherapists, 2010a).

Mission: The organization does not have a clearly articulated mission statement.

Vision: The organization does not have a clearly articulated vision statement.

Organizational structure: It is a membership-based organization. To become a member a person must fulfill the following criteria (American Academy of Psychotherapists, 2010b):

"(a) A doctoral or professional degree in one of the following mental health fields: psychiatry, clinical or counseling psychology, social work, pastoral counseling, marriage and family therapy, counseling, or nursing, and the fulfillment of those requirements deemed necessary by the applicant's academic discipline for the independent practice of psychotherapy.

(b) Specific training in psychotherapy with a minimum of 100 hours of supervision.

(c) At least one year of full-time post graduate clinical experience (or the equivalent in part-time experience) for doctoral level applicants, at least two years for others. In neither case may more than two of these years be in student or training status.

(d) A minimum of 100 hours of personal psychotherapy.

(e) Exceptions to these standards may be made for full membership at the discretion of the Executive Council for the following:

1. A distinguished contributor to the field of psychotherapy, as defined herein, or a person who has achieved a reputation as an outstanding psychotherapist.
2. A person who does not fulfill the above requirements but who is able to document a reasonable claim for eligibility. Such applications will be reviewed by a special committee appointed by the Membership Chair. This committee shall be empowered to request additional information from the candidate and/or reference before formulating its recommendations for the Membership Chair."

> *The American Academy of Psychotherapists is a membership-based national professional organization of psychotherapists with the aims of enhancing psychotherapists, challenging experienced practitioners to professional excellence, and exploring the relationship of person and process to psychotherapy.*

The organization has an Executive Council and officers that include President, President Elect, Secretary, Treasurer, and Immediate Past President. The American Academy of Psychotherapists Central Office is located in Garner, North Carolina and has an Executive Director.

Other details: The organization coordinates several events for its members. It also publishes a newsletter that is published four times a year. The newsletter includes details of American Academy of Psychotherapists business, calendar of events, and a forum for members to exchange perspectives and views.

AMERICAN PUBLIC HEALTH ASSOCIATION–MENTAL HEALTH SECTION

Website: http://www.apha.org

Founded: 1872 (the mental health section was founded over 50 years ago)

History: The **American Public Health Association (APHA)** is among the oldest public health organization founded in 1872. Stephen Smith was the first president of the organization. The aim of the organization is "to protect all Americans, their families and their communities from preventable, serious health threats and strives to assure community-based health promotion and disease prevention activities and preventive health services are universally accessible in the United States" (American Public Health Association, 2010a).

Mission: The mission of the organization is to "improve the health of the public and achieve equity in health status" (American Public Health Association, 2010b). APHA is an association of individuals and organizations that aims to improve the health of the public and aims to achieve equity in health status for all people in the society. APHA promotes scientifically based public health practices and policies and aims to build a healthy global society that promotes prevention and enables its members to promote and protect community and environmental health. The mission of the **Mental Health Section** is to promote public health policy and educational programs aimed at enhancing the mental health of all people and improving the quality of health care for the mentally ill.

> *The American Public Health Association (APHA) is a membership-based national professional organization of individuals interested in public health. The Mental Health Section of this organization promotes public health policy and educational programs aimed at enhancing the mental health of all people and improving the quality of health care for the mentally ill.*

Vision: "A Healthy Global Society" (American Public Health Association, 2010b).

Organizational structure: It is a membership-based organization. Membership is open to health professionals, other career workers in the health field, and any person interested in public health. The governance of the organization is done by the Governing Council.

The Governing Council consists of voting and nonvoting members. The voting members include (1) at least two elected representatives of each section, (2) an additional number of representatives from the unaffiliated membership, (3) one representative designated by each (state) Affiliated Association, (4) the officers of the Association, and (5) the *elected* members of the Executive Board. Nonvoting ex officio members of the Governing Council include (1) the chair of the Science Board, (2) the chair of the Action Board, (3) the chair of the Education Board, (4) the chair of the Committee on Affiliates, (5) the chair of the Inter Sectional Council, (6) the chair of each standing committee of the Association, (7) the executive director, (8) chairs of each Section, and (9) past presidents of the Association.

There are 27 primary sections in APHA that represent salient public health disciplines/programs. One of these sections is the Mental Health Section. The purposes of the Mental Health Section of APHA include the following (American Public Health Association, 2010c):

- "Quality: Identify issues adversely affecting the public's mental health; seek solutions that enhance mental health; provide training, information and support; advocate public mental health needs.
- Participation: Create a mechanism by which interested individuals can participate in the programs, policies, and actions of the Association.
- Coordination: Develop and evaluate programs in conjunction with the APHA Program Development Board, Action Board, and other sections.
- Recommendations: Serve the APHA through making interpretations and recommendations regarding public mental health concerns.

- Collaboration: Identify opportunities for collaboration between professionals and other interested individuals."

Other details: The Mental Health Section has its members as psychiatrists, psychologists, clinicians, policy makers, researchers, postdoctoral students, other students, and all others interested in mental health. Each year the Mental Health Section gives three awards: (1) Carl Taube Award given for significant contributions in the field of mental health services research, (2) Lutterman Award for best student presentation, and (3) Rema Lapouse Award for significant contributions to epidemiology and control of mental disorders.

OTHER ORGANIZATIONS IN MENTAL HEALTH

American Academy of Psychoanalysis and Dynamic Psychiatry (http://aapdp.org/)

The American Academy of Psychoanalysis and Dynamic Psychiatry is an organization of psychiatrists who are interested in using psychodynamic psychotherapy in their clinical practice. The aims of the American Academy of Psychoanalysis and Dynamic Psychiatry (2009) are as follows:

- "To provide a forum for the expression of ideas, concepts, and research in psychodynamic psychiatry and psychoanalysis;
- To constitute a forum for expression of and inquiry into the phenomena of individual motivation and social behavior;
- To encourage and support research in psychodynamic psychiatry and psychoanalysis;
- To advance the development of psychodynamic psychiatry and psychoanalysis in all other aspects;
- To develop communication among psychiatrists, psychoanalysts, and their colleagues in other disciplines in science and in the humanities."

American College of Mental Health Administration (http://www.acmha.org/)

This is a national organization of mental health and substance abuse administrators. The mission of this organization is to (American College of Mental Health Administration, 2010) "be a convener of diverse and emerging leaders concerned with mental health and substance use policy and practice from across systems to:

- Identify and address complex issues of emerging importance;
- Develop consensus through cross discipline dialogs;
- Promote best and evidence-based practices;
- Broker ideas that contribute to the evolution of behavioral health outcomes;
- Promote leadership development and succession; and
- Provide education, networking, and other opportunities to interact with leaders in relevant fields."

American Counseling Association (http://www.counseling.org/)

The American Counseling Association is an association of counselors who also deal with mental health problems. The organization promotes the counseling profession through three-pronged work in advocacy, research, and maintaining professional standards. Founded in 1952, its members come from all counseling settings. It has a current membership of about 45,000 members. The mission of the American Counseling Association (2010) is "to enhance the quality of life in society by promoting the development of professional counselors, advancing the counseling profession, and using the profession and practice of counseling to promote respect for human dignity and diversity."

American College Counseling Association (http://www.collegecounseling.org/)

The American College Counseling Association was founded in 1991 and is a division of the American Counseling Association. It is primarily composed of mental health professionals from the areas of counseling, psychology, and social work who work within higher education settings. "The mission of the American College Counseling Association is to be the interdisciplinary and inclusive professional home that supports emerging and state of the art knowledge and resources for counseling professionals in higher education" (American College Counseling Association, 2009).

American Mental Health Counselors Association (http://www.amhca.org/)

The American Mental Health Counselors Association is a group of approximately 6,000 counselors. The organization's mission is "to enhance the profession of mental health counseling through licensing, advocacy, education and professional development" (American Mental Health Counselors Association, 2010). The vision of the organization is "to be the national organization representing licensed mental health counselors and state chapters, with consistent standards of education, training, licensing, practice, advocacy and ethics" (American Mental Health Counselors Association, 2010).

American Psychiatric Nurses Association (http://www.apna.org/)

American Psychiatric Nurses Association was founded in 1987 and has a current membership of over 7,000 members. Its members comprise registered nurses, nurses with associate degrees, baccalaureate nurses, advanced practice nurses which include clinical nurse specialists and psychiatric nurse practitioners, and nurse scientists and academicians. It publishes the *Journal of American Psychiatric Nurses Association*.

American Psychoanalytic Association (http://www.apsa.org/)

Founded in 1911, the American Psychoanalytic Association is professional organization for psychoanalysts that focuses on education, research, and membership development. It has about 3,500 members. It publishes the peer-reviewed quarterly, *Journal of the American Psychoanalytic Association*. Membership in the American Psychoanalytic Association is only available to candidates and graduates of American Psychoanalytic Association–accredited training institutes and new training facilities and members of the International Psychoanalytical Association or graduates of an institute of an International Psychoanalytical Association component society. In recent years the organization has developed alliances with other psychoanalytic groups, which has led to the creation of the Psychoanalytic Consortium (Margolis, 2001).

International Psychoanalytical Association (http://www.ipa.org.uk/Public/)

This is the world's primary accrediting and regulatory body for psychoanalysis. It has 70 constituent organizations in 33 countries that support over 12,000 members. The aims of the organization include creating new psychoanalytic groups, fostering debate over psychoanalysis, conducting research related to psychoanalysis, developing training policies, and establishing links with other bodies.

International Society for Mental Health Online (https://www.ismho.org/home.asp)

This organization was formed in 1997 and is an online group. The members of this organization include "students, teachers, researchers, clinical practitioners, and others interested in using Internet technologies to sustain positive mental health" (International Society for Mental Health Online, 2010). The mission of the organization is "to promote the understanding, use and development of online communication, information and technology for the international mental health community" (International Society for Mental Health Online, 2010). The yearly membership fee for this organization is $25, and one can access the various forums such as ISMHO Café, ISMHO Academy, Business and Technical Aspects of Online Counseling, Online Support Boards & Groups, Online Counseling and Psychotherapy, International Forum, ISMHO in Second Life, Ethical & Legal Issues, Educators, About ISMHO, Cyberspace News, and Opportunities and Resources.

Mental Health America (formerly National Mental Health Association) (http://www.nmha.org/)

This not-for-profit organization is devoted to helping all people live mentally healthier lives. It has 320 affiliates in 41 states. Mental Health America was founded in 1909 by Clifford W. Beers (see Chapter 1). The mission of the organization is to address the full spectrum of mental and substance abuse conditions by informing, advocating, and enabling access to quality behavioral health services for all Americans. The vision of Mental Health America is "a just, humane and healthy society in which all people are accorded respect, dignity and the opportunity to achieve their full potential through meaningful social inclusion that is free from discrimination" (Mental Health America, 2010).

FOCUS FEATURE 12.1 WORLD HEALTH ORGANIZATION'S MENTAL HEALTH GAP ACTION PROGRAMME (mhGAP)

On October 9, 2008 the World Health Organization launched an action program in Geneva called the Mental Health Gap Action Programme (mhGAP) (World Health Organization, 2010). The purpose of this program is to scale up the services in the area of mental, neurological, and substance use (MNS) disorders for low-income and middle-income countries. Based on epidemiological studies conducted all over the world, it has been determined that lifetime prevalence rates of mental disorders in adults are 12.2% to 48.6% and 12-month prevalence rates are 8.4% to 29.1% (World Health Organization, 2008). Although MNS disorders are prevalent all over the world and approximately 14% of the global burden of disease is attributed to these disorders, up to 75% of people in low-income countries affected with these disorders do not have access to the treatment they need (World Health Organization, 2010). The World Health Organization (2008) found treatment gaps to be 32% for schizophrenia, 56% for depression, and as much as 78% for alcohol use disorders. The World Health Organization (2008) further noted that approximately one-third of countries do not have a specific budget for mental health and of the countries that have a mental health budget, 21% spend less than 1% of their total health budgets on mental health.

It is in this context that mhGAP was launched. The four core strategies identified by the mhGAP are (1) information, (2) policy and service development, (3) advocacy, and (4) research. The objectives of the mhGAP are as follows (World Health Organization, 2008):

- "To reinforce the commitment of governments, international organizations, and other stakeholders to increase the allocation of financial and human resources for care of MNS disorders.
- To achieve much higher coverage with key interventions in the countries with low and lower middle incomes that have a large proportion of the global burden of MNS disorders."

Priority conditions included in mhGAP are depression, schizophrenia and other psychotic disorders, suicide, epilepsy, dementia, disorders due to alcohol use, disorders due to use of illicit drugs, and mental disorders in children. Scaling up in mhGAP involves accomplishing the following tasks (World Health Organization, 2008):

- Identification of key interventions and approaches for delivery of health-services
- Planning a progression for adoption of these actions
- Identification of barriers to success of interventions
- Identification of means to overcome these barriers
- Assessment of the total costs of scaling up
- Sustaining interventions

In 2010, on the mental health day on October 10, the World Health Organization launched the Mental Health Gap Intervention Guide (mhGAP-IG), a practical guide about the implementation of mhGAP.

SKILL-BUILDING ACTIVITY

In this chapter we introduced you to several mental health organizations. Collect information about all these organizations and choose one organization of which you would be eligible to become a member. Establish contact through e-mail or telephone with an office bearer or staff member of that organization. Inquire from that individual the strengths, weaknesses, opportunities, and threats (SWOT) confronting the organization. If you are not able to establish contact, do this analysis based on the information provided on their website. Formulate your SWOT analysis in the form of a 500- to 600-word paper.

SUMMARY

The American Psychological Association (APA) was formed in 1892 and is a professional membership organization of psychologists. Its current membership includes 148,000 individuals. The mission of the APA relates to advancing the creation, communication, and application of psychological knowledge to benefit society and improve people's lives. The American Psychiatric Association was formed in 1844 and is a professional membership organization of psychiatrists. Its current membership includes 38,000 physicians. The mission of the American Psychiatric Association is to ensure the highest quality of care for mentally sick, foster psychiatric education and research, advance the discipline of psychiatry, and cater to the needs of its members. The National Institute of Mental Health (NIMH), formed in1949, is a federal organization with the aim of preventing and treating mental illnesses through basic and clinical research. The National Alliance on Mental Illness (NAMI) was founded in 1979 as a grassroots organization of over 200,000 members and is devoted to improving the lives of individuals and families affected by mental illnesses. The World Federation for Mental Health (WFMH) was founded in 1948 as an international organization composed of members all over the world to prevent mental disorders, ensure proper treatment of mental disorders, and promote mental health.

The American Psychotherapy Association is a membership-based national professional organization of about 6,000 psychotherapists that credentials psychotherapists and advances the profession of psychotherapy. The American Academy of Psychotherapists, founded in 1955, is a membership-based national professional organization of psychotherapists with the aims of enhancing psychotherapists, challenging experienced practitioners to professional excellence, and exploring the relationship of person and process to psychotherapy. The American Public Health Association (APHA)–Mental Health Section was founded in 1872 and is a membership-based national professional organization of individuals interested in public health. The Mental Health Section of this organization promotes public health policy and educational programs aimed at enhancing the mental health of all people and improving the quality of health care for the mentally ill.

Other mental health organizations reviewed here are the American Academy of Psychoanalysis and Dynamic Psychiatry, American College of Mental Health Administration, American Counseling Association, American College Counseling Association, American Mental Health Counselors Association, American Psychiatric Nurses Association, American Psychoanalytic Association, International Psychoanalytical Association, International Society for Mental Health Online, and Mental Health America.

REVIEW QUESTIONS

1. Discuss the mission, vision, and organizational structure of the American Psychological Association.
2. Describe the mission, vision, and organizational structure of the American Psychiatric Association.
3. Summarize the mission, vision, and organizational structure of the National Institute of Mental Health (NIMH).

4. Identify the mission, vision, and organizational structure of the National Alliance on Mental Illness (NAMI).
5. Describe the mission, vision, and organizational structure of the World Federation for Mental Health (WFMH).
6. Explain the mission, vision, and organizational structure of the American Psychotherapy Association.
7. Describe the mission, vision, and organizational structure of the American Academy of Psychotherapists.
8. Explicate the mission, vision, and organizational structure of the American Public Health Association (APHA)–Mental Health Section.

WEBSITES TO EXPLORE

American Psychiatric Association

http://www.psych.org/

This is the website of the American Psychiatric Association. Links have been provided to Psychiatric Practice, Education & Career Development, Research, Advocacy, Newsroom, and Members corner. *Explore these links and learn more about American Psychiatric Association. Visit the links of research and advocacy and find out some of the research and advocacy initiatives of this organization.*

American Psychological Association (APA)

http://www.apa.org/

This is the website of the American Psychological Association (APA). Links have been provided to About APA, Psychology Topics, Publications, Psychology Help Center, News and Events, Research, Education, Careers, and Membership. *Explore these links and learn more about APA. Under the link of careers, browse through jobs. Do you like any job that has been posted? What more qualifications do you need to get that job?*

Mental Health America (formerly National Mental Health Association)

http://www.nmha.org/

This is the website of Mental Health America, formerly known as National Mental Health Association. Links have been provided to Home, About us, Health info, Get help, Action, Our affiliates, Store, and Donate. *Explore these links. In the Health Info Section visit the frequently asked questions (FAQs) link. Read the FAQs. Are there one or more questions you would like to be answered that are not there? Compile a list of such questions and send them to the administrator.*

National Alliance on Mental Illness (NAMI)

http://www.nami.org/

This is the website of National Alliance on Mental Illness (NAMI). Links have been provided for mental illnesses, medications, support and programs, how you can help, find your local NAMI, NAMIWalks, inform yourself, fight stigma, grading the states, legislative action center, online communities, newsroom, NAMI store, Advocate maga-zine, NAMI blog, NAMI on twitter, and NAMI on facebook. *Explore some of these links. Visit the link "fight stigma" and learn more about becoming a "Stigma buster." Is it something you would like to do?*

National Institute of Mental Health (NIMH)

http://www.nimh.nih.gov/index.shtml

This is the website of National Institute of Mental Health (NIMH). Links have been provided to Health Information, Outreach, Research and Funding, Newsroom, and About NIH. The link to Health Information has four tabs: Health info home, clinical trials, statis-tics, and publications. *Explore the Health info home tab. Choose a topic in mental health informa-tion and read more about it. Summarize your readings in a paragraph of key findings on that topic.*

World Federation for Mental Health (WFMH)

http://www.wfmh.org/

This is the website of World Federation for Mental Health (WFMH). Links have been provided for about WFMH, Awareness and Information Services, Center for Fam-ily and Consumer Advocacy and Support, WFMH Center for Transcultural Mental Health, Disaster Response Initiative, International Constituency Development, WFMH Africa Initiative, Mental Health Policy & Human Rights Advocacy, Promotion of Men-tal Health and Prevention of Mental Disorders, Recovery focused interventions, World Mental Health Day, Global Advocacy Directory, Helpful links, and contact us. *Explore these links. Pay special attention to Mental Health Day link and read about the emphasis of this day in the previous three years.*

REFERENCES AND FURTHER READINGS

American Academy of Psychoanalysis and Dynamic Psychiatry. (2009). Mission. Retrieved from http://aapdp.org/.

American Academy of Psychotherapists. (2010a). Purpose of the American Academy of Psychother-apists. Retrieved from http://www.aapweb.com/.

American Academy of Psychotherapists. (2010b). AAP membership. Retrieved from http://www.aapweb.com/membership.html.

American College Counseling Association. (2009). Mission statement. Retrieved from http://www.collegecounseling.org/about/mission-statement.

American College of Mental Health Administration. (2010). About ACHMA. Retrieved from http://www.acmha.org/about.shtml.

American Counseling Association. (2010). About us. Retrieved from http://www.counseling.org/AboutUs/.

American Mental Health Counselors Association. (2010). About AMHCA. Retrieved from http://www.amhca.org/about/default.aspx.

American Psychiatric Association. (2003). APA history. Retrieved from http://www.psych.org/MainMenu/EducationCareerDevelopment/Library/APAHistory.aspx.

American Psychiatric Association. (2007). History of the district branches and of the district branch assembly. Retrieved from http://www.psych.org/MainMenu/EducationCareerDevelopment/Library/APAHis tory/AssemblyDistrictBranchesHistory.aspx.

American Psychiatric Association. (2010a). About APA. Retrieved from http://www.psych.org/FunctionalMenu/AboutAPA.aspx.

American Psychiatric Association. (2010b). Governance. Retrieved from http://www.psych.org/Resources/EarlyCareerPsychiatrists/Governance2.aspx.

American Psychiatric Association. (2010c). APIRE. Retrieved from http://www.psych.org/MainMenu/Research/APIRE.aspx.

American Psychological Association. (2010a). APA history. Retrieved from http://www.apa.org/about/archives/apa-history.aspx.

American Psychological Association. (2010b). About APA. Retrieved from http://www.apa.org/about/index.aspx.

American Psychotherapy Association. (2010a). Mission statement. Retrieved from http://www.americanpsychotherapy.com/about/mission/.

American Psychotherapy Association. (2010b). Goals. Retrieved from http://www.americanpsychotherapy.com/about/goals/.

American Public Health Association. (2010a). Overview. Retrieved from http://www.apha.org/about/.

American Public Health Association. (2010b). Vision/mission. Retrieved from http://www.apha.org/about/gov/execboard/executiveboardvisionmission.htm.

American Public Health Association. (2010c). Mental health section. Retrieved from http://www.apha.org/membergroups/sections/aphasections/mental/.

Brown, E. C. (1989). How the Academy began. *VOICES: The Art and Science of Psychotherapy*, 25(1/2), 70–78.

Brown, T. J. (1998). *Dorothea Dix: New England reformer*. Cambridge, MA: Harvard University Press.

Dewsbury, D. A. (1997). On the evolution of divisions. *American Psychologist, 52*, 733–741.

Evans, R. B., Sexton, V. S., & Cadwallader, T.C. (Eds.). (1992). *The American Psychological Association: A historical perspective*. Washington, DC: American Psychological Association.

Fernberger, S. W. (1932). The American Psychological Association: A historical summary, 1892–1930. *Psychological Bulletin, 29*, 1–89.

Grob, G. N. (1973). *Mental institutions in America: Social policy to 1875*. New York: Free Press.

Grob, G. N. (1996). Creation of the National Institute of Mental Health. *Public Health Reports, 111*(4), 378–381.

Hirschbein, L. D. (2004). History, memory, and profession: A view of American psychiatry through APA presidential addresses, 1883–2003. *American Journal of Psychiatry, 161*(10), 1755–1763.

International Society for Mental Health Online. (2010). International Society for Mental Health online home. Retrieved from https://www.ismho.org/home.asp.

Kirkbride, T. S. (1845). Medical association: Meeting of the Association of the Medical Superintendents of American Institutions for the Insane. *American Journal of Insanity, 1*, 253–258.

Margolis, M. (2001). The American Psychoanalytic Association: A decade of change. *Journal of American Psychoanalytic Association, 49*(1), 11–25.

Mental Health America. (2010). Mission, vision, statement of purpose, guiding principles. Retrieved from http://www.mentalhealthamerica.net/go/mission-vision.

National Alliance on Mental Illness. (2009). Annual report 2009. Retrieved from http://www.nami.org/Content/NavigationMenu/Inform_Yourself/About_NAMI/Annual_Reports/2009AnnualReport.pdf.

National Alliance on Mental Illness. (2010a). About NAMI. Retrieved from http://www.nami.org/template.cfm?section=About_NAMI.

National Alliance on Mental Illness. (2010b). National bylaws. Retrieved from http://www.nami.org/Template.cfm?Section=Governance&Template=/ContentMa nagement/ContentDisplay.cfm&ContentID=17695.

National Alliance on Mental Illness South West. (n.d.). National Alliance on Mental Illness South West. Retrieved from http://namisw.nami.org/.

National Institute of Mental Health. (2010a). The President's budget request. Retrieved from http://www.nimh.nih.gov/about/budget/index.shtml.

National Institute of Mental Health. (2010b). About NIMH. Retrieved from http://www.nimh.nih.gov/about/index.shtml.

World Federation for Mental Health. (2007). About WFMH. Retrieved from http://www.wfmh.org/00about.htm.

World Health Organization. (2008). mhGAP: Mental Health Gap Action Programme: Scaling up care for mental, neurological and substance use disorders. Geneva: Author. Retrieved from http://www.who.int/mental_health/mhgap_final_english.pdf.

World Health Organization. (2010). Launch of the WHO Mental Health Gap Action Programme (mhGAP). Retrieved from http://www.who.int/mental_health/mhgap/en/index.html.

Glossary

abandonment: A type of abuse that includes the desertion of an older person by the individual taking responsibility for providing their care.

acculturation: Psychosocial adjustment and adaptation to a new culture of a person from another culture.

acute stress disorder: A disorder is characterized by reexperiencing, avoidance, and increased arousal, much like posttraumatic stress disorder but the symptoms persist less than a month.

adolescent: A time during the human lifespan that lasts from approximately 12 to 19 years of age.

advance directive: A document that specifies what actions should be taken for an individual's health in case he or she can no longer make such decisions due to sickness or incapacity and appoints a person to make such decisions on their behalf.

affectivity: The range, intensity, responsiveness, and appropriateness of emotional response.

agoraphobia: The feeling of intense anxiety about being in places or situations from which escape might be difficult (or embarrassing) or in which help may not be available in the event of having an unexpected panic attack or panic-like symptoms.

alcohol: A beverage consisting of ethyl alcohol that is usually available as beer, wine, or spirits.

alcohol use: Entails drinking beer, wine, or spirits. In some parts of the world local home-brewed alcoholic beverages are also taken. Typically, one drink consists of 12 ounces of beer, 5 ounces of wine, or 1.5 ounces of 80 proof distilled spirits. According to the U.S. National Institute of Alcohol Abuse and Alcoholism up to two drinks per day for men and one drink per day for women can be considered safe. Consuming 14 drinks per week for men and 7 drinks per week for women is indicative of at-risk behavior.

alcoholism (alcohol dependence): According to DSM-IV-TR, is clinically significant impairment or distress in the presence of three or more of the following: (1) tolerance; (2) withdrawal; (3) a great deal of time spent obtaining alcohol, using alcohol, or recovering from its effects; (4) reducing or giving up important activities because of alcohol; (5) drinking more or longer than intended; (6) a persistent desire or unsuccessful efforts to cut down or control use of alcohol; and (7) continued use.

Alzheimer's disease: A chronic condition that involves parts of the brain that controls thought, memory, and language.

American Academy of Psychotherapists: A membership-based national professional organization of psychotherapists with the goals of enhancing psychotherapists, challenging experienced practitioners to professional excellence, and exploring the relationship of person and process to psychotherapy.

American Psychiatric Association: A membership-based national professional organization of psychiatrists with the goals of promoting the highest quality care for individuals with mental disorders and their families, promoting psychiatric education and research, advancing and representing the profession of psychiatry, and serving the professional needs of its membership.

American Psychological Association: A membership-based national professional organization of psychologists with the goals of advancing the creation, communication, and application of psychological knowledge to benefit society and improve people's lives.

American Psychotherapy Association: A membership-based national professional organization of psychotherapists that credentials psychotherapists and advances the profession of psychotherapy.

American Public Health Association (APHA)–Mental Health Section: A membership-based national professional organization of individuals interested in public health. The Mental Health Section of this organization promotes public health policy and educational programs aimed at enhancing the mental health of all people and improving the quality of health care for the mentally ill.

Americans with Disabilities Act: This comprehensive law prohibits private employers, state and local governments, employment agencies, and labor unions from discriminating against qualified individuals with disabilities in job application procedures, hiring, firing, advancement, compensation, job training, and other terms, conditions, and privileges of employment.

amok: A dissociative episode characterized by a period of brooding followed by an outburst of violent, aggressive, or homicidal behavior directed at people and objects. The episode tends to be precipitated by a perceived slight or insult and seems to be prevalent only among males. The episode is often accompanied by persecutory ideas, automatism, amnesia, exhaustion, and a return to premorbid state after the episode. Some instances of amok may occur during a brief psychotic episode or constitute the onset or an exacerbation of a chronic psychotic process.

amphetamines: Synthetically prepared stimulants of the central nervous system. Common street names for these drugs are "speed," "crank," "crystal," "meth," and "ice." Examples of these drugs are dextroamphetamine (Dexedrine), *d–1-*amphetamine (Benzedrine), and methamphetamine (Methedrine).

analysand: The patient being analyzed in psychoanalysis.

analyst: The psychoanalytic therapist.

anorexia nervosa: A psychiatric illness whereby the patient refuses to maintain ≥85% of his or her ideal body weight, has an intense fear of becoming fat or gaining weight, and has disturbances in the way they assess his or her own body weight.

anterograde amnesia: Memory problems that usually improve within a couple of months.

antianxiety agent (anxiolytic): A drug used for the treatment of anxiety and its attendant psychological and physical symptoms.

antidepressant: A psychotropic agent used to treat mood disorders such as major depression and dysthymia.

antidepressant medications: Medications commonly used in the treatment of depression and help improve the mood and other symptoms of depression like low energy, poor appetite, and insomnia.

antipsychotic medications: Medications used mainly to target symptoms of psychotic conditions such as hallucinations and delusions.

anxiety: The presence of fear or apprehension that is out of proportion to the context of the life situation.

appraisal support: A type of social support that includes people who have given useful feedback for self-evaluation.

Asperger syndrome: A disorder similar to autistic disorder but typically seen as a milder version with less developmental delays.

assertive community treatment (ACT): A service-delivery model that provides comprehensive, locally based treatment to people with serious mental illnesses. It provides highly individualized services directly to consumers. ACT approach takes the multidisciplinary, round-the-clock staffing of a psychiatric unit directly to patients within the comfort of their home and community.

ataque de nervios: A culture bound syndrome mainly reported from the Latino population from the Caribbean but recognized among many other Latin American countries. Ataque de nervios frequently occurs as a direct outcome of a life stressor pertaining to the family and is characterized by amnesia, feelings of being out of control, and other symptoms.

attempted suicide: A nonfatal attempt to kill oneself.

Aulus Cornelius Celsus (25 BCE–50 CE): An important contributor to medicine in the Roman Empire who differentiated between different types of insanity and prescribed humane treatment for insane.

authoritarian parenting style: A parenting styles that is restrictive, places firm boundaries on the child, and does not allow room for discussion. Parents have high control but low responsiveness toward children.

authoritative parenting style: A parenting styles that encourages children to be independent thinkers and gives choices among a defined set a boundaries. Parents have high control and high responsiveness toward children.

autism spectrum disorder: A group of developmental deficits that encompasses three domains: social interaction, communication, and repetitive or stereotypic behavior.

autistic disorder: A disorder in which individuals have significant language delays, social and communication challenges, unusual behaviors and interests, and many have intellectual disabilities.

automatic thought: Thought (which can include both verbal ideas and images) that occurs spontaneously and rapidly, representing an immediate interpretation of a situation.

Ayurveda: Ancient Indian system of medicine that is known as the science of life or health.

baby boomer generation: A generation of children born during the post–World War II era from 1946 to 1964 that was much larger than previous generations.

behaviorism: A philosophy of psychology based on the proposition that all actions taken by organisms can and should be regarded as behaviors. It has also been called the learning perspective.

Benjamin Rush (1745–1813): A physician from United States who wrote, *Medical Inquires and Observations upon the Diseases of the Mind*, considered as the first textbook of psychiatry in America.

binge eating disorder: The most common eating disorder not otherwise specified that is similar to bulimia nervosa; however, after consuming a large amount of calories in one sitting the patient does not engage in a compensatory behavior.

biological psychiatry: An approach to understanding mental disorders in terms of the biological functions of the nervous system.

bipolar disorder: A brain disorder associated with abnormal shifts in mood, energy, activity levels, and the ability to carry out daily activities. Also called manic-depressive illness.

bipolar I disorder: A type of bipolar disorder with distinct manic or mixed episodes that last at least 7 days or manic symptoms that are so intense the individual requires immediate hospital care.

bipolar II disorder: A type of bipolar disorder characterized by an episodic shift between depressive and hypomanic episodes, without full-blown manic or mixed episodes.

brief psychotic disorder: Combination of psychotic symptoms for more than a day but less than a month.

body mass index: An indicator of weight status associated with risk of chronic disease. Can be calculated using a weight-to-height ratio, dividing an individual's weight in kilograms by the square of height in meters.

bulimia nervosa: An illness whereby the patient consumes a large amount of calories at one sitting and then engages in a compensatory behavior (i.e., purging or nonpurging methods) in an attempt to alleviate his or her body from these calories.

capping: The practice of limiting the dollar amount for an individual's lifetime psychiatric care.

catastrophizing: Focusing on the worst possible outcome, however unlikely, without factoring in other possible (and less tragic) outcomes.

Certified Health Education Specialist (CHES): A health educator who meets the required health education training qualifications, successfully passes the certification exam conducted by National Commission for Health Education Credentialing (NCHEC) and meets continuing education requirements.

challenge: A construct of hardiness that refers to a person's willingness to undertake change, confront new activities, and obtain opportunities for growth.

child: A time during the human lifespan that lasts from approximately 4 to 11 years of age.

chronic disease: A type of disease that occurs over a long period of time.

chronic strains: A type of chronic stressors that result from responses of one social group to another, such as overt or covert, intentional or unintentional discriminatory behavior due to race, ethnicity, etc. *See also chronic stressors, community-wide strains, daily hassles, persistent life difficulties, and role strains.*

chronic stressors: Type of stressors that are ongoing and last for a sustained period of time. These include persistent life difficulties, role strains, chronic strains, community wide strains, and daily hassles. *See also chronic strains, community-wide strains, daily hassles, persistent life difficulties, and role strains.*

client-centered therapy (Rogerian psychotherapy): A fairly widely used model of psychotherapy wherein the therapist creates a relaxed, nonjudgmental environment by demonstrating genuineness, empathy, and unconditional positive regard toward their patients while using a nondirective approach. This facilitates the individual undergoing therapy in generating solutions to his or her problems.

Clifford Beers (1876–1943): A Yale graduate and young businessman who was largely responsible for ushering in 20th century reforms in psychiatric care; also credited with the foundation of the Connecticut Society for Mental Hygiene.

cocaine: A stimulant of the central nervous system derived from the coca leaves.

code of ethics for health educators: An ethical code for health educators that includes responsibility to the public, responsibility to the profession, responsibility to employers, responsibility in delivery of health education, responsibility in research and evaluation, and responsibility in professional preparation.

cognition: Mental process of knowing and becoming aware; function is closely associated with judgment.

cognitive behavioral therapy: A form of psychotherapy that attempts to treat problems concerning dysfunctional emotions, behaviors, and cognitions through a goal-oriented, systematic approach.

cognitive distortions: When people experience maladaptive subjective emotional distress, the cognitive behavioral approach links it to their problematic, stereotypic, biased interpretations pertinent to this cognitive triad of self, world, and future. These biased interpretations are often called cognitive distortions.

cognitive triad: A central tenet of the cognitive theory of emotional disorders is its stress on the cognitive triad, the psychological significance of people's beliefs about themselves, their personal world (including significant others), and their future.

commitment: A construct of hardiness that refers to a person's tendency to become involved in whatever he or she encounters or to a feeling of deep involvement in the activities of life.

common-law marriage: A type of marriage that two people enter into informally. In some areas this type of marriage can be legally binding, but in others it is meaningless.

community-based care: The provision of services in the users' own social environment.

community-wide strains: A type of chronic stressors that include stressors which operate at an ecological level, such as residing in a high-crime neighborhood. *See also chronic strains, chronic stressors, daily hassles, persistent life difficulties, and role strains.*

comprehensibility: A construct of sense of coherence that refers to the extent to which one perceives the stressors that confront one make cognitive sense, implying there is some set structure, consistency, order, clarity, and predictability.

compulsions: Repetitive acts, behaviors, or thoughts designed to counteract the anxiety associated with an obsession.

conduct disorder: Repetitive and persistent pattern of behavior in which the basic rights of others or major age-appropriate societal norms or rules are violated.

constructive play: A type of play that combines sensorimotor play, practice play, and symbolic play.

continuum model: Conceptualization of mental health and mental illness where on one end is mental health and on the other end is mental illness.

control: A construct of hardiness that refers to a person's belief that he or she causes the events of his or her life and can influence the environment.

coping: Purposive, psychological mechanism of dealing with stressors. *See also emotion-focused coping and problem-focused coping.*

Corpus Hippocraticum: A body of writings (a compilation of around 70 books) attributed to Hippocrates in the Greek civilization.

cultural competence: Possession of cultural knowledge and respect for different cultural perspectives and having skills and being able to use those skills effectively in cross-cultural situations.

cultural sensitivity: Paying attention to and incorporating the cultural beliefs, attitudes, behaviors, values, historical aspects, social dimensions, and ecological characteristics of different ethnic compositions of target population in planning, implementation, and evaluation of mental health programs.

culture-bound syndromes: Episodic and dramatic reactions specific to a particular community locally defined as discrete patterns of behavior.

cyclothymia: A milder form of bipolar disorder where episodes of hypomania shift back and forth with mild depression for at least 2 years. However, the symptoms fail to meet the diagnostic requirements for any other type of bipolar disorder.

daily hassles: A type of chronic stressors that include everyday problems such as getting stuck in traffic. *See also chronic strains, chronic stressors, community-wide strains, persistent life difficulties, and role strains.*

defense mechanisms: Devices that the mind uses to alter one's perception of situations that disturb the internal milieu or mental balance. These include methods such as introjection, isolation, projection reversal, reaction formation, regression, repression, sublimation, turning against the self, and undoing.

deinstitutionalization: The process of replacing long-stay psychiatric hospitals with less isolated community mental health service for those diagnosed with mental disorder or developmental disability.

delirium tremens: The withdrawal symptoms associated with stopping the regular use of alcohol characterized by delusions or false beliefs, disorientation, delirium, and amnesia or loss of memory. Also involves seizures in a later stage.

delusion: A false belief based on incorrect inferences about reality, at odds with the person's social and cultural background.

delusional disorder: Nonbizarre delusion of at least 1 month's duration.

dementia: A progressive brain impairment that interferes with memory and other cognitive functions that can impede normal daily living activities.

depot injection: A long-acting injectable formulation of an antipsychotic medication.

depressants: Drugs that decelerate the central nervous system, such as barbiturates and benzodiazepines. The three types of depressants are sedatives, which reduce anxiety; tranquilizers, which calm the system; and hypnotics, which induce sleep.

depression: A common mental disorder that presents with depressed mood, loss of interest or pleasure, feelings of guilt or low self-worth, disturbed sleep or appetite, low energy, and poor concentration.

depressive episode: A sad or hopeless state.

depersonalization: Feelings of being detached from oneself.

derealization: Feelings of unreality.

dhat: A culture-bound syndrome seen in India and characterized by vague somatic complaints of fatigue, weakness, anxiety, appetite loss, guilt, and sexual dysfunction attributed by the patient to loss of semen in nocturnal emissions and through urine and/or masturbation.

dialectical behavior therapy: A form of psychotherapy that was originally developed for the treatment of individuals diagnosed with borderline personality disorder. The technique combines standard cognitive behavioral techniques for emotion regulation and reality-testing with concepts of distress tolerance, acceptance, and mindfulness.

disorganized speech: Loss of the orderliness of one's speech characterized by impairments in speech production, the pace, lucidity, and content.

distress: Negative effects experienced as a result of encountering stressors and not managing them effectively.

divorce: A legal dissolution of a marriage by a court or other authoritative body.

Dorothea Lynde Dix (1802–1887)**:** An American activist who is credited with the creation of the first generation of American mental asylums. Through a vigorous program of lobbying state legislatures and the U.S. Congress she was able to effect legislation for better care of the mentally ill.

double bind theory of schizophrenia: A theory describing the "double bind" situation in which no matter what an individual did, they could not "win." It was hypothesized that a person caught in the double bind could develop schizophrenic symptoms.

drug abuse (substance abuse): The use of a substance in a way, quantity, or circumstances so as to cause problems or increase the propensity of occurrence of problems.

drug dependence (substance dependence): Becoming habituated to use of a drug to the extent that it is required in higher and higher doses and stopping it causes physical and psychological symptoms that require it to be used again and again.

drug misuse: Using a drug for a purpose other than the one prescribed by a licensed health care provider or using amounts of a drug in greater quantity than normally used.

eating disorder not otherwise specified: Any disordered eating behaviors that have not been classified by the DSM-IV-TR.

electroconvulsive therapy: A controversial psychiatric treatment in which seizures are electrically induced in anesthetized patients for therapeutic effect. Also known as ECT or electroshock therapy.

Emil Kraepelin (1856–1926): A German psychiatrist who classified mental disorders and advocated that the origins of mental illnesses were rooted in biology and genetics.

emotion-focused coping: Method of dealing with a stressor where the focus is inward on altering the way one thinks or feels about a situation or an event. *See also coping and problem–focused coping.*

emotional or psychological abuse: A type of abuse that includes severe mental or physical pain suffered through verbal or nonverbal acts, such as verbal assaults, threats, intimidation, or harassment.

eustress: Positive effects experienced as a result of encountering stressors and managing them effectively.

event-based models: Model of stress that underscores the role of life events in causation of stress. *See also life events or life change events.*

extinction: Lack of any consequence after a behavior that leads to a decline in the frequency of that behavior.

eye movement desensitization and reprocessing: A comprehensive, integrative psychotherapy approach described as an eclectic approach that combines elements of many different psychotherapy styles in structured protocols that are designed to maximize treatment effects. These include psychodynamic, cognitive behavioral, interpersonal, experiential, and body-centered therapies.

family-focused therapy: Therapy involving the entire family unit and assisting in developing and enhancing coping strategies, such as early recognition of new mood episodes. It also helps improve communication by recognizing new episodes early and helping the loved one.

family planning: The practice of controlling the number of children a couple desires and the spacing (or timing) between those children.

family therapy (family systems therapy or couple and family therapy): A kind of psychotherapy that focuses on families and couples to foster change and development. This branch of psychotherapy emphasizes family relationships as an important factor in psychological health.

financial or material exploitation: A type of abuse that includes any illegal or improper use of an older person's money, property, or other asset, including unauthorized credit card purchases or stealing money from an older person's account.

flashbacks: Psychological phenomenon where an individual has a sudden, usually powerful, and reexperiencing of a past experience or elements of a past experience.

flat or blunted affect: Reduction in the normal range of facial expressions.

Frank Mesmer (1733–1815): An Austrian physician who postulated that mental illnesses were due to misdistribution or deficiency of magnetism and suggested the mentally ill could be cured by holding rods filled with iron filings in water. His technique was later proved to be wrong.

games: Activities that can be played alone or with others and typically include a defined set of rules and competition with other.

gender: The social dimensions of being a man or woman.

gender identity: A sense of belongingness to one sex.

gender role: A set of expectations one believes a certain sex should fulfill.

general adaptation syndrome: When any organism encounters nonspecific stimuli it responds physiologically in three stages: alarm reaction, stage of resistance, and stage of exhaustion.

General Educational Diploma (GED): A high school equivalency diploma that evaluates an adult's high school level skills and knowledge in five core academic areas: math, reading, writing, science, and social studies.

generalized anxiety disorder: An anxiety disorder characterized by frequent and lasting worry and anxiety that is inconsistent with the actual events or circumstances on which the anxiety is focused.

generic drug: A drug identical, or bioequivalent, to a brand name drug in dosage form, safety, strength, route of administration, quality, performance characteristics, and intended use.

group psychotherapy: An approach that uses a professionally trained therapist who organizes and guides a group of members to work together toward the maximal attainment of the goals for each individual in that group and for the group itself.

hallucination: A false sensory perception occurring in the absence of any relevant external stimulation of the sensory modality involved.

hallucinogens: Type of psychoactive drugs that cause hallucination or alteration of perception of tactile sensation, visual sensation, or auditory sensation. Examples include LSD (lysergic acid diethylamide), "magic mushrooms" or psilocybin, morning glory seeds, dimethyltryptamine, mescaline or peyote cactus (*Lopophora williamsii*) derivative, DOM (2,5-dimethoxy–4-methylamphetamine) or STP (serenity, tranquility, and peace), Ecstasy, PCP (Phencyclidine), and anticholinergic hallucinogens.

hardiness: A set of personality traits comprising commitment, control, and challenge that lead to better coping with stressors and improved mental health.

health: A means to achieve desirable goals in life while maintaining multidimensional (physical, mental, social, political, economic, spiritual) equilibrium that is operationalized for individuals as well as for communities.

health education: Systematic application of a set of techniques to voluntarily and positively influence health through changing the antecedents of behavior (awareness, information, knowledge, skills, beliefs, attitudes, and values) in individuals, groups, or communities.

health promotion: Process of empowering people to improve their health by providing educational, political, legislative, organizational, social, and community supports.

humane treatment: A scientific understanding of schizophrenia as a human brain disease started developing around the 19th century. The "humane" treatment often prescribed for "insanity" was a method that advocated care, protection, and human understanding for those afflicted.

hyperprolactinemia: Abnormally high levels of prolactin, a hormone primarily associated with lactation, in the blood.

infant: A time during the human lifespan that lasts from approximately 0 to 3 years of age.

informational support: Any support an individual receives regarding sharing knowledge that could benefit them, such as information about available resources.

insight: A conscious recognition of one's own condition. In psychiatry, it refers to the conscious awareness and understanding of one's own symptoms of maladaptive behavior; highly important in effecting changes in the personality and behavior of a person.

instrumental support: Any support an individual receives directly from someone else, such as transportation or help with daily living activities.

interpersonal and social rhythm therapy: A form of therapy that helps people with bipolar disorder improve their relationships with others and manage their daily routines. Regular daily routines and sleep schedules may help protect against manic episodes.

interpersonal deficits: Refer to patients who are socially isolated or who are in chronically unfulfilling relationships.

interpersonal psychotherapy: A time-limited psychotherapy that focuses on the interpersonal dynamics and on building interpersonal skills. The basic premise upon which interpersonal psychotherapy is based is the belief that interpersonal factors may contribute significantly to psychological problems. Interpersonal psychotherapy aims to change an individual's interpersonal behavior by promoting adaptation to current interpersonal roles and situations.

interpersonal role disputes: Conflicts with a significant other (e.g., a partner, other family member, coworker, or close friend) that emerge from differences in expectations about the relationship.

involuntary commitment: The practice of placing a person in a psychiatric hospital or ward against his or her will, in compliance with mental health laws of the country. Commitment is normally time-limited and requires reevaluation at fixed intervals.

Jahoda's model of mental health: According to this model mental health comprises the (1) ability to be realistic, (2) ability to accept self, (3) ability to invest in living, (4) ability to make independent decisions, and (5) ability to demonstrate mastery of environment as demonstrated by ability to love, show adequacy in work, love, and play, adequacy in interpersonal relationships, efficiency in situational necessities, ability to adjust and adapt and efficiency in problem solving.

Jean-Martin Charcot (1825–1893): A French neurologist who is nicknamed "the Napoleon of the neuroses." He is well known for his work on hypnosis and hysteria.

joint custody: A type of child custody after divorce whereby both parents share legal and physical decisions pertaining to that child.

launch: A stage in life when a young adult leaves the security of his or her family and becomes more independent and self-sustaining.

legal custody: A type of custody that allows a parent to make any decision regarding the needs of the child (i.e., education, health care, and religion).

life events or life change events: A distinct category of stressors that are discrete, major happenings affecting or having the potential to influence one's body, mind, family, or community, for example, death of a family member. *See also event-based model, chronic stressors, recent life events, remote life events, and stressors.*

life expectancy: The average number of years an individual is expected to live beyond his or her current age, if death rates remain constant.

living wills: A type of advance directive in which an individual's instructions for health care and medical emergencies are formally stated.

locus of control: Belief of an individual regarding the location of happenings in life, whether from an outside source or the self.

lobotomy: A psychosurgical procedure that entails the removal or severing of certain connections in the brain as treatment of mental illnesses. This technique was popular from 1936 to 1950s and then discontinued. *Also see psychosurgery.*

magnification: Distorting aspects of a memory or situation through magnifying them such that they no longer correspond to objective reality.

manageability: A construct of sense of coherence that refers to the extent to which one believes the resources under one's control are adequate to meet the demands posed by the stressors.

managed care: A system of financing and providing health care that seeks to cut costs and improve quality of care.

manic episode: A euphoric, overexcited state.

marijuana: Derived from the plant *Cannabis sativa*, *C. indica*, or *C. ruderalis* in which the active ingredient is THC (tetrahydrocannabinol). Various products are available such as *Charas* (pure resin extracted from surface of leaves and stem), *Hashish* (less pure: 5–15% THC), *Ganja or sinsemilla* (dried pistillate of female flowers before pollination: 5–10% THC), *Bhang* (powder from the entire plant: 1% THC), and hash oil (boiled in alcohol: 50% THC).

marriage: A legal union between one man and one woman as husband and wife.

McCollum's model of mental health education: A six-step model developed in 1981 for mental health education that includes the following steps: (1) population selection, (2) need identification, (3) goal setting, (4) selection of resources, (5) selection of instructional techniques, and (6) evaluation.

meaningfulness: A construct of sense of coherence that refers to the extent to which one believes life makes sense emotionally and that at least some of the stressors in life are worth investing energy in and are worthy of commitment and engagement.

mental disorder: A clinical condition that affects the mind (behavioral or psychological) and that leads to significant suffering or disability in any sphere of life. *Same as mental illness.*

mental health: The ability of an individual to fulfill his or her obligations to self and society while living in mutual harmony with the physical and social environment.

mental health educator: One who works in the area of mental health education by voluntarily modifying health behaviors that are conducive to making a person be in harmony with his or her environment.

mental health promoter: A person who develops policies, regulations, and environments that are conducive to making an individual be in harmony with his or her environment.

mental illness: A clinical condition that affects the mind (behavioral or psychological) and that leads to significant suffering or disability in any sphere of life. *Same as mental disorder.*

middle-old: A time periods in an individual's life that spans from ages 75 to 84 years.

midlife crisis: A time in middle adulthood in which individuals question their sense of life accomplishments, have an overwhelming sense of self-doubt, and begin to fear their eventual death.

migration: Phenomenon of individuals moving from one country, place, or locality to another.

mind reading: Assuming knowledge of the intentions or thoughts of others without explicit communication of the same.

mindfulness: Derives from both Western Christian contemplative and Eastern meditative traditions and refers to the practice of paying attention in a particular way to the present moment and without any judgment. Patients learn their behavior is a function of current emotions (emotion mind) or logical analysis (reasonable mind).

minimization: Distorting aspects of a memory or situation through minimizing them such that they no longer correspond to objective reality.

minor: An individual under the age of adulthood, which is commonly 18 years of age.

mixed state: A mood episode in which symptoms of both depression and mania are present.

Montgomery GI Bill: A monetary benefit for active duty servicemen and women to provide money for college and/or vocational training after completion of active duty service.

mood episode: Intense emotional states in distinct periods experienced by people with bipolar disorder.

mood stabilizer: A psychotropic agent used to treat mood disorders characterized by sustained and extreme shifts in mood states, seen usually in bipolar disorders.

mood-stabilizing medications: Medications that help control the abnormal mood episodes; usually the first line of treatment for bipolar disorder.

National Alliance on Mental Illness (NAMI): A grassroots membership-based organization devoted to improving the lives of individuals and families affected by mental illnesses.

National Commission for Health Education Credentialing (NCHEC): A national body that develops and administers a national competency-based examination for health educators, sets standards for professional preparation of health educators, and fosters professional development for health educators through continuing education.

National Institute of Mental Health (NIMH): A federal organization with the aim of preventing and treating mental illnesses through basic and clinical research.

negative symptom: Affects and behaviors that are lacking in persons with schizophrenia.

neglect: A type of abuse in which any individual refuses or fails to fulfill any part of his or her obligation or duty to serving an older person.

neglectful parenting style: A parenting style in which parents are uninvolved with their children, have no control, and are not responsive.

neuroleptic drugs: Drugs used to treat psychotic conditions, such as chlorpromazine, haloperidol, and molindone. Also known as antipsychotic drugs.

new couple: The second stage of the *Family Life Cycle* that pertains to the joining of families through marriage.

nonevents: Absence of events that have the potential to cause stress and includes situations when desired or anticipated events do not occur or when desired events do not occur even though their occurrence is normative for people of a certain group or not having anything to do. *See also stressors.*

normal weight: A body mass index of 18.5 to 24.9 kg/m^2.

obese: A body mass index greater than 30 kg/m^2.

obsessions: Persistent ideas, thoughts, impulses, or images that are experienced as intrusive and inappropriate

obsessive-compulsive disorder: An anxiety disorder characterized by obsessions and compulsions.

old-old: A time period in an individual's life that spans from age 85 and older.

operant conditioning: Use of a behavior's antecedent and/or its consequence to influence the occurrence and form of behavior.

opioids: Drugs derived from opium and its derivatives from the plant *Papaver somniferum*. Examples include morphine, codeine, and heroin.

oppositional defiant disorder: Recurrent pattern of negativistic, defiant, disobedient, and hostile behavior toward authority figures that persists for at least 6 months.

optimism: The tendency to expect the best possible outcome or to believe the most hopeful aspects of any situation.

overgeneralization: Taking isolated cases and using them to make far-reaching generalizations.

overweight: A body mass index of 25 to 29.9 kg/m^2.

panic attack: A discrete period of intense fear or discomfort along with several other physical symptoms.

paresthesias: Sensation of tingling, pricking, or numbness of a person's skin.

partial hospitalization: A type of mental health program used to treat mental illness and substance abuse in which the individual patient continues to reside at his or her home but commutes to a treatment center up to 7 days a week. Also known as PHP (partial hospitalization program).

perceived emotional support: A type of support that includes any emotional support an individual believes he or she has available, whether in need of support or not.

permissive parenting style: A parenting style in which parents are highly involved in their children's life but place few demands on them. Parents are responsive but show no control toward the child.

persistent life difficulties: A type of chronic stressors that include life events lasting more than 6 months, such as long-term disability. *See also chronic strains, chronic stressors, community-wide strains, daily hassles, life events, persistent life difficulties, and role strains.*

personality disorders: An enduring pattern of inner experience and behavior that deviates markedly from the expectations of the individual's culture.

personalization: Attribution of personal responsibility (or causal role) for events over which the individual has no control.

pervasive developmental disorder not otherwise specified: A disorder that describes individuals who only meet some of the criteria for autistic disorder or Asperger syndrome.

phase I studies: The initial introduction of the new drug in humans. The studies are closely monitored, conducted usually in healthy volunteers, and identify the properties of the drug and overt toxicities. These studies also establish tolerable doses for further testing.

phase II studies: Studies that include carefully chosen patients with the disease or condition being studied. Phase II studies are closely monitored and optimized for the collection of efficacy data. Optimal doses of the drug and safety data regarding common short-term side effects is also obtained during this phase.

phase III studies: These studies help expand the information on the effectiveness and safety of the drug to assess the overall risk-to-benefit ratio. The study subjects are selected from a broader pool in comparison with phase II studies to help select a population that is more representative of the patients who will be exposed to the drug during marketing. Phase III studies may include from several hundred to several thousand subjects, including individuals with a broad range of typical comorbid conditions and concomitant medications seen in the target population.

phase IV studies: Refers to the postmarketing activities conducted subsequent to the FDA approval of a drug. Active surveillance for rare adverse events and studies designed to look into approval for additional indications are two examples of phase IV studies.

Philippe Pinel (1745–1826): A French physician who introduced simple and humane psychological treatments and wrote *Traité médico-philosophique sur l'aleniation mentale; ou la manie* (Medico-Philosophical Treatise on Mental Alienation or Mania). His approach can be considered as the first psychotherapeutic approach to mentally ill patients.

phobia: An excessive fear of a specific object, circumstance, or situation.

physical abuse: The use of any physical force that may result in bodily injury, physical pain, or impairment, such as hitting, beating, pushing, and shoving.

physical activity: Any bodily movement produced by skeletal muscles resulting in energy expenditure.

physical custody: A type of custody that refers to the amount of time a child lives or visits both parents.

physical fitness: A multicomponent trait related to the ability to perform physical activity.

positive symptom: When a symptom involves an addition to an individual's normal experiences, it is said to be a "positive" symptom. Examples include auditory and visual hallucinations (hearing voices and seeing things).

postmodern family: A description of the changing dynamic of families, which today includes a larger female workforce, declining birth rate, rising rates of divorce, cohabitation, and nonmarital childbearing.

postpartum depression: The period immediately after childbirth in which the risk of depression is increased, with approximately 10% of women developing this incapacitating illness, which can have devastating effects on the patient and her family if not recognized and treated in a timely fashion.

posttraumatic stress disorder: An anxiety disorder characterized by the onset of psychiatric symptoms immediately after exposure to a traumatic event and which includes symptoms associated with a reexperiencing of the trauma, those related to avoidance of the stimuli associated with the trauma, and finally symptoms of increased autonomic arousal.

poverty: A status that is determined by comparing an individual's annual income to a set of dollar values (or thresholds) that vary by family size, number of children, and age of household members.

power of attorney: A type of advance directive for which someone is appointed by the individual to make decisions on his or her behalf when he or she is unable.

practice play: Similar to sensorimotor play in infancy but starts in childhood. Includes any repetition of behavior when learning new skills or when physical or mental mastery is needed for games or sports.

pretense of symbolic play: A type of play whereby children transform their surroundings into symbols.

primary prevention: Preventive actions that are taken before the onset of disease or an injury with a view of removing the possibility of their ever occurring.

problem-focused coping: Method of dealing with a given stressor by one's ability to think and alter the environmental event or situation. *See also coping and emotion-focused coping.*

prodromal period: The early symptoms and signs of an illness that pave the way for the characteristic manifestations of the acute, fully developed illness.

psychoanalysis (Freudian psychology): A body of ideas developed by Austrian neurologist Sigmund Freud and that continually evolved in the decades that followed. The major application of psychoanalysis is the study of human psychological functioning and mental illnesses.

psychoanalytic psychotherapy: Based fundamentally on the application of techniques that derive from psychoanalysis. Also called psychodynamic psychotherapy or expressive psychotherapy.

psychoeducation: An approach that helps impart education about mental illnesses and their treatment both to the individual and the family. This approach helps people identify early signs of relapse so they can seek treatment early, thereby averting a full-blown mood episode. It can be delivered in group or individual settings and may also prove helpful for family members and caregivers.

psychopharmacology: The use of medications for the treatment of mental disorders.

psychosis: Delusions and prominent hallucinations, with the hallucinations occurring in the absence of insight into their pathological nature.

psychosurgery: A surgical procedure that entailed the removal or severing of certain connections in the brain as treatment of mental illnesses. This technique was popular from 1936 to 1950s and then discontinued. *Also see lobotomy.*

psychotic disorder due to a medical condition: Delusions/hallucinations occurring as the direct consequence of a general medical condition.

punishment: A consequence that causes a behavior to occur with less frequency.

qi: A concept in Chinese medicine; the basis of the activities of body and mind and the primordial entity of both material (body) and nonmaterial (mind) things, gross and subtle.

reality testing: The ability to differentiate between the external world and the internal world and to accurately judge the relation between the self and the environment.

recent life events: Discrete major life happenings that have occurred within the past one year. *See also life events and remote life events.*

reinforcement: A consequence that causes a behavior to occur with greater frequency.

remote life events: Discrete major life happenings that have occurred in distant past beyond 1 year. *See also life events and recent life events.*

René Descartes (1596–1650): A French mathematician and philosopher who dichotomized mind and the body. He advocated that the mind was under the purview of religion and the body was to be treated by physicians.

resilience: The ability to rebound back in the face of adversity.

response-based models: Model of stress that underscores the role of responses arising out of stress. *See also event-based model and transactional model.*

retirement: The act of leaving a job and ceasing to work.

retrograde amnesia: Trouble remembering events that occurred before treatment began.

role strains: A type of chronic stressors that include either strain from performing specific roles (such as parenting, working, being in a relationship, etc.) or performing multiplicity of roles at the same time. *See also chronic stressors.*

role transition: Any difficulties resulting from a change in life status.

same-sex marriage: A type of marriage that recognizes the legal union between members of the same sex.

schizoaffective disorder: A combination of schizo (psychotic) + affective (mood) symptoms.

schizophrenia: As a disturbance lasting at least 6 months (if untreated) not due to substance use or a general medical condition such as a brain tumor and in which two or more of the following symptoms are present for at least 1 month: delusions or hallucinations, disorganized speech, disorganized or catatonic behavior, or negative symptoms. The symptoms of schizophrenia have been divided into positive, negative, and cognitive types.

schizophreniform disorder: An episode of schizophrenia lasting more than 1 month but less than 6 months.

seasonal depression: The name given to the specific kind of depression that is precipitated by the circadian rhythms during the winter months.

secondary prevention: A type of prevention that attempts to identify individuals afflicted with a disease at an early stage (sometimes called prodromal stage) and seeks to reduce morbidity through prompt treatment.

secondary prevention: Actions that block the progression of an injury or disease at its incipient stage.

self-efficacy: Confidence a person has in his or her ability to pursue a behavior.

self-esteem: An individual's sense of one's own worth or the extent of an individual's approval, value, appreciation, or liking of oneself.

self-neglect: A type of self-abuse that includes any behavior that threatens one's own life, health, or safety, including refusal or failure to provide him- or herself with adequate food, water, clothing, or shelter.

sense of coherence: A theory about a way of seeing the world that enhances mental health and comprises three constructs, namely comprehensibility, manageability, and meaningfulness.

sensorimotor play: Any behavior in infancy that derives pleasure from exercising the existing sensorimotor schema.

sex: The biological factors of being a man or a woman.

sexual abuse: A type of abuse that includes nonconsensual sexual contact, such as unwanted touching, rape, sodomy, and coerced nudity.

shared psychotic disorder: A delusion that develops in an individual in the context of a close relationship with another person(s), who has an already established delusion.

Sigmund Freud (1856–1939)**:** An Austrian physician who founded the psychoanalytic school of psychology. Freud is best known for his theories of the unconscious mind.

social capital: All characteristics of social life such as networks, norms, and trust that enable members to act together in pursuing shared objectives.

social phobia: Marked or persistent fear of one or more social or performance situations in which the person is exposed to unfamiliar people or to possible scrutiny by others.

social play: Any type of play performed with peers or friends.

Social Security: A federal entitlement program paid to people who have already retired, are disabled, survivors of workers who have died, or are dependents of beneficiaries.

social stigma: A set of deeply discrediting attributes, related to negative attitudes and beliefs toward a group of people, likely to affect a person's identity and thus leading to a damaged sense of self through social rejection, discrimination, and social isolation.

social support: Real or perceived resources provided by others that enable a person to feel cared for, valued, and part of a network of communication and mutual obligation.

socioeconomic status: A measure of an individual's economic and social position in society.

sole custody: A type of child custody after divorce whereby only one parent can make all legal and physical decisions pertaining to that child.

specific phobia: A marked and persistent fear that is excessive or unreasonable, cued by the presence or anticipation of a specific object or situation (e.g., flying, heights, animals, receiving an injection, seeing blood).

spirituality: An individual's connection to self, family members, and surrounding community; does not necessary imply the involvement of organized or other types of religions.

split treatment: A model of care where instead of a single mental health practitioner who can deliver comprehensive holistic mental health care (i.e., the psychiatrist), fragmented care is encouraged by two or more providers.

spouse: A person of the opposite sex who is a husband or a wife.

Stafford loans: A form of needs-based aid provided by the federal government that consists of unsubsidized loans, for which the beneficiary pays interest while in college, and subsidized loans, for which the government pays interest while the student is enrolled in college.

stimulants: Category of psychoactive drugs that stimulate the central nervous system, such as cocaine and amphetamines.

stress: The response of the body and mind, including behaviors, as a result of encountering stressors, interpreting them, and making judgments about controlling or influencing the outcomes of these events.

stressors: Various external events that pose actual or perceived threat to the body or mind. *See also life events and chronic stressors.*

substance-induced psychotic disorder: Development of psychotic symptoms as a direct outcome of substance abuse or withdrawal from a substance.

suicidality: All suicide-related behaviors and thoughts, including completing or attempting suicide, suicidal ideation, or suicide-related communications.

suicide: An act of deliberately killing oneself.

suicidal ideation: Thoughts of harming or killing oneself.

systematic desensitization: Consists of two components: relaxation therapy and the presentation of fear-producing stimuli arranged within a hierarchy. The hierarchy consists of a series of situations (real or imagined) that represent successive approximations to the feared object, situation, or event. Conceptually, a hierarchy may be considered to be a ladder in which each rung brings one closer to the fearful stimulus.

Taoism: Chinese philosophy developed by Lao Tse (Lao Tzu) and based on *Tao* (or the *Way*), which refers to reality that naturally exists from primordial time and gives rise to all other things. *Tao* can be found by experiencing oneness in all things.

telepsychiatry: A specifically defined form of video conferencing that can provide psychiatric services to patients living in remote locations or otherwise underserved areas via the electronic transmission of images.

Tengland's model of mental health: According to this model the criteria for mental health are (1) ability to have high degree of correct memory, (2) ability to correctly perceive various stimuli, (3) ability to exhibit high degree of rationality, (4) ability to have self-knowledge, (5) ability to exhibit flexibility, (6) ability to experience emotions, (7) ability to feel empathy, (8) ability to have self esteem and self confidence, (9) demonstrate ability to communicate cognitive information, (10) ability to identify what is appropriate in a communication, and (11) ability to cooperate.

tertiary prevention: Those actions that are taken after the onset of disease or an injury with a view of assisting diseased or disabled people.

testator: An individual who leaves a will upon his or her death.

The mental health parity law (The Wellstone-Domenici Parity Act): The Act ensures that mental illnesses be treated just like physical illnesses by insurance plans covering 50 or more employees.

therapeutic milieu: A structured group setting in which the existence of the group is a key force in the outcome of treatment.

thought blocking: A sudden interruption in the thinking process leading to a blank state.

thought broadcasting: A symptom of psychosis in which the patient believes that his or her thoughts are being transmitted beyond the head so that other people can hear them.

tobacco use: The act of smoking cigarettes, cigars, pipes, bidis or kreteks (clove cigarettes), hookahs, or using smokeless tobacco (snuff and chewing tobacco).

transactional analysis: Conceived by Eric Berne, a psychiatrist trained in the psychoanalytic tradition, in which the underlying premise is that human beings seek intimacy, comfort, or recognition through social interactions. They get such intimacy and recognition through mutual exchanges that Berne called "strokes."

transactional model: Model of stress and coping characterized by interaction of a person in an environment that goes through four stages of primary appraisal, secondary appraisal, coping, and reappraisal.

transcranial magnetic stimulation: The application of a rapidly changing magnetic field to the superficial layers of the cerebral cortex, thereby inducing small electric currents called "eddy" currents. Transcranial magnetic stimulation exemplifies noninvasive stimulation of focal regions of the brain and can be used for research or therapeutically without the need for anesthesia.

transference: A phenomenon in psychoanalysis characterized by unconscious redirection of feelings from one person to another.

trephining: A technique practiced by primitive tribes to treat the mentally ill by drilling holes in the skulls to let the evil spirits out.

tridosha theory of disease: In the system of *Ayurveda*, an ancient Indian medical system, diseases were explained as disturbances in the three *doshas*, or humors, which were *vata* (wind), *pitta* (gall), and *kapha* (mucus).

type A personality: Personality type characterized by hurrying nature, exercising control over people and things, sense of urgency, and challenging nature. *See also type B personality.*

type B personality: Personality type characterized by more laid-back lifestyle and a more relaxed disposition. *See also type A personality.*

Unani system of medicine: Arabic system of medicine that originated in Middle Ages and utilizes herbs and folk remedies.

underweight: A body mass index less than 18.5 kg/m^2.

unemployment: A status given to those who are currently available to work but have been unable to find work for over 4 weeks.

widowhood: A time for women (widow) or men (widower) when their spouse has died and they have not remarried.

will: A legal document by which a testator names one or more individuals to manage his or her estate and outlines who receives which properties of the testator.

World Federation for Mental Health (WFMH): An international membership-based organization composed of members all over the world to prevent mental disorders, ensure proper treatment of mental disorders, and promote mental health.

work-related stress: Stress that results directly or indirectly from experiences at work.

yang: The masculine principle in Chinese medicine. It should be in balance with feminine principle, *yin*, for good health.

yin: The feminine principle in Chinese medicine. It should be in balance with masculine principle, *yang*, for good health.

yoga: A practice from Ancient India that attempts to establish balance between body, mind, and environment. This practice has been found to be useful for mental health.

young-old: A time period in an individual's life that spans from age 65 to 74.

youth violence: Any form of behavior that leads to serious injury, emotional harm, or death among youth.

Index

Lightning Source UK Ltd.
Milton Keynes UK
UKOW02f1700160114

224756UK00012B/71/P